STATISTICAL METHODS
FOR HEALTH CARE RESEARCH

THIRD EDITION

STATISTICAL METHODS
FOR HEALTH CARE RESEARCH

THIRD EDITION

BARBARA HAZARD MUNRO, PhD, FAAN

Dean and Professor
School of Nursing
Boston College
Chestnut Hill, Massachusetts

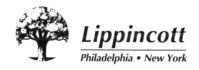

Lippincott
Philadelphia • New York

Acquisitions Editor: Margaret Zuccarini
Assistant Editor: Emily Cotlier
Project Editor: Gretchen Metzger
Production Manager: Helen Ewan
Production Coordinator: Patricia McCloskey
Design Coordinator: Melissa Olson
Indexer: Lynne Mahan

Edition 3

9 8 7 6 5 4 3 2 1

Library of Congress Cataloging in Publications Data

Munro, Barbara Hazard.
    Statistical methods for health care research / Barbara Hazard
Munro. — 3rd ed.
        p.   cm.
    Includes bibliographical references and index.
    ISBN 0-397-55365-X (alk. paper)
    1. Nursing—Research—Statistical methods.   2. Medical care—Research—
Statistical methods.   I. Title.
    [DNLM: 1. Statistics.   2. Health Services Research—methods.   WA 950 M968s
1997]
RT81.5.M86 1997
610′.72—dc21   96-46123
DNLM/DLC   CIP
for Library of Congress

Care has been taken to confirm the accuracy of the information presented and to describe generally accepted practices. However, the authors, editors, and publisher are not responsible for errors or omissions or for any consequences from application of the information in this book and make no warranty, express or implied, with respect to the contents of the publication.

The authors, editors, and publisher have exerted every effort to ensure that drug selection and dosage set forth in this text are in accordance with current recommendations and practice at the time of publication. However, in view of ongoing research, changes in government regulations, and the constant flow of information relating to drug therapy and drug reactions, the reader is urged to check the package insert for each drug for any change in indications and dosage and for added warnings and precautions. This is particularly important when the recommended agent is a new or infrequently employed drug.

Some drugs and medical devices presented in this publication have Food and Drug Administration (FDA) clearance for limited use in restricted research settings. It is the responsibility of the health care provider to ascertain the FDA status of each drug or device planned for use in their clinical practice.

Contributors

Leonard Braitman, PhD

Biostatistician
Office for Research Development
Albert Einstein Medical Center
Philadelphia, Pennsylvania

Jane Karpe Dixon, PhD

Professor
Yale University School of Nursing
New Haven, Connecticut

Barbara S. Jacobsen, MS

Professor (Retired)
The University of Pennsylvania School of Nursing
Philadelphia, Pennsylvania

Anne E. Norris, PhD, RN

Associate Professor
Boston College School of Nursing
Chestnut Hill, Massachusetts

Preface

The purpose of the first edition of *Statistical Methods for Health Care Research* was to acquaint the reader with the statistical techniques most commonly reported in the research literature of the health professions. We attempted to make the book user friendly by keeping mathematical symbolism to a minimum, and by using computer print-outs and examples from the literature to demonstrate specific techniques. In the second edition, we further reduced mathematical equations, moved from mainframe to personal computer examples, and added new techniques such as logistic regression.

In this third edition, we continue to strive to present complex statistical techniques in the most understandable way possible. We continue to underplay the role of mathematical calculations, assuming that readers will be using a personal computer for statistical analyses. We have updated all chapters and provided examples from the most up-to-date software.

Text Organization

We have organized the text into two sections:

Section I includes four chapters that present content essential to Understanding the Data, including chapters on organizing and displaying data, univariate descriptive statistics, inferential statistics and hypothesis testing, and lastly, confidence interval estimates and significance tests for percentages.

Section II presents 12 chapters that address Specific Statistical Techniques including nonparametric techniques, *t* tests, one-way and multifactorial analysis of variance, analysis of covariance, repeated measures analysis of variance, correlation, regression, logistic regression, factor analysis, path analysis, and structural equation modeling.

New to This Edition

Professor Barbara S. Jacobson from The University of Pennsylvania School of Nursing has provided even more detail on knowing one's data, covering such issues as dealing with outliers and missing values.

Dr. Jane Karpe Dixon, from Yale University School of Nursing, has added more content on confirmatory factor analysis to Chapter 14, Grouping Techniques.

Dr. Anne E. Norris, from Boston College School of Nursing, has completely revised two chapters: Chapter 15, Path Analysis, and Chapter 16, Structural Equation Modeling.

We have strengthened the content on sample size determination and evaluation.

New Features

APPLICATION EXERCISES at the end of each chapter provide the student with the opportunity to work with specific statistical techniques described in the text.

FREE COMPUTER DISK containing datasets provides data to use in completing the Application Exercises and encourages practice in applying the techniques outlined in Section II of the text.

GLOSSARY offers a quick and easy reference defining terms used throughout the text and in health care statistics.

Once again, we would like to thank the users and reviewers of the first two editions who made very helpful suggestions for this third edition. The students at Boston College, The University of Pennsylvania, and Yale University who have taken courses taught by authors of this text have most definitely played a role in the continuing development of this text, and we thank them too.

Contents

SECTION I   *Understanding the Data*

CHAPTER **1**   *Organizing and Displaying Data*   •   *3*
Barbara S. Jacobsen

CHAPTER **2**   *Univariate Descriptive Statistics*   •   *30*
Barbara S. Jacobsen

CHAPTER **3**   *Introduction to Inferential Statistics and Hypothesis Testing*   •   *53*
Barbara Hazard Munro, Barbara S. Jacobsen, and Leonard Braitman

CHAPTER **4**   *Confidence Interval Estimates and Significance Tests for Percentages: Examples to Aid Understanding of Statistical Inference*   •   *84*
Leonard Braitman

SECTION II   *Specific Statistical Techniques*

CHAPTER **5**   *Selected Nonparametric Techniques*   •   *99*
Barbara Hazard Munro

CHAPTER **6**   *t Tests: Measuring the Differences Between Group Means*   •   *122*
Barbara Hazard Munro

CHAPTER **7**   *Differences Among Group Means: One-Way Analysis of Variance*   •   *138*
Barbara Hazard Munro

CHAPTER **8**   *Differences Among Group Means: Multifactorial Analysis of Variance*   •   *162*
Barbara Hazard Munro

CHAPTER 9   *Analysis of Covariance* • *188*
Barbara Hazard Munro

CHAPTER 10   *Repeated Measures Analysis of Variance* • *202*
Barbara Hazard Munro

CHAPTER 11   *Correlation* • *224*
Barbara Hazard Munro

CHAPTER 12   *Regression* • *246*
Barbara Hazard Munro

CHAPTER 13   *Logistic Regression* • *287*
Barbara Hazard Munro

CHAPTER 14   *Grouping Techniques* • *310*
Jane Karpe Dixon

CHAPTER 15   *Path Analysis* • *342*
Anne E. Norris

CHAPTER 16   *Structural Equation Modeling* • *368*
Anne E. Norris

Glossary • *397*

Appendices

APPENDIX A   *Percent of Total Area of Normal Curve Between a z-Score and the Mean* • *407*
APPENDIX B   *Distribution of χ^2 Probability* • *409*
APPENDIX C   *Distribution of t* • *411*
APPENDIX D   *The 5% and 1% Points for the Distribution of F* • *413*
APPENDIX E   *Critical Values of the Correlation Coefficient* • *417*
APPENDIX F   *Transformation of r to z_r* • *419*
APPENDIX G   *Survey for Exercises* • *421*

Bibliography • *426*

Index • *434*

I

Understanding the Data

Organizing and Displaying Data

Barbara S. Jacobsen

OBJECTIVES FOR CHAPTER 1

After reading this chapter, you should be able to do the following:

1 • Discuss levels of measurement and their relationship to statistical analysis.

2 • Interpret a frequency distribution created by a computer program.

3 • Organize data into a table.

4 • Interpret data presented in a graph.

Research problems are questions that can be answered by collecting facts. The field of study concerned with obtaining, describing, and interpreting facts is called statistics; thus, the raw materials of research are data, and a major portion of scientific research involves statistical thinking about data. To proceed with obtaining facts to answer research questions, scientists must first measure characteristics of people or objects.

Measurement, in the broadest sense, is the assignment of numerals to objects or events according to a set of rules (Stevens, 1946). For example, the width of a piece of paper can be measured by following a set of rules for placing a graduated straightedge and then reading the numeral that corresponds to the concept of width. This definition can be broadened to include the assignment of numerals to abstract, intangible concepts, such as empathy. After a method of measurement for a concept is chosen, the concept then is called a *variable,* that is, a measured characteristic that takes on different values.

MEASUREMENT SCALES

Stevens (1946) noted four types of measurement scales for variables: nominal, ordinal, interval, and ratio. When analyzing data, the first task is to be aware of the type of measurement scale for each of the variables, because this knowledge helps in deciding how to organize and display data.

Nominal Scales

This type of scale allows a researcher to classify characteristics of people or objects into categories. Sometimes nominal variables are called categorical or qualitative. Numeric values may be assigned to the categories as labels for computer storage, but the choice of numerals for those labels is absolutely arbitrary. Some examples follow:

Variable	Values
Group membership	1 = Experimental 2 = Placebo 3 = Routine
Gender	1 = Male 2 = Female
Adherence to scheduled appointment	1 = Kept appointment 2 = Did not keep appointment

Ordinal Scales

In this case, the characteristics can not only be put into categories, but the categories also can be ordered; that is, the assignment of numerals is not arbitrary. The distance between the categories, however, is unknown. For example, in a horse race the results are reported in terms of which horse was first, which was second, and which was third. For the record books and for the bettor, it is irrelevant whether the winning horse won by a nose or by several lengths. Some other examples follow:

Variables	Values
Rank in army	1 = Private 2 = Corporal 3 = Sergeant 4 = Lieutenant
Socioeconomic status	1 = Low 2 = Middle 3 = High
Global opinion of instructor	1 = Very poor 2 = Poor 3 = Fair 4 = Good 5 = Excellent

Interval Scales

For this type of scale, the distances between the values are equal because there is some accepted physical unit of measurement. In a Fahrenheit thermometer, mercury rises in equal intervals called degrees. However, the zero point is arbitrary, chosen simply because Daniel Gabriel Fahrenheit, the inventor, decided that the zero point on his scale would be 32° below the freezing point of water. Because the units are in equal intervals, it is possible to add and subtract across an interval scale. You can say that 100°F is 50° warmer than 50°F, but you cannot say that 100°F is twice as hot as 50°F.

Interval variables may be continuous (i.e., in theory there are no gaps between the values) or discrete (i.e., there are gaps between the values). The Fahrenheit scale is considered to be continuous because only our eyesight or the quality of the measuring instrument prevents us from reading the scale in more finely graduated divisions. In contrast, parity of a woman is a discrete variable, because the number of children borne is obtained by counting indivisible units (children).

Ratio Scales

The zero point for these variables is not arbitrary but determined by nature. On the Kelvin temperature scale, zero represents the absence of molecular motion. Weight and blood pressure are other examples of ratio variables. Because the zero point is not arbitrary, it is possible to multiply and divide across a ratio scale; thus, it is possible to say that 100°K is twice as hot as 50°K. The distinction between interval and ratio variables is interesting, but for the purposes of this text, those two types of variables are handled the same way when analyzing data.

Issues Concerning Measurement Scales

What type of measurement scale involves variables resulting from psychological inventories and tests of knowledge? Certainly they have arbitrary zero points as determined by the inventor of each scale, and they have no accepted unit of measurement comparable to the degree on a temperature scale. Technically, these variables are ordinal, yet in practice researchers often think of them as interval. This has been a controversial issue in the research literature for years. Gardner (1975) reviewed the early literature on this conflict, and Knapp (1990) has commented on more recent literature. In his original article on measurement (1946) and in a later article (1968), Stevens noted that treating ordinal scales as interval or ratio scales may violate a technical canon, but in many instances, the outcome had demonstrable usefulness. More recently, Knapp (1990) pointed out that such considerations as measurement perspective, the number of categories that comprise an ordinal scale, and the concept of *meaningfulness* may all be important in deciding whether to treat a variable as ordinal or interval. We recommend the articles by Stevens (1946), Gardner (1975), and Knapp (1990) for further reading on this topic.

Interval or ratio variables can be converted to ordinal or nominal variables. For example, diastolic blood pressure, as measured by a sphygmomanometer, is a ratio variable. However, if, for research purposes, blood pressure is recorded as controlled or uncontrolled, then it is a nominal variable. In this case, there is a physiological basis for such a dichotomous division, but when no such reason exists, converting interval or ratio variables to nominal or ordinal variables can be unwise because information is lost. Cohen (1983) detailed the amount of degradation of measurement as a consequence of dichotomization and urged researchers to exploit fully all of the original measurement information.

UNIVARIATE ANALYSIS

As the first step, researchers should examine each variable separately, whether those variables are demographic, prognostic, group membership, or outcomes. Univariate analyses are helpful in cleaning and checking the quality of data. The data values must be scanned for each variable visually or via computer. If the data indicate that a pregnant woman is 99 years old, then an error may have occurred in data entry. Perhaps "99" represents a missing value, and the programmer forgot to inform the computer. Univariate analyses are also helpful in examining the variability of data, describing the sample, and checking statistical assumptions prior to more complex analyses. In some cases, data analysis may end here; your research questions may be answered solely by univariate analyses.

Tables

When data are organized into values or categories and then described with titles and captions, the result is a statistical table. A researcher begins to construct a table by tabulating data into a frequency distribution, that is, by counting how frequently each value or category occurs.

For nominal and ordinal variables, the categories should be listed (in some natural order if possible) and then the frequencies indicated for each category. Table 1-1 is an example of such a table, as produced by a computer, for the ordinal variable of stage of breast cancer at diagnosis. It is helpful to state the percentage in each category. Then the reader can quickly see that the majority of subjects in this sample were either stage 1 or stage 2A.

For interval or ratio variables, an ordered array of values (Table 1-2) is usually the first step in constructing a table. This frequency distribution table might be termed a *working table*. If the difference between the maximum and the minimum value is greater than 15, you may want to group the data into classes or categories before forming the final table (this may also be true for some ordinal variables). In Table 1-2, the range in days is 1 to 54; therefore, grouping the values will make the data more comprehensible (the period under the value of 54 denotes missing data).

As the next step, the computer printout for Table 1-3 shows a frequency distribution for the same data, with the values grouped into 11 classes, each having an interval (or width) of 5 days. Two of the 11 classes were not listed by the computer because the frequencies were zero. Note that the bottom class began with 0, although everyone in the sample was in the hospital for at least 1 day. This was done to keep the lower limit for each interval divisible by 5 and to keep the classes of equal width. Again, it is most helpful to know the percentage falling into each class.

It is clear from Table 1-3 that the category of 5 to 9 days included the largest frequency. In this computer printout, the column labeled "Valid Percent" gives the per-

TABLE 1-1
Example of Frequency Distribution Produced by SPSS:
Stage of Breast Cancer in a Sample of 189 Patients

Program

FREQUENCIES VARIABLES=STAGE.

Output

STAGE   Stage of disease

Value Label	Value	Frequency	Percent	Valid Percent	Cum. Percent
Zero	1	8	4.2	4.2	4.1
Stage 1	2	94	49.7	49.7	53.9
Stage 2A	3	50	26.5	26.5	80.4
Stage 2B	4	15	7.9	7.9	88.3
Stage 3A	5	7	3.7	3.7	92.0
Stage 3B	6	9	4.8	4.8	96.8
Stage 4	7	6	3.2	3.2	100.0
	TOTAL	*189*	*100.0*	*100.0*	
Valid Cases	189	Missing cases	0		

(Lowery, B. J., Jacobsen, B. S., & Ducette, J. [1992]. Causal attributions, control, and adjustment to breast cancer. Psychosocial Oncology, 10:4.)

centages for each category with missing data excluded. The column labeled "Cum Percent" refers to cumulative percentages, again with missing values excluded; these columns enable the reader to see quickly that approximately 83% of this sample stayed 9 days or less.

Computer programs can group values for you; however, some programs have defaults for the interval width and the number of classes that can result in an inconveniently constructed table. Most statistical programs allow you to control the choice of interval and the number of classes. Using a multiple of 5 for the interval width is helpful because it is easy to think about numbers that are divisible by 5. Authorities differ somewhat in their recommendations for the number of classes: Freedman, Pisani, Purves, and Adhikari (1991) suggest 10 to 15 classes; Freund (1988) suggests 6 to 15 classes; and Ott and Mendenhall (1990) suggest 5 to 20 classes. Too few or too many classes will obscure important features of a frequency distribution. Some detail is lost by grouping the values, but information is gained about clustering and the shape of the distribution.

The final presentation of the data from Table 1-3 depends on the format requirements of each journal or of the dissertation. Table 1-4 illustrates one possible way of presenting the frequency distribution for length of stay of a sample in a research report. Note that the categories of "45–49" and "35–39," although containing no patients, were included in the table for completeness. Once you have decided

TABLE 1-2
Example of Frequency Distribution (Condensed) Produced by SPSS:
Length of Stay for 218 Elderly Patients

Program

FREQUENCIES VARIABLES=LENGTH.

Output

LENGTH   Length of stay

Value Label	Frequency	Value Label	Frequency	Value Label	Frequency
1	2	11	19	24	1
2	8	12	5	25	1
3	11	13	6	26	1
4	16	14	6	27	1
5	18	15	4	28	1
6	20	16	4	30	2
7	19	17	2	40	1
8	21	18	3	54	1
9	26	20	1	•	1
10	16	22	1		

Data collected in grant funded by the National Institute for Nursing Research, NR-02095-07. P.I., M. Naylor (University of Pennsylvania School of Nursing), Comprehensive Discharge Planning for the Elderly.

that you need a table to present your data, that table should be mentioned in the text of the research report. The discussion of a table should reinforce the major points for which the table was developed (Burns & Grove, 1987). You should comment on the important patterns in the table and the major exceptions (Chatfield, 1988) but should not rehash every fact in the table.

Suggestions for the Construction of Tables for Research Reports

1. Use tables only to highlight major facts. Most of the tables examined by researchers while analyzing their data do not need to be published in a journal. If a finding can be described well in words, then a table is unnecessary. Too many tables can overwhelm the rest of a research report (Burns & Grove, 1987).
2. Make the table as self-explanatory as possible. The patterns and exceptions in a table should be obvious at a glance once the reader has been told what they are (Ehrenberg, 1977). With this goal in mind, the title should state the variable; when and where the data were collected, if pertinent; and the size of the sample. Headings within the table should be brief but clear.
3. Find out the required format for tables in your research report. If you are aiming for a particular journal, examine tables in past issues. Follow the advice about

TABLE 1-3
Example of Frequency Distribution Produced by SPSS:
Length of Stay for 218 Elderly Patients

Program

RECODE LENGTH (50 THRU 54=1)(45 THRU 49=2)(40 THRU 44=3)(35 THRU 39=4)
(30 THRU 35=5)(25 THRU 29=6)(20 THRU 24=7)(15 THRU 19=8)(10 THRU 14=9)
(5 THRU 9=10)(0 THRU 4=11).
VALUE LABELS LENGTH 1 '50–54' 2 '45–49' 3 '40–44' 4 '35–39' 5 '30–34' 6 '25–29' 7 '20–24'
8 '15–19' 9 '10–14' 10 '5–9' 11 '0–4'.
FREQUENCIES VARIABLES=LENGTH.

Output

LENGTH   Length of stay

Value Label	Value	Frequency	Percent	Valid Percent	Cum. Percent
50–54	1	1	.5	.5	.5
40–44	3	1	.5	.5	.9
30–34	5	2	.9	.9	1.8
25–29	6	4	1.8	1.8	3.7
20–24	7	3	1.4	1.4	5.1
15–19	8	13	6.0	6.0	11.1
10–14	9	52	23.9	24.0	35.0
5–9	10	104	47.7	47.9	82.9
0–4	11	37	17.0	17.1	100.0
	•	1	.5	Missing	
	Total	218	100.0	100.0	
Valid cases	217	Missing cases		1	

Data collected in grant funded by the National Institute for Nursing Research, NR-02095-07. P.I., M. Naylor (University of Pennsylvania School of Nursing), Comprehensive Discharge Planning for the Elderly.

table format for publication in a manual of style, such as the *Publication Manual of the American Psychological Association* (1994).

Graphs

Wainer and Thissen (1981) aptly quote two 19th century scientists as saying, "Getting information from a table is like extracting sunlight from a cucumber." Graphs, on the other hand, can quickly reveal facts about data that might only be gleaned from a table after careful study. They are often the most effective way to describe, explore, and summarize a set of numbers (Tufte, 1983). Graphs are the visual representations of frequency distributions. They provide a global, bird's-eye view of the data and help us to gain insight.

TABLE 1-4
Frequency Distribution for Length of Stay in a Sample of Elderly Patients From an Urban Medical Center (N = 217)

Days	Frequency	Percent
50–54	1	0.5
45–49	0	0.0
40–44	1	0.5
35–39	0	0.0
30–34	2	0.9
25–29	4	1.8
20–24	3	1.4
15–19	13	6.0
10–14	52	24.0
5–9	104	47.9
0–4	37	17.1
	217	100.0

Note: *Length of stay was not recorded in the medical chart for one patient.*
Data collected in grant funded by the National Institute for Nursing Research, NR-02095-07. P.I., M. Naylor (University of Pennsylvania School of Nursing), Comprehensive Discharge Planning for the Elderly.

There were 33 graphs of data published in *Nursing Research, Research in Nursing and Health,* and *Western Journal of Nursing Research* in 1994 (excluding charts and diagrams). These 33 graphs were contained in 18 articles, representing 19% of all the research articles published in those journals during that time. For the same period, there were 230 tables in 85 articles representing 89% of the research articles. Although tables are published much more frequently than graphs, researchers examine many "working" graphs of their data without necessarily attempting to publish them. Some of the most commonly used types of graphs for univariate analysis are discussed in this chapter. More complex graphs are discussed in subsequent chapters.

Bar Graph

Bar graphs are the proper type of graph for nominal or ordinal data. When constructing such graphs, the category labels usually are listed horizontally in some systematic order, and then vertical bars are drawn to represent the frequency or percent in each category. A space separates each of the bars to emphasize the nominal or ordinal nature of the variable. The choices of spacing and width of the bars are at the discretion of the researcher, but once chosen, all the spacing and widths should be equal. Figure 1-1 is an example of a bar graph for ordinal data. If the category labels are lengthy, it can be more convenient to list the categories vertically and draw the bars horizontally, as in Figure 1-2.

Bar graphs also facilitate comparisons between univariate distributions. Two or more univariate distributions can be compared by means of a cluster bar graph. Fig-

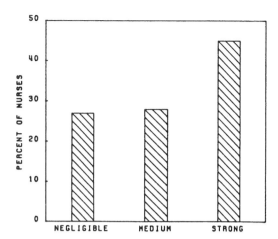

FIGURE 1-1

Degree of emphasis on the nurse as a sex object in motion pictures, 1930–1980 ($N = 211$). (From Kalisch, B. J., Kalisch, P. A., & McHugh, M. L. [1982]. *Research in Nursing and Health, 5,* 150.)

ure 1-3 is an example of such a graph. Current computer graphics, statistics, and spreadsheet programs offer many tempting patterns for filling in the bars, but the researcher should stay away from shading and cross-hatchings that weary the eye or cause illusion effects (Tufte, 1983). Note that the legend explaining Figure 1-3 is outside the graph to avoid clutter (Cleveland, 1985).

Histogram

Histograms are appropriate for interval and ratio variables and sometimes ordinal variables. These graphs appear similar to bar graphs, but the bars are placed side-by-side. The area of each bar represents frequency or percent; therefore, each histogram has a

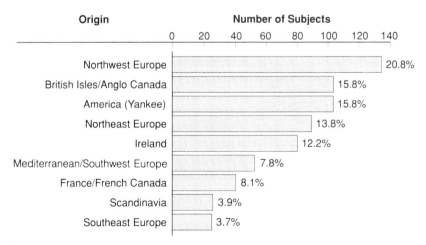

FIGURE 1-2

Claimed region of ethnic origin ($N = 645$). (From Clinton, J. [1982]. The development of an empirical construct for cross-cultural health research. *Western Journal of Nursing Research, 4,* 281.)

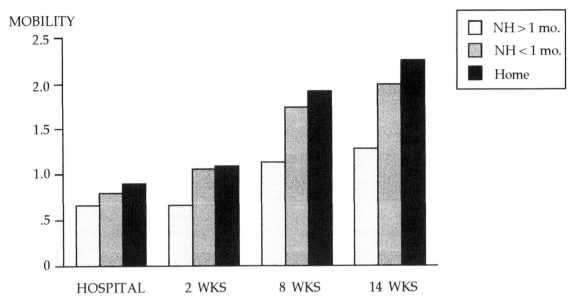

FIGURE 1-3

Mobility after hip fracture among women discharged home and to nursing homes. (Data from Williams, M. A., Oberst, M. T., & Bjorklund, B. C. [1994]. Early outcomes after hip fracture among women discharged home and to nursing homes. *Research in Nursing and Health, 17,* 175–183.)

total area of 100%. The first decision when constructing a histogram is to decide on the number of bars. With too few bars, the data will be clumped together; with too many, the data will be overly detailed. Figure 1-4 shows how the choice of the number of bars affects the appearance of a histogram. The top graph presents a jagged appearance; the bottom graph clumps the data into only four bars and makes the distribution seem quite skewed. The middle graph, with 10 bars, presents a smoother appearance.

Computer programs are handy for a preliminary graph of a variable, but a researcher should be aware of built-in defaults and think about the adjustments that are necessary. The advice in the previous section about constructing frequency distributions for interval or ratio variables is helpful here. For example, if the difference between the maximum and minimum values is larger than 15, consider grouping the data. Try to choose an interval and a starting point that are divisible by 5. You will find that most histograms have 5 to 20 bars.

For interval or ratio variables that are discrete, the numerals representing the values should be centered below each bar to emphasize the discrete nature of the variable. Figure 1-5 illustrates a histogram for the discrete variable of number of pregnancies. For continuous variables, the numerals representing the values should be placed at the sides of the bars to emphasize the continuous nature of the distribution.[1]

---

[1] *The grouping interval of "25–29" has a lower limit of 25 and an upper limit of 29. These are called the written limits. The real or mathematical limits are understood to extend half a unit above and below the written class limits. For convenience, researchers almost always use the written class limits in tables and graphs.*

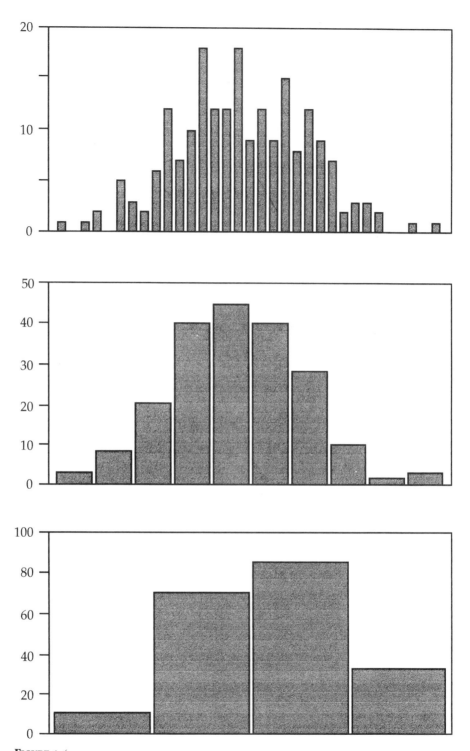

FIGURE 1-4

Illustration of the importance of the number of bars when designing a histogram for a set of data.

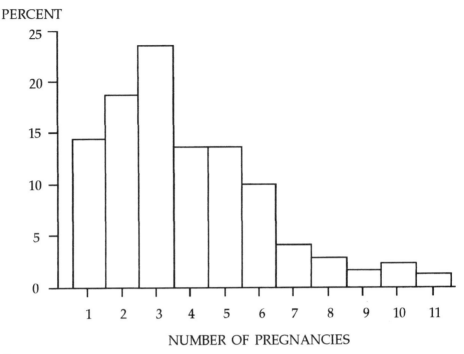

PERCENT

NUMBER OF PREGNANCIES

FIGURE 1-5

Number of previous pregnancies in a sample of high-risk pregnant women ($N = 176$). (Data collected with a grant funded by the National Institute for Nursing Research, NR-02867. P.I., D. Brooten, University of Pennsylvania School of Nursing, *Nurse Home Care for High Risk Pregnant Women: Outcome and Cost.*)

Figure 1-6 illustrates a histogram for the continuous variable of length of stay given previously in Table 1-4. Note that tick marks are placed outside the data region to avoid clutter (Cleveland, 1985).

Once the number of bars has been determined, the next decision concerns the height of the vertical axis. If the graphic is horizontal, Tufte (1983) recommends a height of approximately half the width. Other authorities, such as Schmid (1983), recommend a height approximately two-thirds to three-fourths the width. The reason for these recommendations is the different effect that can be produced by altering the height of a graph.

Figure 1-7 shows the different impressions that can be created for the same data set by a tall, narrow graph and a flat, wide graph. The tall, narrow graph seems to emphasize the clustering of the data in the middle, while the flat, wide graph seems to emphasize the scatter of the data to the right.

Polygon

A graph for interval or ratio variables, which is the equivalent of the histogram but appears smoother, is the polygon. For any set of data, the histogram and the poly-

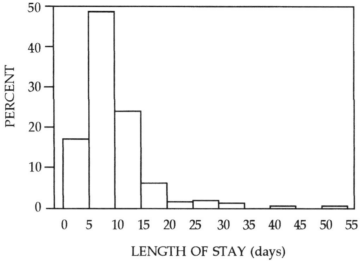

FIGURE 1-6

Length of stay in a sample of 217 elderly patients from an urban medical center. (Data collected with a grant funded by the National Institute for Nursing Research, NR-02095-07. P.I., M. Naylor. University of Pennsylvania School of Nursing, *Comprehensive Discharge Planning for the Elderly.*)

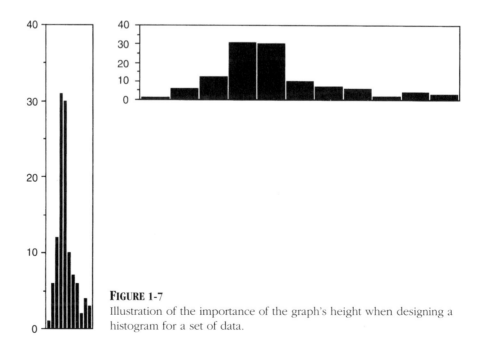

FIGURE 1-7

Illustration of the importance of the graph's height when designing a histogram for a set of data.

gon have equivalent total areas of 100%. The polygon is constructed by joining the midpoints of the top of each bar of the histogram and then closing the polygon at both ends by extending lines to imaginary midpoints at the left and right of the histogram. Figure 1-8 illustrates a polygon superimposed on a histogram. In the process of construction, triangles of area are removed from the histogram, but congruent triangles are added to polygon. Two such congruent triangles are shaded in Figure 1-8 to show why the areas of the two types of graphs are equivalent.

Polygons are especially appropriate for comparing two univariate distributions by superimposing them. Figure 1-9 shows such a comparison. Note that percentages were used on the vertical scale because the sizes of the two samples were different.

What to Look for in a Histogram or Polygon

A graph can help us see quickly the shape of a distribution. Frequency distributions have many possible shapes. Often they have a bell-shaped appearance as in the computer printout in Figure 1-10. In this case, heart attack patients were rated for denial on a summated inventory of 24 items, with each item rated for evidence of denial

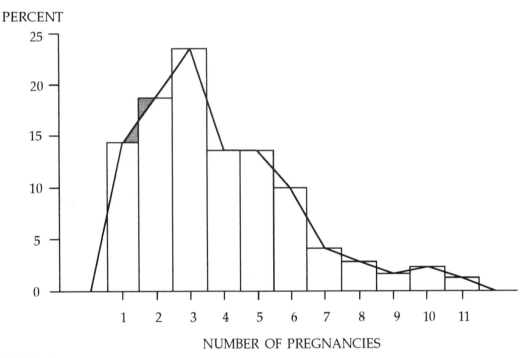

FIGURE 1-8
Polygon superimposed on histogram shown in Figure 1-5. The two shaded triangles are congruent. (Data collected with a grant funded by the National Institute for Nursing Research, NR-02867. P.I., D. Brooten, University of Pennsylvania School of Nursing, *Nurse Home Care for High Risk Pregnant Women: Outcome and Cost.*)

PERCENT

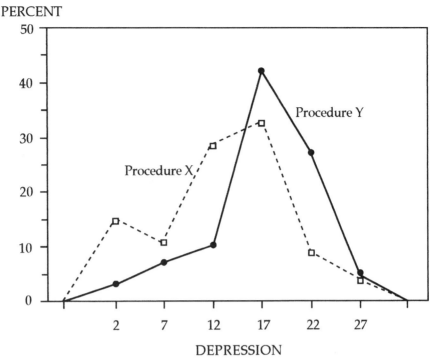

FIGURE 1-9

Comparison of depression scores for patients having surgical procedure X ($N = 104$) and patients having surgical procedure Y ($N = 61$).

on a seven-point scale. Technically, such a scale is ordinal, because there is no accepted physical unit of "denial," and the zero point is arbitrary. An ordinal scale with such a large range, however, is usually treated as interval in the research literature. In Figure 1-10, the frequency count is given at the left, and the midpoint of each class is listed directly beside each bar. The programmer chose an interval width of 5 with a starting point of 10. Thus, the first class is 10 to 15, and the midpoint of that class is 12.5. In addition, the programmer instructed the computer to plot the bell-shaped (normal) curve atop the histogram with a series of dots. The reader can then visually compare the distribution of denial with the theoretical bell-shaped curve. Distributions also may be skewed, as in Figures 1-11 and 1-12. Occasionally, data may clump at several places, as in Figure 1-13.

Graphs also can be helpful in spotting where the data cluster, how the data are scattered around the clustering points, whether there are far-out observations that may be outliers, and whether there are gaps in the data. These are the kinds of features that researchers need to know, and they become immediately evident with simple graphic representation (Cohen, 1990). With the assistance of a computer, researchers have no excuse for failing to know their data (Jacobsen, 1981). As with

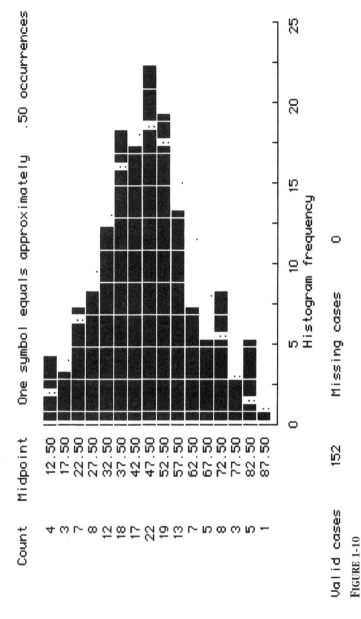

FIGURE 1-10

Example of a histogram produced by SPSS: Denial scores from a sample of 152 heart attack patients. (Jacobsen, B., & Lowery, B. [1992]. Further analysis of the psychometric characteristics of the Levine Denial of Illness Scale. *Psychosomatic Medicine, 54, 372–381*).

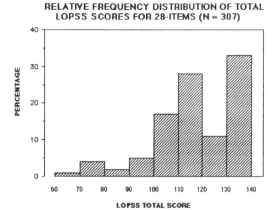

FIGURE 1-11

Relative frequency distribution of patient satisfaction scores (LOPPS) for 28-items ($N = 307$). (From Munro, B. H., Jacobsen, B. S., & Brooten, D. A. [1994]. Re-examination of the psychometric characteristics of the La Monica-Oberst patient satisfaction scale. *Research in Nursing and Health, 17,* 122.)

tables, all graphs included in a research report should be cited in the accompanying text, and the important features of the distribution should be discussed in the text.

General suggestions for constructing graphs

The purpose of graphing is to promote understanding without distorting the facts; therefore, your graph should make the point you want to make *fairly.* Because gross misuses of graphs are not generally found in respected research journals, some researchers believe that attention to the construction of their graphs is not really necessary because editors and reviewers will tell them how to fix their graphs. We urge you to read some of the references on graphing listed at the end of this book and to

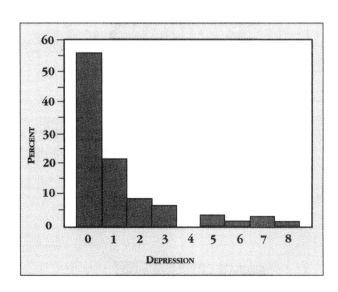

FIGURE 1-12

Relative frequency distribution of state depression (MAACL-R) in a sample of 112 hysterectomy patients. (From Jacobsen, B. S., Munro, B. H., & Brooten, D. A. [1996]. Comparison of original and revised scoring systems in the Multiple Affect Adjective Check List. *Nursing Research, 45,* 58.)

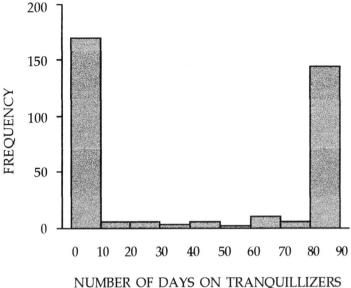

FIGURE 1-13

Number of days on tranquillizers in a sample of 350 nursing home patients during a 3-month period. (Data from grant funded by the National Institute for Nursing Research, R01-AG-08324. P. I., L. Evans, University of Pennsylvania School of Nursing. Reducing restraints in nursing homes: A clinical trial.)

follow their advice to avoid having your research report rejected. Schmid (1985) lists the following five characteristics of a good graph:

1. *Accuracy*—If you are using computer graphics software, be sure the data have been entered properly. The graph should not be misleading in any way nor be susceptible to misinterpretation. The best advice is to try out the graph on several people, including some who are not involved in your study. Ask them what the graph says to them.
2. *Simplicity*—The graph should be straightforward, not a puzzle. It should not present a cluttered appearance and should not have any "chartjunk" (Tufte, 1983). Grid lines and tick marks should be kept to a minimum, and elements such as odd lettering or ornate patterns should be avoided.
3. *Clarity*—The graph should be unambiguous and easily understood. The title and axes should be clearly labeled and the scale carefully chosen.
4. *Appearance*—The graph should not be sloppy but should be appealing.
5. *Well-designed structure*—The graph should conform to certain basic principles of perception. The more important elements should be emphasized visually, and the less important should be in the background. For example, grid lines should be comparatively light. Tufte (1983) suggests that the bars be dark and the grid lines

be white (see Fig. 1-10). Tufte (1983) also recommends, if possible, that all lettering be horizontal because it is easier to read.

SUMMARY

The first steps toward understanding data are univariate analyses. The researcher should study each variable separately by means of tables and graphs. The type of table or graph varies according to the type of measurement scale. For nominal data, the table should be a simple listing of categories with corresponding frequencies and percents, and the bar graph is appropriate for further display. For interval and ratio variables, it may be necessary first to group the data into appropriate numerical intervals before constructing a frequency table, histogram, or polygon. For ordinal variables, the researcher must decide whether the values need to be grouped into intervals and whether a bar graph or a histogram is appropriate. The best tables and graphs are self-explanatory and present data in a straightforward manner.

APPLICATION EXERCISES AND RESULTS

GENERAL INTRODUCTION

Appendix G contains a survey instrument that was developed at Boston College for doctoral students to collect data with for use in a statistics class. Each student is responsible for getting 10 people to fill out the questionnaire. Students are asked to have variety in terms of respondents' gender, age, and so forth. We also ask them to try to keep missing data to a minimum by checking questionnaires to be sure they are complete.

Each student then enters the data from their 10 subjects into a data file. They examine a printout of file information, run frequencies, and examine the output carefully to be sure they have entered their data correctly. The students make corrections as necessary, and then their datasets are merged and we provide them with a dataset they can use for all their homework assignments.

The disk at the back of this book contains data collected by these students on 177 subjects. If the same survey is used for several years, a fairly substantial dataset can be developed. The reader may use our survey form, collect data, and add it to the dataset we have provided.

When the students collect and enter data and then clean the datasets, they attain a much better understanding of data and its management. Although our students use their dataset for all homework exercises, for the midsemester and final exams larger datasets are used that are available from researchers in the school. Each student is provided with data from a randomly drawn subset of a large dataset. Thus, although they are answering the same questions using the same variables, their output depends on their sample.

The major dataset for the exercises throughout the book is named SURVEY.SAV and was created in SPSS for Windows, version 7.0. For the purpose of this book, we have asked specific questions for students to answer. In daily practice, we often just ask the students to state a research question or hypothesis that can be answered using their dataset and the statistical technique being studied that week. They then run the analysis and write up the results. We have found that students need more guidance in how to write the results in a manner that would be acceptable for a research journal than in how to run the analysis. We have not provided step-by-step guidance in the use of software because so many options are available.

INTRODUCTION TO EXERCISES IN CHAPTERS 1 AND 2

The exercises for Chapters 1 and 2 are fairly extensive. They reflect the amount of work that is necessary to set up a data base, be sure everything is correct, and understand what type of data you have collected. You may be thinking that if the data collection instrument were planned carefully, you would already know what type of data you have; however, we have learned and hope to demonstrate that what you collect may not be what you anticipated. For example, you may have inadequate subjects in some categories, and some of your continuous variables may be badly skewed.

EXERCISES

1. Access a small data set named CHAPTER1.SAV, and bring it into your computer software package. This data set was created to provide you the opportunity to do some data cleaning. First, run frequencies on this data set. You do not need to run statistics. Look at the three variables. Is there anything wrong with them?

2. Access SURVEY.SAV, which contains data collected using the survey form contained in Appendix G, and either bring it into SPSS or convert it into a file for SAS or whatever software you are using. Print the dictionary, which contains a list of the variables in the working file, formats, and labels. In SPSS for Windows 7.0, this is done by clicking on Utilities, then on File Info. Once the file is on the screen, it can be printed from the File menu.

3. Compare the file information with the survey form in Appendix G. Note that the variable names have been selected to reflect each variable, making it easy to recognize them when working with the file. Variable labels and value labels have been added to enhance the output. Are there any discrepancies between the survey form and the file information?

4. Produce graphs. Many options are available for producing graphs in statistical software programs. They may be produced within specific techniques and in separate graphics sections. We will confine ourselves to requesting graphics that are available with the specific techniques. The following can be requested as part of the output from frequencies in most software programs.

   Within the frequencies program, request a bar graph for GENDER, a histogram for SATCURWT, and a histogram with a polygon (normal curve) for SATCURWT.

RESULTS

1. Exercise Figure 1-1 contains output produced by SPSS for Windows Version 7.0. The first of the three variables is Gender, which was coded as 1 = Male and 2 = Female. Is there anything wrong with it? Yes; of the 10 subjects, four are males, five are females, and one subject is coded a 3.

   Now you need to find out which subject was coded a 3. In this small data set, you can simply look at the data and fix the 3. See Exercise Figure 1-2 for a picture of the data in the file. In larger data sets, you may want to list out the cases for variables that are incorrect. In SPSS for Windows, you can search for data through the data editor. For example, select the first cell in the column for Gender; that is, click on the 1 for subject 1. Next, click on

Gender

		Frequency	Percent	Valid Percent	Cumulative Percent
Valid	Male	4	40.0	40.0	40.0
	Female	5	50.0	50.0	90.0
	3.00	1	10.0	10.0	100.0
	Total	10	100.0	100.0	
Total		10	100.0		

Self-esteem

		Frequency	Percent	Valid Percent	Cumulative Percent
Valid	8.00	1	10.0	10.0	10.0
	10.00	1	10.0	10.0	20.0
	15.00	1	10.0	10.0	30.0
	21.00	1	10.0	10.0	40.0
	28.00	1	10.0	10.0	50.0
	32.00	1	10.0	10.0	60.0
	45.00	1	10.0	10.0	70.0
	47.00	1	10.0	10.0	80.0
	50.00	1	10.0	10.0	90.0
	65.00	1	10.0	10.0	100.0
	Total	10	100.0	100.0	
Total		10	100.0		

Age

		Frequency	Percent	Valid Percent	Cumulative Percent
Valid	12.00	1	10.0	10.0	10.0
	24.00	1	10.0	10.0	20.0
	25.00	1	10.0	10.0	30.0
	27.00	1	10.0	10.0	40.0
	28.00	1	10.0	10.0	50.0
	32.00	1	10.0	10.0	60.0
	34.00	1	10.0	10.0	70.0
	35.00	1	10.0	10.0	80.0
	38.00	1	10.0	10.0	90.0
	70.00	1	10.0	10.0	100.0
	Total	10	100.0	100.0	
Total		10	100.0		

EXERCISE FIGURE 1-1. Frequencies of three variables.

	Gender	SE	Age
1	1.00	8.00	28.00
2	1.00	10.00	32.00
3	2.00	45.00	25.00
4	1.00	21.00	35.00
5	2.00	32.00	38.00
6	2.00	47.00	12.00
7	3.00	28.00	34.00
8	1.00	65.00	27.00
9	2.00	15.00	24.00
10	2.00	50.00	70.00

EXERCISE FIGURE 1-2. Data in the file.

the Edit menu, then on Find. Type in a 3 and click on Search Forward. You should find that subject 7 was coded a 3.

If you had collected the data, you would check to see whether subject number 7 was a male or female and enter the correct code. Because you do not have the data, what else could you do? You could assign 3 to the missing values category. You do that in SPSS by changing the 3 to a period or to the value that has been defined as a missing value. (To define a missing value, highlight the variable, then click on Data Menu, Define Variable, and Missing Values.) Please correct the code for Gender for subject 7 by assigning 3 to the missing values category.

The second variable is Self-Esteem. It is based on a 10-item scale, in which each item is scored from 1 to 5. Is there anything wrong with this scale? Given the description of the scale, the potential range of scores is 10 to 50, but two subjects have scores outside this range. There is one 8 and one 65. Again, you must first determine which subjects have the incorrect scores. You should find that subject 1 is scored an 8, and subject 8 is scored a 65. Please correct the scores for these two subjects by giving subject 1 an 18, and subject 8 a 36.

The third variable is Age. Is there anything wrong with that variable? Two scores do not fit with the others. All but two subjects are in their 20s or 30s. The two outliers are one 12 year old and one 70 year old. You should find that subject 6 is listed as 12 years old,

	Gender	SE	Age
1	1.00	18.00	28.00
2	1.00	10.00	32.00
3	2.00	45.00	25.00
4	1.00	21.00	35.00
5	2.00	32.00	38.00
6	2.00	47.00	22.00
7	.	28.00	34.00
8	1.00	36.00	27.00
9	2.00	15.00	24.00
10	2.00	50.00	.

EXERCISE FIGURE 1-3. Corrected data.

Gender

		Frequency	Percent	Valid Percent	Cumulative Percent
Valid	Male	4	40.0	44.4	44.4
	Female	5	50.0	55.6	100.0
	Total	9	90.0	100.0	
Missing	System Missing	1	10.0		
	Total	1	10.0		
Total		10	100.0		

Self-esteem

		Frequency	Percent	Valid Percent	Cumulative Percent
Valid	10.00	1	10.0	10.0	10.0
	15.00	1	10.0	10.0	20.0
	18.00	1	10.0	10.0	30.0
	21.00	1	10.0	10.0	40.0
	28.00	1	10.0	10.0	50.0
	32.00	1	10.0	10.0	60.0
	36.00	1	10.0	10.0	70.0
	45.00	1	10.0	10.0	80.0
	47.00	1	10.0	10.0	90.0
	50.00	1	10.0	10.0	100.0
	Total	10	100.0	100.0	
Total		10	100.0		

Age

		Frequency	Percent	Valid Percent	Cumulative Percent
Valid	22.00	1	10.0	11.1	11.1
	24.00	1	10.0	11.1	22.2
	25.00	1	10.0	11.1	33.3
	27.00	1	10.0	11.1	44.4
	28.00	1	10.0	11.1	55.6
	32.00	1	10.0	11.1	66.7
	34.00	1	10.0	11.1	77.8
	35.00	1	10.0	11.1	88.9
	38.00	1	10.0	11.1	100.0
	Total	9	90.0	100.0	
Missing	System Missing	1	10.0		
	Total	1	10.0		
Total		10	100.0		

EXERCISE FIGURE 1-4. Corrected frequencies.

```
                    List of variables on the working file

     Name                                                          Position

     CODE       subject's identification number                        1
                Print Format: F3
                Write Format: F3

     GENDER     gender                                                  2
                Print Format: F1
                Write Format: F1

                Value     Label

                    0     male
                    1     female

     AGE        subject's age                                           3
                Print Format: F3
                Write Format: F3

     MARITAL    marital status                                          4
                Print Format: F1
                Write Format: F1

                Value     Label

                    1     Never Married
                    2     Married
                    3     Living with Significant Other
                    4     Separated
                    5     Widowed
                    6     Divorced
```

```
     DEPRESS    depressed state of mind                                 9
                Print Format: F1
                Write Format: F1

                Value     Label

                    1     Rarely
                    2     Sometimes
                    3     Often
                    4     Routinely
```

```
     IPA1       energy level                                           19
                Print Format: F8
                Write Format: F8

                Value     Label

                    1     very low
                    7     very high
```

```
     IPA2       reaction to pressure                                   20
                Print Format: F1
                Write Format: F1

                Value     Label

                    1     I get tense
                    7     I remain calm
```

EXERCISE FIGURE 1-5. A portion of the dictionary.

and subject 10 is listed as 70 years old. Please correct these scores by entering 22 for subject 6, and assigning subject 10's age to the missing values category.

Your data should now look like Exercises Figure 1-3. Rerun the frequencies on the three variables to be sure you have made the changes correctly. Your output should look like Exercises Figure 1-4.

```
IPA3      characterization of life as a whole                    21
          Print Format: F1
          Write Format: F1

          Value    Label

             1     dull
             7     vibrant

IPA4      daily activities                                       22
          Print Format: F1
          Write Format: F1

          Value    Label

             1     not a source of satisfaction
             7     a source of satisfaction
```

```
  CONFID    Confidence during stressful situations               49
            Print Format: F8.2
            Write Format: F8.2

            Value    Label

            13.00    lowest score
            91.00    highest score


  LIFE      Life purpose and satisfaction                        50
            Print Format: F8.2
            Write Format: F8.2

            Value    Label

            17.00    lowest score
           119.00    highest score

 IPPATOT    Positive Psychological Attitudes                     51
            Print Format: F8.2
            Write Format: F8.2

            Value    Label

            30.00    Lowest score
           210.00    Highest score
```

EXERCISE FIGURE 1-5. (CONTINUED)

2. Exercises Figure 1-5 contains a portion of the dictionary.

3. If you have looked carefully, you should note the following:

   a. The value labels for the following items from the Inventory of Personal Attitudes (IPPA) have been reversed: 1, 2, 4, 6, 8, 13, 15, 20, 22, 24, 27, and 29. These items need to be recoded for scoring of the scale. For example, look at item 1. On the questionnaire, we see that a very high level of energy is scored 1 and a very low level is scored 7. Because the inventory measures **positive** attitudes, the originators (Kass, et al., 1991) reverse this item before adding it to the scale. We have already done the reverse scoring for you. We recoded all of these items so that 1 = 7, 2 = 6, 3 = 5, 4 = 4, 5 = 3, 6 = 2, and 7 = 1. Thus, with item 1, if someone checked a 1, they would now be scored a 7. We also reversed the value labels to reflect the new scoring.

   If you add your own data to our data set, be sure to recode these items, and be sure the value labels are correct before adding them to our data set.

   b. You should also note that there are three "extra" variables listed in the dictionary. These new variables follow the 30 IPPA items.

CONFID is the sum of the following items: 2, 5, 7, 10, 14, 15, 16, 17, 18, 22, 24, 26, and 29. It is defined as self-confidence during stressful situations. Because it includes 13 questions and each question is rated on a scale from 1 to 7, the potential range of scores for CONFID is 13 to 91.

LIFE is the sum of the following items: 1, 3, 4, 6, 8, 9, 11, 12, 13, 19, 20, 21, 23, 25, 27, 28, and 30. It is defined as life purpose and satisfaction and includes 17 questions, with a potential range of scores of 17 to 119.

IPPATOT is the sum of all 30 items and is the total score on the IPPA. The potential range of scores is 30 to 210.

4. Exercises Figure 1-6 contains the frequencies for gender and the associated bar graph. Exercises Figure 1-7 contains the frequencies for satisfaction with current weight, the histogram, and the histogram with the normal curve superimposed.

Gender

		Frequency	Percent	Valid Percent	Cumulative Percent
Valid	male	58	32.8	33.3	33.3
	female	116	65.5	66.7	100.0
	Total	174	98.3	100.0	
Missing	System Missing	3	1.7		
	Total	3	1.7		
Total		177	100.0		

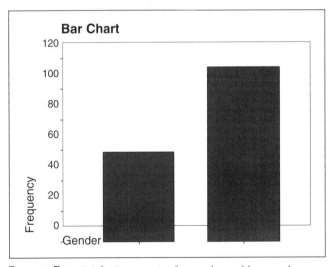

EXERCISE FIGURE 1-6. Frequencies for gender and bar graph.

Satisfaction with current weight

		Frequency	Percent	Valid Percent	Cumulative Percent
Valid	Very Dissatisfied	9	5.1	5.1	5.1
	2	6	3.4	3.4	8.6
	3	27	15.3	15.4	24.0
	4	21	11.9	12.0	36.0
	5	14	7.9	8.0	44.0
	6	8	4.5	4.6	48.6
	7	21	11.9	12.0	60.6
	8	25	14.1	14.3	74.9
	9	25	14.1	14.3	89.1
	Very Satisfied	19	10.7	10.9	100.0
	Total	175	98.9	100.0	
Missing	System Missing	2	1.1		
	Total	2	1.1		
Total		177	100.0		

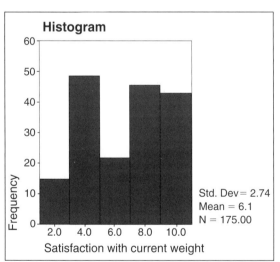 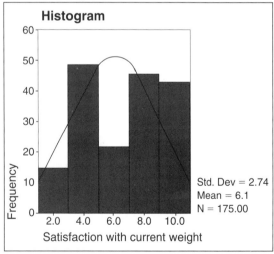

EXERCISE FIGURE 1-7. Frequencies for satisfaction with current weight and two histograms.

Univariate Descriptive Statistics

Barbara S. Jacobsen

Objectives for Chapter 2

After reading this chapter, you should be able to do the following:

1 • Define measures of central tendency and dispersion.

2 • Select the appropriate measures to use for a particular data set.

3 • Discuss methods to identify and manage outliers.

Graphs may bring facts to life vividly, but the information they offer is often inexact. Frequency distribution tables provide many details, but often a researcher wants to condense a distribution further. After the data have been organized, quantitative measures are frequently calculated to capture the essence of the four basic characteristics of a distribution: central tendency, variability, skewness, and kurtosis. These statistics may be used not only in a descriptive summary but also in statistical inference. Symbols and formulas for descriptive statistics vary depending on whether one is describing a sample or a population. A *population* includes all members of a defined group; a *sample* is a subset of a population. It is important to distinguish between these. An instructor who is grading an exam given to a class of students ordinarily views that class as a population. A researcher who plans to publish a report on denial in heart attack patients may interview patients from a single urban hospital but may view those patients as a sample of all heart attack patients from that type of hospital or that geographic area.

Characteristics of populations are called *parameters;* characteristics of samples are called *statistics.* To distinguish between them, different sets of symbols are used. Usually, lower case Greek letters denote parameters, and Roman letters denote statistics.

MEASURES OF CENTRAL TENDENCY

These statistics, commonly called averages, describe where the values of a distribution cluster. The three measures of central tendency that are discussed in this text are the mean, median, and mode.

Mean

The mean, the most widely used average, locates the center of gravity or fulcrum of a distribution. This measure of central tendency does not necessarily imply that 50% of the data are below average, because a center of gravity may not be located in the middle.

The mean of a sample[1] is represented symbolically by $\bar{X}$, which is read "X bar." Many journals simply use "M" to represent the mean.

To compute the mean, simply add up all the values and divide by the number of values. Expressed as a formula, the sample mean is defined as:

$$\bar{X} = \frac{\Sigma X}{N}$$

The upper case Greek letter sigma (Σ) means "the sum of." If the letter X represents a single quantitative value in a distribution, then ΣX means "sum of all the values."

For example, the following list of values for length of stay (in hours) for a sample of cesarean delivery mothers has 10 entries: 61, 70, 112, 74, 104, 97, 85, 132, 125, 70. The mean is:

$$\frac{61 + 70 + 112 + 74 + 104 + 97 + 85 + 132 + 125 + 70}{10} = \frac{930}{10} = 93 \text{ hours}$$

In this example, the mean is located near the middle of the 10 values. It is clear from the formula and the example that each value in the distribution contributes to the mean. Because the mean is influenced by all of the data points, it is not appropriate as a descriptive statistic for a variable when all the data points are not known. For instance, not everyone with cancer may have a recurrence of that disease; therefore, some of the values of the variable "time to recurrence" may be absent or "censored."

Any extreme values in the distribution also influence the mean. For example, in the previous distribution relating to length of stay in hours for a group of women who underwent cesarean delivery, suppose the value of 132 hours was instead 702. The new mean would be:

$$\frac{61 + 70 + 112 + 74 + 104 + 97 + 85 + 702 + 125 + 70}{10} = \frac{1,500}{10} = 150 \text{ hours}$$

---

[1]*The mean of a population is represented by the lower case Greek letter mu (μ). The formula is the same as that for the sample mean.*

TABLE 2-1
Demonstration of Several Important Properties of the Mean

X	X − $\bar{X}$	(X − $\bar{X}$)²
4	4 − 6 = −2	(−2)² = 4
4	4 − 6 = −2	(−2)² = 4
10	10 − 6 = +4	(+4)² = 16
5	5 − 6 = −1	(−1)² = 1
7	7 − 6 = +1	(+1)² = 1
$\Sigma X = 30$	$\Sigma(X − \bar{X}) =$ 0	$\Sigma(X − \bar{X})^2 = 26$
$N =$ 5		sum of squares
$\bar{X} =$ 6		

This mean would not be located in the middle of the 10 values. Only one pa-tient would have a length of stay greater than the mean. Thus, the mean works best as an average for symmetrical frequency distributions that have a single peak.

The mean has several other interesting properties. First, for any distribution, the sum of the deviations of the values from the mean always equals zero. This helps to explain why the mean is the center of gravity or fulcrum of a distribution. Table 2-1 demonstrates this property. The mean (6) is subtracted from each value to form *de-viations* (X − $\bar{X}$). These deviations from the mean sum to zero. If any value other than the mean is subtracted from each value, the $\Sigma(X − \bar{X})$ will not be zero. The reader is invited to try subtracting other values, such as the median or the mode, and summing these deviations.

A second property of the mean relates to the sum of the squared deviations, that is, $\Sigma(X − \bar{X})^2$. In Table 2-1, each of the deviations from the mean has been squared, and the sum of these squared deviations is 26. This sum, referred to in statistics as the *sum of squares,* is at a minimum; that is, it is smaller than the sum of squares around any other value. If any value other than the mean (6) is subtracted from each value and squared, the total will be greater than 26. Again, the reader is invited to try subtracting other values, such as the median or the mode. This characteristic of the mean underlies the idea of *least squares,* which is important in later chapters.

Third, because the mean has a formula, it is algebraic and can be manipulated in equations. For example if two or more means are available from samples of dif-ferent sizes, a mean of the total group can be calculated. By transposing terms in the formula for the mean, the following shows that the sum of the values is equal to the mean multiplied by the size of the sample.

$$\bar{X}N = \Sigma X$$

Therefore, a formula for a combined mean for two samples (which can be eas-ily extended to include more than two samples) weighted according to sample size, logically follows:

$$\bar{X}_{total} = \frac{\bar{X}_1 N_1 + \bar{X}_2 N_2}{N_1 + N_2}$$

Finally, when repeatedly drawing random samples from the same population, means will vary less among themselves and less from the true population mean than other measures of central tendency. Thus, the mean is the most reliable average when making inferences from a sample to a population.

The mean is intended for interval or ratio variables when values can be added, but many times it is also sensible for ordinal variables. Computers, of course, do not know whether variables are interval, ordinal, or nominal and will compute means for a nominal variable reporting such uninterpretable facts for a sample as "the mean religion = 2.34."

Median

The median is the middle value of a set of ordered numbers. It is the point or value below which 50% of the distribution falls. Thus, 50% of the sample will be below the median, regardless of the shape of the distribution. The median is sometimes called the 50th percentile and symbolized as P_{50}. It may also be thought of as the bisector of the total area of the histogram or polygon. There is no formula for the median, simply a procedure:

1. Arrange the values in order.
2. If the total number of values is odd, count up (or down) to the middle value. If there are several identical values clustered at the middle, the median is that value.
3. If the total number of values is even, compute the mean of the middle values.

In the example relating to length of stay in cesarean delivery mothers, the 10 values, arranged in order, are:

61, 70, 70, 74, 85, 97, 104, 112, 125, 132

Counting to the center of these 10 entries, the two middle values are 85 and 97. Thus, the median is $(85 + 97) \div 2 = 91$. Note that the mean for these data is 93, quite similar to the median.

From the procedure, it is clear that every value does not enter into the computation of the median; only the number of values and the values near the midpoint of the distribution enter into the computation. If the value of 132 is changed to 702 in the previous example, the new distribution is:

61, 70, 70, 74, 85, 97, 104, 112, 125, 702

The median of this distribution is still located midway between 85 and 97 and is still 91 hours. Thus, the median is not sensitive to extreme scores. It may be used with symmetrical or asymmetrical distributions, but is especially useful when the data are skewed. Of course, this property of not reflecting all of the values in a distribution can also be a disadvantage in that the median is nonalgebraic. Hence, there is no formula for a weighted median.

The median is appropriate for interval and ratio data and for ordinal data but not for nominal data. It can be used for open-end or censored data, such as "time to recurrence," if more than half of the sample have contributed a value to the distribution.

Mode

The mode is the most frequent value or category. It may be interpreted as the fashionable score, as in "a la mode." In the previous example of length of stay in hours, the 10 entries were: 61, 70, 70, 74, 85, 97, 104, 112, 125, 132. The mode for this distribution is 70 because that score occurs most frequently. The mode is not calculated but simply spotted by inspection, which is easy with a graph or table of ordered values.

If all of the scores are different, the mode does not exist. If several values occur with equal frequency, then there are several modes. If the values of a distribution cluster in several places but with unequal frequency, then there are primary and secondary modes. For example, when discussing Figure 1-13 in the previous chapter, it would be helpful to note that the primary mode was 5 days (the midpoint of the first bar) with a secondary mode of 85 days (the midpoint of the last bar). Alternatively, the primary mode for Figure 1-13 could be reported as less than 10 days and the secondary mode as at least 80 days.

The mode can be used with interval, ratio, or ordinal variables as a rough estimate of central tendency. If it is used as an average for nominal data, it is reported as the modal category. For instance, in Figure 1-2 in the previous chapter, the modal category for ethnic origin is "Northwest Europe."

Comparison of Measures of Central Tendency

The mean is the most common measure of central tendency. It has a formula and is the most trustworthy estimate of a population average. Generally, researchers prefer to use it, unless there is a good reason for not doing so. The most compelling reason for not using the mean is a distribution that is badly skewed. The effect of extreme values on the mean lessens as the size of the sample increases; therefore, another good reason for not using the mean is a small sample with a few extreme values. The mean is best when used with distributions that are reasonably symmetrical and have one mode.

The median is easy to understand as the 50th percentile of a distribution or the bisector of the area of a histogram. It has no formula but is calculated by a counting procedure. The median may be used with distributions of any shape but is especially useful with very skewed distributions.

The main use of the mode is to call attention to a distribution in which the values cluster at several places. It can also be used for making rough estimates. In addition, the mode is the only average available for nominal data.

Figure 2-1 illustrates the relative positions of these three averages for a polygon that is very skewed. The mode is the value under the high point of the polygon, the mean is pulled to the right by the extreme values in the tail of the distribution, and the median usually falls in between. Thus, if the mean is greater than the median, then the distribution is positively skewed. Consider how Figure 2-1 would be different if the distribution were negatively skewed.

Weisberg (1992) points out that it is not always necessary to select only a single

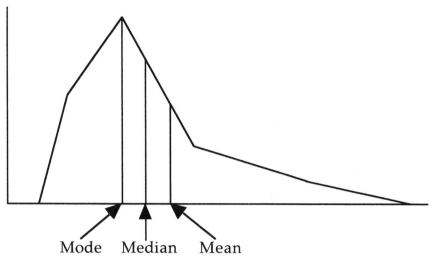

FIGURE 2-1

Sketch of frequency polygon for a distribution skewed to the right, indicating the relative positions of mean, median, and mode.

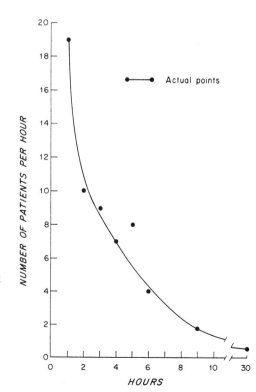

FIGURE 2-2

Graph illustrating a distribution (rate at which patients seek medical care for coronary symptoms as a function of time from onset of symptoms) in which mean, median, and mode are quite different. (From Hackett, T. P., & Cassem, N. H. [1969]. Factors contributing to delay in responding to the signs and symptoms of acute myocardial infarction. *American Journal of Cardiology, 24,* 653.) Mean, 10.6 hours; median, 4 hours; mode, 1 hour.

measure of central tendency because these statistics provide different information. Sometimes it is useful to examine multiple aspects of a distribution. An example from a research journal is presented in Figure 2-2. In this case, the mode for delay in seeking treatment was 1 hour, the median was 4 hours, and the mean was 10.6 hours. If the objective of reporting an average is to present a fair view of the data, consider which average (or averages) should be used here.

MEASURES OF VARIABILITY OR SCATTER

Reporting only an average without an accompanying measure of variability is a good way to misrepresent a set of data. A common story in statistics classes tells of the woman who had her head in an oven and her feet in a bucket of ice water. When asked how she felt, the reply was, "On the average, I feel fine." Researchers tend to focus on measures of central tendency and neglect how the data are scattered, but variability is at least equally important (Tulman & Jacobsen, 1989). Two data sets can have the same average but very different variabilities (Fig. 2-3). The three measures of variability discussed in this text are the standard deviation (SD), interpercentile measures, and range. Unlike averages, which are points representing a central value, measures of variability should be interpreted as distances on a scale of values.

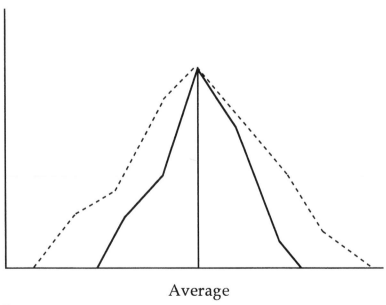

Average

FIGURE 2-3
Two frequency distributions with equal averages but different variabilities.

TABLE 2-2
Demonstration of the Calculation of the Sample
Standard Deviation for Length of Stay (in Hours)
of Cesarean Birth Mothers

X	X − X̄	(X − X̄)²
61	$61 - 93 = -32$	$(-32)^2 = 1{,}024$
70	$70 - 93 = -23$	$(-23)^2 = 529$
112	$112 - 93 = +19$	$(+19)^2 = 361$
74	$74 - 93 = -19$	$(-19)^2 = 361$
104	$104 - 93 = +11$	$(+11)^2 = 121$
97	$97 - 93 = +4$	$(+4)^2 = 16$
85	$85 - 93 = -8$	$(-8)^2 = 64$
132	$132 - 93 = +39$	$(+39)^2 = 1{,}521$
125	$125 - 93 = +32$	$(+32)^2 = 1{,}024$
70	$70 - 93 = -23$	$(-23)^2 = 529$

$\Sigma X = 930$ $\Sigma(X - \bar{X}) = 0$ $\Sigma(X - \bar{X})^2 = 5{,}550 = $ Sum of squares
$\bar{X} = 93$

$$\text{Variance} = \frac{5{,}550}{9} = 616.67 \text{ square hours}$$

$$\text{SD} = \sqrt{\frac{5{,}550}{9}} = 24.8 \text{ hours}$$

Standard Deviation

This is the most widely used measure of variability. The sample[2] SD is defined as:

$$\text{SD} = \sqrt{\frac{\Sigma(X - \bar{X})^2}{N - 1}}$$

The reason for dividing by the quantity $(N - 1)$ involves a theoretical consideration called *degrees of freedom*. This concept is discussed later in this text. Briefly, it can be shown that using $(N - 1)$ produces, for a random sample, an unbiased estimate of a population variance. This consideration assumes more importance, of course, with small samples.

Table 2-2 illustrates the calculation of the SD for the list of 10 values for length of stay in a sample of cesarean deliveries. The first step is to calculate the mean and then subtract it from each value, making sure that the sum of the deviations is zero. Next, each deviation is squared. The sum of the squared deviations (or "sum of

[2]*The SD of a population is represented symbolically by the lower case Greek letter sigma (σ). The formula differs from the sample SD in that the denominator is simply* N, *not* N − 1.

squares") is then divided by ($N - 1$). This quantity is called the *variance*. Although it is a measure of variability, the variance is not used as a descriptive statistic because it is not in the same unit as the data. For example, the variance of the data in Table 2-2 is 616.67 square hours. Most people would have difficulty interpreting a square hour. Therefore, the square root is taken to return the statistic to its original scale of measurement. The resulting statistic of 24.8 hours is the SD. Again, as with the mean, it is clear that every value in the distribution enters into the calculation of the SD. It is also clear from the formula that the SD is a measure of variability around the mean. The example in Table 2-2 provides the basic understanding of the SD.

The SD, like the mean, is sensitive to extreme values. For example, in Table 2-2, if the value of 132 is changed to 702, the new SD is 195.1, a large inflation from the original SD of 24.8. Therefore, the SD is best for distributions that are symmetrical and have a single peak. In general, if it is appropriate to calculate a mean, then it is also appropriate to calculate the SD.

The SD has a straightforward interpretation if the distribution is bell shaped or normal (the normal curve is discussed in detail in the next chapter). If the distribution is perfectly bell shaped, 68% of the values are within 1 SD of the mean, 95% of the values are within 2 SDs of the mean, and more than 99% of the data will be within 3 SDs of the mean. For instance, Table 2-3 is a computer printout of basic statistics for the approximately bell-shaped distribution of denial scores given in Figure 1-10 in the previous chapter. The mean for denial is 46.5, and the SD is 16.4. By actual count, 70% of the denial values fall within the interval of mean ± 1 SD, and 94% of the values are within the interval of mean ± 2 SDs.

Even if the distribution is not bell shaped, however, these percentages hold fairly well. Chebyshev's theorem states that even in oddly shaped distributions, at least 75% of the data will fall within 2 SDs of the mean (Freund, 1988). Figure 1-6 displays

TABLE 2-3
Descriptive Statistics Produced by SPSS for the Data in Figure 1-10: Denial Scores From a Sample of 152 Heart Attack Patients

Program

FREQUENCIES VARIABLES = DENIAL/FORMAT = NOTABLE/STATISTICS = ALL.

Output

Mean	46.533	Std err	1.328	Median	45.500
Mode	45.000	SD	16.374	Variance	286.092
Kurtosis	−.249	S E Kurt	.391	Skewness	.195
S E Skew	.197	Range	76.000	Minimum	11.000
Maximum	87.000	Sum	7073.000		
Valid cases	152	Missing cases	0		

(Jacobsen, B. S., & Lowery, B. J. [1992]. Further analysis of the psychometric properties of the Levine Denial of Illness Scale. Psychosomatic Medicine, 54, 372–381.)

a skewed distribution, with a mean of 9.1 and an SD of 6.3. By actual count, 86% of the values lie within the interval of mean ± 1 SD. Because this distribution is decidedly not bell shaped, the percentage in this interval is different from the expected 68%. Note that subtracting 2 SDs from the mean of 9.1 leads to the absurd conclusion that some patients had a negative length of stay!

Based on the rationale of 95% expected to be within 2 SDs of the mean for a bell-shaped distribution, Freedman, Pisani, Purves, and Adhikari (1991) suggest a "quick and dirty" method of roughly estimating the SD: Compute the difference between the maximum and minimum values and divide by 4. For the denial distribution (see Fig. 1-10), this produces an estimated SD of 19, a bit larger than the actual SD of 16.4, but within reason for a rough estimate.

The SD, like the mean, is algebraic. There is, for example, a formula for combining SDs from several distributions with different sample sizes (Glass & Stanley, 1970).

To compare SDs between several investigators who have examined the same variable, the coefficient of variation (CV) is useful (Daniel, 1987). This statistic is defined as:

$$CV = 100(SD/\bar{X})$$

For example, Spielberger (1983) reported the following statistics on the State-Trait Anxiety Inventory for a sample of depressed patients: mean = 54.43 and SD = 13.02. For general medical or surgical patients without depression, the statistics were mean = 42.68 and SD = 13.76. The CV for the depressed group was 24%, and the same coefficient for the nondepressed group was 32%. Thus, the nondepressed group was more variable relative to their mean than the depressed group.

Interpercentile Measures

There are several interpercentile measures of variability. Perhaps the most common is the interquartile range (IQR). The first quartile is the 25th percentile, and the third quartile is the 75th percentile. The IQR is defined as the range of the values extending from the 25th percentile to the 75th percentile. To locate the first quartile, first locate the median of the distribution. The first quartile is the middle value of all the data points below the median, and the third quartile is the middle value of all the data points above the median. In the example considered previously, the set of ordered values was 61, 70, 70, 74, 85, 97, 104, 112, 125, 132. The 50th percentile was noted to be 91; there are five values below 91. The median of those five values is 70, and the median of the five values above the 50th percentile is 112. Thus the IQR is 112 − 70.

This statistic tells how the middle 50% of the distribution is scattered. Other frequently used interpercentile ranges are (P_{10} to P_{90}) and (P_{3} to P_{97}). Note that the latter interpercentile range identifies the middle 94% of a distribution, a percentage similar to that identified in a bell-shaped distribution by the interval of mean ± 2 SDs.

TABLE 2-4
Selected Percentiles Produced by SPSS for the Data in Figure 1-6: Length of Stay for a Sample of 217 Elderly Patients From an Urban Medical Center

Program

FREQUENCIES
VARIABLES=INILOS/FORMAT=NOTABLE/PERCENTILES=3, 10, 25, 50, 75, 90, 97.

Output

INILOS   LENGTH OF INITIAL HOSPITAL STAY

Percentile	Value	Percentile	Value	Percentile	Value
3.00	2.000	10.00	3.900	25.00	5.000
50.00	8.000	75.00	11.000	90.00	15.000
97.00	26.430				

Valid cases   217   Missing cases   1

Table 2-4 contains a printout of selected computer percentiles for the variable of length of stay in a sample of elderly patients.

These interpercentile ranges, like the median, are not sensitive to very extreme values. If a distribution is badly skewed, and your judgment is that the median (P_{50}) is the appropriate average, then the IQR (or other interpercentile measure) is also appropriate. One of the most common uses of interpercentile measures is for growth charts.

Range

The range is the simplest measure of variability. It is the difference between the maximum value of the distribution and the minimum value. In Table 2-2, the range is $(132 - 61) = 71$. If the range is reported in a research journal, it would ordinarily be given as a maximum and a minimum, without the subtracted value.

The range can be unstable because it is based on only two values in the distribution and because it tends to increase with sample size. It is sensitive to very extreme values. For example, in Table 2-2, if the single value of 132 is changed to 702, the range would be $702 - 61 = 641$, a tremendous increase.

The main use of the range is for making a quick estimate of variability; however, the range can be informative in certain situations. For example, an engineer planning a dam may want to know about the *worst* flood that ever occurred in the surrounding area. Also, an investigator who is considering a case study may be interested in knowing the most extreme values. A researcher who intends to report an SD or an IQR may also choose to report the range for the additional information it provides about the two endpoints of a distribution.

Comparison of Measures of Variability

The SD is the most widely reported measure of variability. It has a formula and is the most reliable estimate of population variability. Generally, researchers prefer to use the SD, unless there is a good reason for not doing so. Like the mean, the most compelling reason for not using the SD is a distribution that has extreme values. The SD is best with distributions that are reasonably symmetric and have one mode.

Interpercentile measures are easy to understand. In a histogram, they mark off a certain percentage of area around the median. For instance, the IQR, extending from P_{25} to P_{75}, delineates the middle 50% of a distribution. These measures have no formulas but are calculated by a counting procedure. They can be used with distributions of any shape, but are especially useful with very skewed distributions.

The main uses of the range are to call attention to the two extreme values of a distribution and for quick, rough estimates of variability. To choose the appropriate measures, you must know the distribution. All of the above measures of variability are intended for use with interval or ratio variables, and often they are sensible for ordinal values. There are no measures of variability for nominal data in common use (Weisberg, 1992).

MEASURES OF SKEWNESS OR SYMMETRY

In addition to central tendency and variability, symmetry is an important characteristic of a distribution. Two sets of data can have the same mean and SD but different skewness (Fig. 2-4). Two measures of symmetry are considered: Pearson's measure and Fisher's measure.

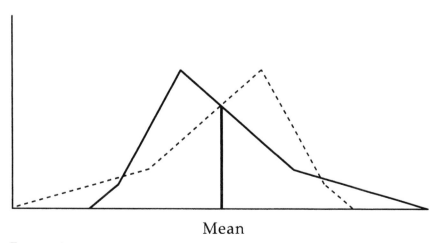

Mean

FIGURE 2-4
Two frequency distributions with the same mean and standard deviation but different symmetry.

Pearson's Skewness Coefficient

This measure of skewness is nonalgebraic but is easily calculated and is useful for quick estimates of symmetry. It is defined as:

$$\text{Skewness} = \frac{(\text{mean} - \text{median})}{\text{SD}}$$

For a perfectly symmetrical distribution, the mean will equal the median, and the skewness coefficient will be 0. If the distribution is positively skewed, as in Figure 2-1, the mean will be greater than the median, and the coefficient will be positive. If the coefficient is negative, then the distribution is negatively skewed. In general, the values will fall between −1 and +1. It would certainly be an odd distribution in which the mean differed from the median by more than 1 SD.

For the denial data of Table 2-3, the coefficient is (46.5 − 45.5) ÷ 16.4. The resulting value of .06 is close to zero. Hildebrand (1986) states that skewness values above 0.2 or below −0.2 indicate severe skewness. Therefore, the value of .06 indicates little skewness. The reader should verify this result visually by means of the graph of the denial data in the previous chapter (Fig. 1-10). For the data in Figure 1-5, the story is different. The mean number of pregnancies for that distribution is 3.7, the median is 3.0, and the SD is 2.1. Therefore, the coefficient is (3.7 − 3.0) ÷ 2.1, resulting in a value of 0.33, indicating severe skewness.

Fisher's Measure of Skewness

This statistic is based on deviations from the mean to the third power. The formula can be found in Hildebrand (1986). The calculation is tedious and is ordinarily done by a computer program. A symmetrical curve will result in a value of 0. If the skewness value is positive, then the curve is skewed to the right, and vice versa for a distribution skewed to the left. For the denial data in Table 2-3, Fisher's skewness measure is 0.195, a value close to zero. Dividing the measure of skewness by the standard error for skewness (0.195 ÷ 0.197 = 0.99) results in a number that is interpreted in terms of the normal curve. (This concept is explained further in the next chapter.) Values above +1.96 or below −1.96 are significant at the .05 level because 95% of the scores in a normal distribution fall between +1.96 and −1.96 SDs from the mean. Our value of 0.99 indicates that this distribution is not significantly skewed. Because this statistic is based on deviations to the third power, it is very sensitive to extreme values.

MEASURES OF KURTOSIS OR PEAKEDNESS

Fisher's Measure of Kurtosis

This statistic indicates whether a distribution has the right bell shape for a normal curve. It measures whether the bell shape is too flat or too peaked. Fisher's measure is based on deviations from the mean to the fourth power. The formula can be found in Hildebrand (1986). Again, the calculation is tedious and is ordinarily done by a computer program. A curve with the correct bell shape will result in a value of zero.

If the kurtosis value is a large positive number, the distribution is too peaked to be normal (leptokurtic); if the kurtosis value is a large negative number, the curve is too flat to be normal (platykurtic). For the denial data in Table 2-3, the kurtosis statistic is given as -0.249, a value close to zero. Dividing this value by the standard error for kurtosis ($-0.249 \div 0.391 = -0.64$), our distribution is not sufficiently kurtosed; that is, the value is not beyond ±1.96. The shape of the bell for this distribution can be called "normal." Because this statistic is based on deviations to the fourth power, it is very sensitive to extreme values. If a distribution is asymmetric, there is no particular need to examine kurtosis—obviously the distribution is not normal.

ROUNDING DESCRIPTIVE STATISTICS FOR TABLES

When reporting descriptive statistics in a table, too many digits are confusing. Even though a computer program has provided the statistic to the fourth decimal place, you do not have to report all the digits. If diastolic blood pressure is measured to the nearest whole number, why report descriptive statistics for blood pressure to the nearest 10,000th?

Chatfield (1988) suggests rounding summary statistics to two "effective" digits. An effective digit varies over the full range of digits from 0 to 9. For example, a set of diastolic blood pressures is recorded as 70, 74, 85, 96, 100, 102, and 108. The digit in the hundreds place is either 0 or 1, and the digit in the tens place is either 0, 7, 8, or 9. Neither of these digits is an effective digit. The remaining digit in the ones place is an effective digit—0, 2, 4, 5, 6, 8. Therefore, a descriptive statistic for blood pressure should be rounded to one decimal place. The mean for the previous example should be reported as 90.7 and the SD as 14.6. These statistics now have two effective digits—those representing ones and tenths.

In rounding to the nearest 10th (or 100th), if the last digit to be dropped is less than 5, round to the lower number; if it is higher than 5, round to the higher number. If the last digit to be dropped is exactly 5, no change is made in the preceding digit if it is even, but if it is odd, it is increased by one. Thus, 4.25 to the nearest tenth is 4.2, but 4.35 becomes 4.4.

GRAPHS USING DESCRIPTIVE STATISTICS

Line Graphs

A frequently used graph in health care research is the line graph, which is often used to display longitudinal trends. Time points in equal intervals are placed on the horizontal axis, and the scale for the statistic on the vertical axis. Dots representing the statistic (e.g., means, medians, or percentages) at each time point are then connected. This type of graph presents a smoother appearance than drawing bars over each time point. Frequently, vertical error bars are added to each time point to indicate the accuracy of the statistic as an estimate of a population parameter. These error bars represent standard errors, which are discussed in detail later in this text. Exam-

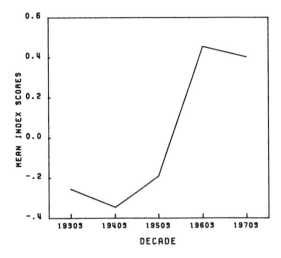

FIGURE 2-5

Mean sex object index scores by decade ($N = 211$). (From Kalisch, B. J., Kalisch, P. A., & McHugh, M. L. [1982]. The nurse as a sex object in motion pictures, 1930–1980. *Research in Nursing and Health, 5,* 151.)

ples of line graphs from research journals showing change over time are given in Figure 2-5 through Figure 2-7. When several groups are being compared in the same line graph, Tufte (1983) recommends that labels be integrated into the graph rather than having a separate legend so the eye is not required to go back and forth.

We are frequently told that graphs should include zero on the vertical axis, but sometimes this wastes a lot of space (Cleveland, 1985). For example, the graph for Figure 2-6 has been redrawn in Figure 2-8 so that zero is included on the vertical

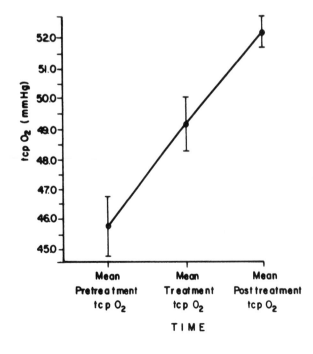

FIGURE 2-6

Effect of non-nutritive sucking on tcp O_2 level as demonstrated by 26 sets of measurements on preterm neonates. Values (means ± standard errors) are the averaged readings for each 8-minute observation period. (From Burroughs, A. K,. Asonye, U. O., Anderson-Shanklin, G. C., & Vidyasagar, D. [1978]. The effect of non-nutritive sucking on transcutaneous oxygen tension in noncrying, preterm neonates. *Research in Nursing and Health, 1,* 69–75.)

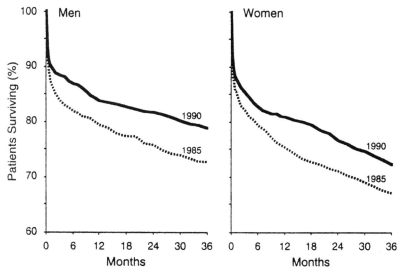

FIGURE 2-7

Trends in survival in the 3 years after hospitalization for definite acute myocardial infarction in 1985 and 1990 among residents of the Twin Cities area who were 30 to 74 years of age. [From McGovern, P. G., Pankow, J. S., Shahar, E., Doliszny, K. M., Folsom, A. R., Blackburn, H., & Leupker, R. V. [1996]. Recent trends in acute coronary heart disease. *New England Journal of Medicine, 34,* 887.)

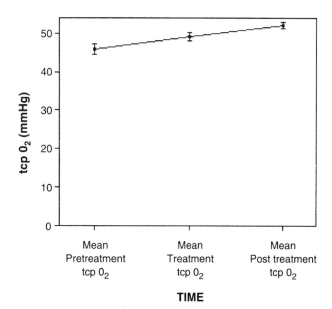

FIGURE 2-8

Data from Figure 2-6 with vertical scale re-drawn to include zero.

axis. Editors of research journals do not appreciate such graphs as Figure 2-8, which have a lot of blank space. Choose the scale for the vertical axis so that the data "fill up" the graph. You may assume that the reader of a scientific journal will look at tick mark labels and breaks in the axes or line plot and understand them (Cleveland, 1985).

Box Plots

A box plot is a graphical display that uses descriptive statistics based on percentiles (Tukey, 1977). The first step in constructing this plot is to draw the box. Its length corresponds to the IQR, that is, the box begins with the 25th percentile and ends with the 75th percentile (Fig. 2-9). A line (or other symbol) within the box indicates the location of the median or 50th percentile. Thus, the box provides information about central tendency and the variability of the middle 50% of the distribution.

The next step is to locate the wild values of the distribution, if any. Calculate the IQR ($P_{75} - P_{25}$), and then multiply this value by 3. Individual scores that are more than three times the IQR from the upper and lower edges of the box are extreme outlying values and are denoted on the plot by a symbol such as E. Next, multiply the IQR by 1.5. Individual scores between 1.5 times the IQR and three times the IQR away from the edges of the box are minor outlying values. Denote them on the box plot with a different symbol, such as O.

Finally, draw the whiskers of the box. These lines should extend to the smallest and largest values that are not minor or extreme outlying values. Thus, the whiskers and designation of the outlying values provide more detail about how the lower 25% and upper 25% of the distribution are scattered. The box plot is well suited for comparisons among several groups. Examples of box plots are given in Figure 2-10 comparing psychological adjustment to illness in a sample of breast cancer patients according to stage of cancer. From this figure, you can see that as the stage of cancer became higher, adjustment worsened (that is, the average score increased). Also, it is clear that the variability of the adjustment scores was greater as the stage became higher. Note that the subject identification numbers can be placed on the plot for convenient reference.

OUTLIERS

Outliers are values that are extreme relative to the bulk of the distribution. They appear inconsistent with the rest of the data. The source of an outlier may be any of the following:

1. An error in the recording of the data
2. A failure of data collection, such as not following sample criteria (e.g., inadvertently admitting a disoriented patient into a study), a subject not following instructions on a questionnaire, or equipment failure
3. An actual extreme value from an unusual subject

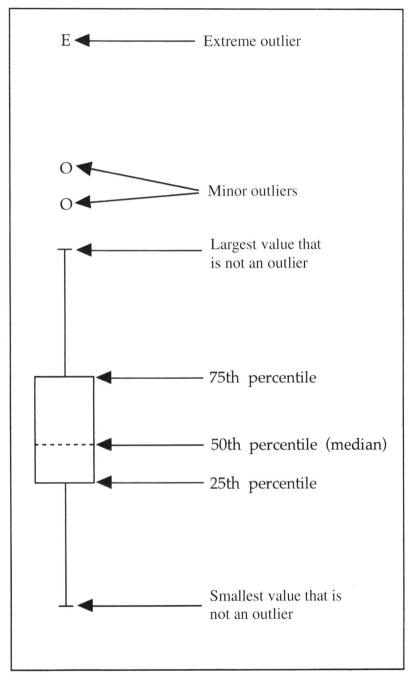

FIGURE 2-9
Schematic diagram of the construction of a box plot.

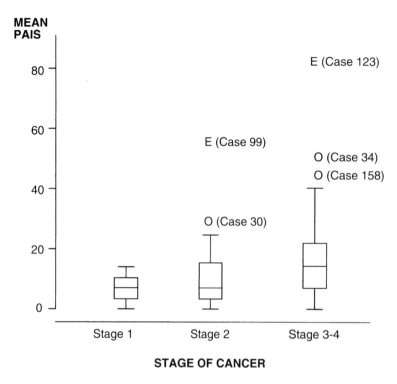

FIGURE 2-10
Box plots of psychological adjustment to illness (PAIS) in a sample of breast cancer patients by stage of cancer (hypothetical data): Higher scores indicate poorer adjustment.

Outliers must first be identified by an objective method. A traditional way of labeling outliers has been to locate any values that are more than 3 SDs from the mean. The problem with this method is that outliers inflate the SD, making it less likely that a value will be 3 SDs away from the mean. A more recent recommendation by Tukey (1977) was described earlier in connection with the box plot. Values that are more than 3 IQRs from the upper or lower edges of the box are extreme outliers. Values between 1.5 IQRs and 3 IQRs from the upper and lower edges of the box are minor outliers. The reason for having an objective method is to prevent undue (perhaps unethical) data manipulation, such as pruning very high or very low values that are not really outliers.

Once outliers have been identified, the next step is to try to explain them. If they represent errors in coding or a failure in the data collection, then those observations are either discarded or corrected. If the outliers represent actual values or the explanation is unknown, then a researcher must decide how to handle them. One frequent suggestion is to analyze the data two ways: with the outliers in the distribution and with the outliers removed. If the results are similar, as they are apt to be if the sample size is large, then perhaps the outliers may be ignored.

If the results are not similar, then a statistical analysis that is resistant to outliers can be used (e.g., median and IQR). If a researcher wants to use a mean with outliers, then the *trimmed mean* is an option. This statistic is calculated with a certain percentage of the extreme values removed from both ends of the distribution. For example, if the sample size is 100, then the 5% trimmed mean is the mean of the middle 90% of the observations. Special formulas for using the trimmed mean in statistical inference are given in Koopmans (1987).

Another alternative is a *winsorized mean*. In the simplest case, the highest and lowest extremes are replaced, respectively, by the next to highest value and the next to lowest value. If the sample size is 100, the resulting 100 data points are then processed as if they were the original data. Winer (1971) outlines the special techniques for handling statistics computed from winsorized samples. Further details on the treatment of outliers can be found in Barnett and Lewis (1985). A researcher can also view these actual outliers as case material and adopt the advice of Skinner (1972): "When you run onto something interesting, drop everything else and study it."

SUMMARY

Descriptive statistics based on the mean are best for distributions that are reasonably symmetrical and have a single peak. These measures include the mean, the SD, and Fisher's measures of skewness and kurtosis. For distributions that are very skewed, the median and the IQR are less influenced by extreme scores. The range, the mode, and Pearson's coefficient of skewness are useful for quick estimates. In addition, the mode is informative when a distribution has several peaks, and the range is useful for locating the most extreme values. Outliers are extreme values that meet objective criteria, and researchers must consider carefully how to handle them in data analysis. Two graphs that make use of summary statistics are the line graph and the box plot. A line graph uses statistics such as means at various time points to display longitudinal trends. Box plots emphasize the extremes of a distribution and are handy for displaying outliers.

APPLICATION EXERCISES AND RESULTS

EXERCISES

1. Access the data set named SURVEY.SAV. Run frequencies and include statistics for all variables. Examine the output for outliers, marked skewness, unequal groups, and so forth.

2. Construct a table that includes some of the categorical variables in this dataset. Write a description of the table.

3. Construct a table that includes some of the continuous variables in this dataset. Write a description of the table.

4. Construct a boxplot (sometimes called a box and whiskers plot) for the variable EDUC.

RESULTS

1. Generally, when you first look at output, you will find invalid numbers, that is, a number that is not valid for a particular variable. We provided you with some examples of that in Chapter 1. With SURVEY.SAV we tried to remove all invalid numbers, so unless we missed one, you should not have found any.

Current Work Status

		Frequency	Percent	Valid Percent	Cumulative Percent
Valid	Unemployed	29	16.4	16.4	16.4
	Part-time	47	26.6	26.6	42.9
	Full-time	101	57.1	57.1	100.0
	Total	177	100.0	100.0	
Total		177	100.0		

Political Affiliation

		Frequency	Percent	Valid Percent	Cumulative Percent
Valid	Republican	41	23.2	23.3	23.3
	Democrat	54	30.5	30.7	54.0
	Independent	81	45.8	46.0	100.0
	Total	176	99.4	100.0	
Missing	System Missing	1	.6		
	Total	1	.6		
Total		177	100.0		

Choosing a Winter Vacation

		Frequency	Percent	Valid Percent	Cumulative Percent
Valid	Beachfront condo in Hawaii	69	39.0	39.4	39.4
	Chalet in Swiss Alps	34	19.2	19.4	58.9
	Luxury hotel at Disney World in Florida	27	15.3	15.4	74.3
	Ocean cruise through Caribbean Islands	45	25.4	25.7	100.0
	Total	175	98.9	100.0	
Missing	System Missing	2	1.1		
	Total	2	1.1		
Total		177	100.0		

EXERCISE FIGURE 2-1. Tables of categorical variables.

For an example of an outlier, look at the frequencies for age. You should see one 83 year old and one 95 year old. I questioned the 95 year old but was assured by the student who collected the data that the individual was indeed 95 years old.

Skewness is often a problem and violates the assumptions underlying parametric tests. Look at the variable HEALTH, overall state of health. It was scored from 1 = very ill to 10 = very healthy. Note that only 20.5% of the distribution falls between the scores of one and five. Only two subjects rate themselves a one or two. This is understandable, because the students are not likely to request data from someone who is quite ill. You can tell by looking at the distribution that it is negatively skewed (i.e., the values tail off at the negative end). The value for skewness (−.821) divided by the standard error of skewness (.183) yields −4.49, indicating significant skewness beyond the .01 level (critical value = 2.58).

There are a number of examples of uneven groups. Males comprise only 33% of the sample. Fortunately, only 13% of the sample is still smoking, and only 2% are routinely depressed. Perhaps unfortunately, only 2% would donate an entire $500,000 gift to charity. What other examples can you find?

2. Exercise Figure 2-1 contains a sample table of categorical variables. Often, variables are combined into one table, but because SPSS for Windows presents these separate tables, which can be copied into a manuscript, we have them as three separate tables. Tables are used to present data clearly and succinctly. One does not repeat all the information in the text; generally just the highlights are presented.

We could describe these three variables by stating that more than half of the sample is employed full time, and 46% list their political affiliation as independent. When choosing a winter vacation, the most popular choice was a beachfront condo in Hawaii, followed by a Caribbean cruise. Sixty-five percent of the respondents selected one of those choices. A chalet in the Swiss Alps and a trip to Disney World were not as popular.

3. Exercise Figure 2-2 contains a sample table of continuous variables. We created the table using the descriptives program in SPSS. We could describe the table by stating that the subjects ranged in age from 15 to 95 with a mean age of 38. They were a well-educated group with a mean of 16 years of education. On the Inventory of Positive Psychological Attitudes, in which scores can range from 30 to 210, the actual scores ranged from 51 to 208.

4. Exercise Figure 2-3 contains the boxplot that we ran in SPSS for Windows 7.0 by clicking on Graphics, then Boxplot. The box encloses the data from the 25th to the 75th percentile

Descriptive Statistics

	N	Minimum	Maximum	Mean	Std. Deviation
Subject's age	170	15	95	38.06	12.84
Education in years	168	4	26	16.15	3.65
Positive psychological attitudes	174	51.00	208.00	152.5805	31.8289
Valid N (listwise)	162				

EXERCISE FIGURE 2-2. A table describing continuous variables.

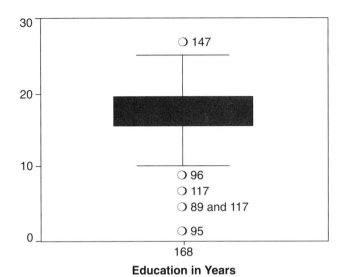

Education in Years

EXERCISE FIGURE 2-3. A boxplot of the variable years of education.

(50% of the data). The median is represented by the horizontal line within the box. In SPSS, extreme outlying values are defined as those that are more than 3 box-lengths from the upper or lower edge of the box and are designated by asterisks (*). Cases with values between 1.5 and 3 box-lengths from the edges of the box are called outliers and are designated by a circle. The number next to the circle is the subject number. For example, we see that subject number 147 has been designated as an outlier. Looking at our data, we find that subject 147 reported 26 years of education. The plot is very helpful because it helps us determine quickly which subjects are associated with the outlying values. In this example, there are no extreme outlying values.

Introduction to Inferential Statistics and Hypothesis Testing

BARBARA HAZARD MUNRO • BARBARA S. JACOBSEN
LEONARD E. BRAITMAN

OBJECTIVES FOR CHAPTER 3

After reading this chapter, you should be able to do the following:

1 • Describe the characteristics of the normal curve.

2 • Explain statistical probability.

3 • Differentiate between a type I and a type II error.

4 • Explain the relationship between one- and two-tailed tests and the power of a test.

5 • Interpret a confidence interval.

NORMAL CURVE

The *normal curve* is a theoretically perfect frequency polygon in which the mean, median, and mode all coincide in the center and that takes the form of a symmetrical bell-shaped curve (Fig. 3-1). De Moivre, a French mathematician, developed the notion of the normal curve based on his observations of games of chance. Many human traits, such as intelligence, attitudes, and personality, are distributed among the population in a fairly "normal" way. That is, if you measure something, such as an intelligence test, in a representative sample of sufficient size, the resulting scores will assume a distribution that is similar to the normal curve. Most of the scores will fall around the mean (an IQ of 100), and there will be relatively few extreme scores, such as an IQ below 55 or one above 145.

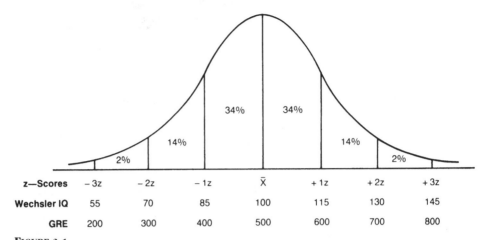

z—Scores	− 3z	− 2z	− 1z	X̄	+ 1z	+ 2z	+ 3z
Wechsler IQ	55	70	85	100	115	130	145
GRE	200	300	400	500	600	700	800

FIGURE 3-1
The normal curve.

The concept of the normal curve is useful. For example, when we discuss hypothesis testing, we talk about the probability (or the likelihood) that a given difference or relationship could have occurred by chance alone. Understanding the normal curve prepares you for understanding the concepts underlying hypothesis testing.

The baseline of the normal curve is measured off in standard deviation (SD) units. These are indicated by the lower case letter z in Figure 3-1. A score that is 1 SD above the mean is symbolized by $+1z$, and $-1z$ indicates a score that is 1 SD below the mean. For example, the Wechsler IQ test has a mean of 100 and a SD of 15. Thus, 1 SD above the mean $(+1z)$ is 115, and one SD below the mean $(-1z)$ is 85.

In a normal distribution, approximately 34% of the scores fall between the mean and 1 SD above the mean. Because the curve is symmetrical, 34% also fall between the mean and 1 SD below the mean. Therefore, 68% of the scores fall between $-1z$ and $+1z$. With the Wechsler IQ test, this means that 68%, or approximately two thirds of the scores, will fall between 85 and 115. Of the one third of the scores remaining, one sixth will fall below 85, and one sixth will be above 115.

Of the total distribution, 28% fall between 1 and 2 SDs from the mean; 14% fall between 1 and 2 SDs above the mean; and 14% fall between 1 and 2 SDs below the mean. Thus, 96% of the scores (14 + 34 + 34 + 14) fall between ±2 SDs from the mean. For the Wechsler IQ test, this means that 96% of the population receive scores between 70 and 130.

Most of the last 4% fall between 2 and 3 SDs from the mean, 2% on each side. Thus, 99.7% of those taking the Wechsler IQ test score between 55 and 145.

Two other z-scores are important because we use them when constructing confidence intervals (CIs). They are $z = \pm 1.96$ and $z = \pm 2.58$. Of the scores in a distribution, 95% fall between $\pm 1.96z$, and 99% fall between $n \pm 2.58z$. For additional practice with the normal curve, look at the graduation requirement examination

(GRE) scores in Figure 3-1. Each section of the GREs was scaled to have a mean of 500 and a SD of 100. Someone who scored 600 on this test would be 1 SD above the mean, or at the 84th percentile. (The 50th percentile is the mean, and 34% above the mean equals the 84th percentile.)

PERCENTILES

Percentiles allow us to describe a score in relation to other scores in a distribution. A percentile tells us the relative position of a given score. It allows us to compare scores on tests that have different means and SDs. A percentile is calculated as:

$$\frac{\text{number of scores less than a given score}}{\text{total number of scores}} \times 100$$

Suppose you received a score of 90 on a test given to a class of 50 people. Of your classmates, 40 had scores lower than 90. Your percentile rank would be:

$$\frac{40}{50} \times 100 = 80$$

You achieved a higher score than 80% of the people who took the test, which also means that almost 20% of those who took the test did better than you.

The 25th percentile is called the *first quartile;* the 50th percentile, the *second quartile,* or more commonly, the *median;* and the 75th percentile, the *third quartile.* The quartiles are points, not ranges like the interquartile range. Therefore, the third quartile is not from 50 to 75, it is just the 75th percentile. One does not usually say that a score fell within a quartile, because the quartile is only one point.

As demonstrated with the GRE score of 600, we also can determine percentile rank by using the normal curve. For another example, note Figure 3-1. The IQ score of 85 exceeds the IQ score of 16% of the population, so a score of 85 is equal to a percentile rank of 16. To test your understanding, determine the percentile rank of a GRE score of 700.

Tables make it possible to determine the proportion of the normal curve found between various points along the baseline. They are set up as in Appendix A. To understand how to read the table, go down the first column until you come to 1.0. Note that the percent of area under the normal curve between the mean and a standard score (z-score) of 1.00 is 34.13. This is how the 34% was determined in Figure 3-1. Moving down the row to the right, note that the area under the curve between the mean and 1.01 is 34.38, between the mean and 1.02 is 34.61, and so forth.

Suppose you have a standard score of +1.86 (the next section discusses how to calculate the z-scores). Finding this score in the table, we see that the percent of the curve between the mean and 1.86 is 46.86. A plus z-score is above the mean, so 50% of the curve is on the minus z side, and another 46.86% is between the mean and +1.86; the percentile rank is 96.86 (50 + 46.86). If the z-score were −1.86, the score would fall below the mean, and the percentile rank would be 3.14 (50 − 46.86).

In summary, to calculate a percentile when you have the standard score, you

TABLE 3-1
*Relationship of Scores to Percentiles
at Varying Distances from the Mean*

Subject	Scores	GRE-Q	Percentile
1	1st score	500	50
	2nd score	510	54
2	1st score	600	84
	2nd score	610	86
3	1st score	700	97.7
	2nd score	710	98.2

first look up the score in the table to determine the percent of the normal curve that falls between the mean and the given score. Then, if the sign is positive, you add the percentage to 50. If the sign is negative, you subtract the percentage from 50.

When using percentiles to determine relative position, remember the following factors:

1. Because so many scores are located near the mean and so few at the ends, the distance along the baseline in terms of percentiles varies a great deal.
2. The distance between the 50th and 55th percentile is much smaller than the distance between the 90th and the 95th.

What this means in practical terms is that if you raise your score on a test, there will be more impact on your percentile rank if you are near the mean than if you are near the ends of the distribution.

As an example, suppose three people retook the GRE quantitative examination in hopes of raising their score and thus their percentile rank (Table 3-1). All three subjects raised their score by 10 points. For subject one, who was right at the mean, that meant an increase of 4 points in percentile rank, whereas for subject three, who was originally 2 SDs above the mean, the percentile rank only went up 0.5 of a point.

STANDARD SCORES

Standard scores are a way of expressing a score in terms of its relative distance from the mean. A z-score is one such standard score. The meaning of an ordinary score varies, depending on the mean and the SD of the distribution from which it was drawn. In research, standard scores are used more often than percentiles. Thus far, we have used examples when the z-score was easy to calculate. The GRE score of 600 is 1 SD above the mean, so the z-score is +1. The formula used to calculate z-scores follows:

$$z = \frac{X - \bar{X}}{\text{standard deviation}}$$

As you can see, the numerator is a measure of the deviation of the score from the mean of the distribution. The following is for the GRE example:

$$z = \frac{600 - 500}{100} = \frac{100}{100} = 1$$

As another example, suppose an individual obtained a score of 48 on a test in which the mean was 35 and the SD was 5:

$$z = \frac{48 - 35}{5} = \frac{13}{5} = 2.6$$

Using the table in Appendix A, we find that 49.53% of the curve is contained between the mean and 2.6 SDs above the mean, so the percentile rank for this score would be 99.53 (50 + 49.53).

Suppose the national mean weight for a particular group is 120 lb, and the SD is 6 lb. An individual from the group, Mary, weighs 112 lb. What is Mary's z-score and percentile rank?

$$z = \frac{112 - 120}{6} = \frac{-8}{6} = -1.33$$

Mary's percentile rank is 50 − 40.82, or 9.18.

If all the raw scores in a distribution are converted to z-scores, the resulting distribution will have a mean of zero and an SD of 1. If several distributions are converted to z-scores, the z-scores for the various measures can be compared directly. Although the new distributions have a new SD and mean (1 and 0), the shape of the distribution is not altered.

Transformed Standard Scores

Because calculating z-scores results in decimals and negative numbers, some people prefer to transform them into other distributions. One distribution that has been widely used is one with a mean of 50 and a SD of 10. Such *transformed standard scores* are generally called *T-scores,* although some authors call them *Z-scores.* Some standardized test results are given in *T*-scores. To convert a z-score to a *T*-score, use the following formula:

$$T = 10z + 50$$

For example, with a z-score of 2.5, the *T*-score would be:

$$T = (10)(2.5) + 50$$
$$T = 25 + 50$$
$$T = 75$$

In the new distribution, the mean is 50 and the SD is 10, so a score of 75 is still 2.5 SDs above the mean.

In the same way, other distributions can be established. This is the technique used to transform z-scores into GRE scores with a mean of 500 and an SD of 100.

The basic formula for transforming z-scores is to multiply the z-scores by the desired SD and add the desired mean.

transformed z-scores = (new standard deviation)(z-score) + (new mean)

Suppose you wanted to transform your z-scores into a scale with a mean of 70 and a SD of 5. Then your formula would be $5z + 70$. Transforming scores in this way does not change the original distribution of the scores. In some circumstances, however, a researcher may want to change the distribution of a set of data. This might occur with a set of data that is not normally distributed.

CORRECTING FAILURES IN NORMALITY THROUGH DATA TRANSFORMATIONS

Although data transformations are often recommended for data that do not meet the assumptions of normality, linearity, and homoscedasticity, such transformations should be approached with caution, because they make interpretation of results more difficult. The transformed scales are not in the same metric as the original; thus, measures of central tendency and dispersion are not clear in relation to the original measure. Often it is necessary to try several approaches to transformation. After each attempt, recalculate the measures of skewness, and so forth, to determine whether or not the transformation was successful. Tabachnick and Fidell (1996, p. 82) suggest the following for positively skewed distributions: For moderately skewed distributions, try a square root transformation first; for substantially skewed distributions, try a log transformation; and for severely skewed distributions, try an inverse transformation.

If a variable is negatively skewed, you can reverse score it first to make it positively skewed and then apply the appropriate transformation. For example, if the variable was scored from a low of 1 to a high of 3, you would create a variable in which 3 = 1, 2 = 2, and 1 = 3.

You can accomplish that through recode procedures or through a compute statement in which you subtract each value from the largest value in the distribution plus one. In our example, this would result in $4 - 3 = 1, 4 - 2 = 2, 4 - 1 = 3$.

If transformations are not successful, you should consider creating a categorical, rather than continuous, variable.

CENTRAL LIMIT THEOREM

If you draw a sample from a population and calculate its mean, how close have you come to knowing the mean of the population? Statisticians have provided us with formulas that allow us to determine just how close the mean of our sample is to the mean of the population.

It has been shown that when many samples are drawn from a population, the *means* of these samples tend to be normally distributed; that is, when they are graphed along a baseline, they tend to form the normal curve. The larger the number of samples, the more the distribution approaches the normal curve. Also, if the average of the means of the samples is calculated (the mean of the means), this average (or mean) is very close to the actual mean of the population. Again, the larger the number of the samples, the closer this overall mean is to the population mean.

If the means form a normal distribution, we can then use the percentages under the normal curve to determine the probability statements about individual means. We would know, for example, that the probability of a given mean falling between $+1$ and -1 SD from the mean of the population is 68%.

To calculate the standard scores necessary to determine position under the normal curve, we need to know the SD of the distribution. You could calculate the SD of the distribution of means by treating each mean as a raw score and applying the regular formula. This new SD of the mean is called the *standard error of the mean.* The term *error* is used to indicate the fact that due to sampling error, each sample mean is likely to deviate somewhat from the true population mean.

Fortunately, statisticians have used these techniques on samples drawn from known populations and have demonstrated relationships that allow us to estimate the mean and SD of a population given only the data from *one sample*. They have demonstrated that there is a constant relationship between the SD of a distribution of sample means (the standard error of the mean), the SD of the population from which the samples were drawn, and the size of the samples. We do not usually know the SD of the population. If we had measured the entire population, we would have no need to infer its parameters from measures taken from samples. The formula for the standard error of the mean can be written as:

$$\frac{\text{standard deviation}}{\sqrt{n}}$$

The formula indicates that we are estimating the standard error given the SD of a sample of n size. It has been shown that a sample of 30 is enough to estimate the population mean with reasonable accuracy.

Given the SD of a sample and the size of the sample, we can estimate the standard error of the mean. For example, given a sample of 100 and an SD of 20, we would estimate the standard error of the mean to be:

$$\frac{20}{\sqrt{100}} = \frac{20}{10} = 2$$

Two factors influence the standard error of the mean: the SD of the sample and the sample size. Note that the sample size has a large impact on the size of the error, because the square root of n is used in the denominator. As the size of n increases, the size of the error decreases. Suppose we had the same SD as just demonstrated, but a sample size of 1,000 instead of 100. Now we have

$$\frac{20}{\sqrt{1000}} = \frac{20}{31.62} = 0.63,$$

a much smaller standard error. This shows that the larger the sample, the less error there is. If there is less error, we can estimate more precisely the parameters of the population.

If there is more variability in the sample, the standard error increases. If there is much variability, it is harder to draw a sample that is representative of the population. Given wide variability, we need larger samples. Note the effect of variability (SD) on the standard error of the mean.

$$\frac{20}{\sqrt{100}} = \frac{20}{10} = 2$$

$$\frac{40}{\sqrt{100}} = \frac{40}{10} = 4$$

As is shown in a later section in this chapter, the standard error of the mean underlies the calculation of CIs.

PROBABILITY

Ideas about probability are of fundamental importance for health care researchers. The use of data in making decisions is a hallmark of our information world, and probability provides a means for translating observed data into decisions about the nature of our world (Kotz & Stroup, 1983). For example, probability helps us to evaluate the accuracy of a statistic and to test a hypothesis. Thus, research findings in journals often are stated in probabilistic terms and often communicated to patients using probabilistic language. The approach to probability in this chapter is practical, with special attention given to concepts that are important later in this text.

In the life of a health care professional, questions about probability frequently occur in connection with a patient's future. For example, suppose patient X's mammogram revealed a cluster of five calcifications with no other signs of breast abnormality. The patient is told she should have a breast biopsy based solely on these x-ray findings. If the patient inquires about the probability that the biopsy will reveal a malignancy, health care professionals refer to the literature. Powell, McSweeney, and Wilson (1983) studied 251 patients who received a breast biopsy with mammographic calcifications as the only reason for the biopsy. Everyone in the sample had at least five microcalcifications in a well-defined cluster; cancer was found in 45 of these patients (17.9%). Consequently, the health care professional might tell patient X that the probability of cancer was 17.9%.

What has really been stated? The health care practitioner has presumably imagined that the names of the 251 patients in the study were placed in a hat, and one name was drawn by lot. The chances of drawing the name of one of the 45 patients with cancer is 45 in 251, or 17.9%. Patient X, of course, is not one of the 251 names in the hat, but the practitioner is thinking along the lines of, "What if she were?" This way of thinking, while hypothetical, is reasonable if patient X is similar to the group of 251 patients in the study. Powell et al. (1983) described the sample of 251 patients as consecutively chosen over a period of 18 years from the practice of one surgeon at one hospital. While this information implies a fairly broad sample, it does not provide any breakdown by prognostic variables.

An outcome may vary according to membership in a certain subset of a total group. For example, in 1982, a male patient was diagnosed with a rare form of abdominal cancer (Gould, 1985). The patient read that the median mortality was 8 months after diagnosis; therefore, he reasoned that his chances of living longer than 8 months were 50%. On reading further, he decided that his chances of being in that 50% who lived longer were good: He was young, the disease was discovered early, and he was receiving the best treatment. Not only that, he realized that the survival distribution was undoubtedly skewed to the right (some patients lived for years with the disease); therefore, if he was in the upper 50%, his chances of living a lot longer than 8 months were very good.

Self-Evident Truths (Axioms) About Probabilities

All probabilities are between 0% and 100%, as illustrated in Figure 3-2. There are no negative probabilities. If the probability of something happening is 0%, then it is impossible. One has to be careful about assigning probabilities of 0% to an event; after all, the Titanic was advertised as an unsinkable ship! However, it does appear that the probability is 0% for a 90 year old to run a 4-minute mile. If the probability of an event is 100%, then we are absolutely certain that it will occur. The eventual death of a person has a probability of 100%.

The probability of an event is 100% minus the probability of the opposite event. Perhaps a different health care worker would have preferred to report the probability for the biopsy of patient X as an 82.1% chance that the calcifications would *not* be malignant. This would be accurate, because 100% − 17.9% = 82.1%.

Table 3-2 lists the four possibilities for the sample of 45 women who were diagnosed with cancer after a biopsy based on a suspicious mammogram, as given by

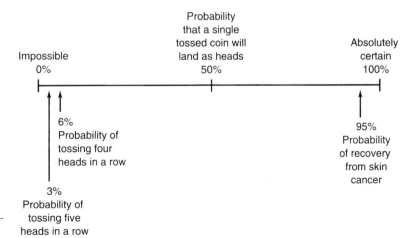

FIGURE 3-2
Diagram of the scale of probabilities.

TABLE 3-2
Malignant Pathology of X-Ray Calcifications

Pathology	N
Duct cancer, in situ	25
Lobular cancer, in situ	9
Duct, invasive	9
Lobular, invasive	2
	45
	(100%)

(Data from Powell, R. W., McSweeney, M. B., & Wilson, C. E. [1983]. X-ray calcifications as the only basis for breast biopsy. Annals of Surgery, 197, 555–559. Modified slightly to represent individual patients rather than 47 breasts from 45 patients.)

Powell et al. (1983). The sum of all the possibilities for an event is 100%. Note that the sum of the four outcomes in Table 3-1 is 100%, indicating that it is certain that one of these possibilities will occur.

Definitions of Probability

Frequency Probability

If scientists were asked about the meaning of probability, they would give many different answers (Carnap, 1953). Most health care professionals, however, think of probability in the sense of a frequency or statistical probability. That is, they think of probability as a percentage based on empirical observation, which allows them to make an intelligent guess about the future. Their definition for such a probability, based on observations from a sample, is given below:

$$\text{sample probability} = \frac{\text{number of times the event occurred}}{\text{total number of people in the sample}} \times 100$$

In the previously noted case of patient X with the suspicious mammogram, the health care worker would substitute as follows:

$$\text{probability of cancer} = \frac{45}{251} \times 100 = 17.9\%$$

Patient X was not a member of the group of 251 patients, but the hypothetical type of thinking "What if patient X were from that group?" is at least reasonable as a practical type of probability. It helps to be able to argue logically that patient X might have been a member of the total group of 251 patients.

In mathematical theory, however, probabilities are only meaningful in the context of chance. In the previous example, we also have to imagine that patient X was chosen "by lot" from the total sample, which implies a random choice. There are two criteria for a random process. First, every item must have an equal chance of being chosen. In the case of drawing from a hat, this means that attention must be given to details, such as whether each name was written on the same size slip of paper, whether the slips were well stirred, whether the person who drew from the hat was blindfolded, and so forth.[1] Second, each choice must be independent of every other choice. This means that we must not be able predict whose name will be drawn after patient X.

These criteria for a random process also are important when we consider the larger question of whether the 17.9% probability of cancer would still be the same if more patients were followed. The mathematical definition for a frequency probability invokes the law of averages. That is, we must think of drawing more patients at random. As the sample becomes larger and larger, the percentage will converge to the true or population value.

$$\text{population probability} = \frac{\text{total number of times the event occurred}}{\text{total number of people in the population}} \times 100$$

Thus, the sample probability is an estimate of the population probability. A random sample provides, in theory, a better estimate of the population probability.

In a brief discussion section following the article by Powell et al. (1983), A. H. Letton reported on a second sample of 269 patients collected for 10 years. A mammogram indicated calcium deposits, and subsequent biopsies revealed that 46 patients (17.1%) had cancer. Thus, a second study, again with a nonrandom sample, produced results remarkably similar to those of Powell et al.

The reader might protest, "but this has no connection to mathematical theory because there was no random process." The 251 women in the first sample were not chosen at random, nor were the 269 women in the second sample, nor was patient X. Random sampling or random assignment to groups is infrequently used in health care research (Brown, Tanner, & Padrick, 1984; Fletcher & Fletcher, 1979; Jacobsen & Meininger, 1985). Patients who arrive for care become the sample, and health care researchers take all they can get rather than drawing random samples. These sample probabilities, though not based on a chance process, remain the only estimates of the true or population probabilities.

Frequency probabilities are based on empirical observations and can thus be termed objective. However, not all probabilities that can be considered objective are determined empirically. For example, when tossing a fair coin, the probabilities of heads or tails can be deduced logically without ever actually tossing the coin. These are called a priori (before the fact) probabilities. Derdiarian and Lewis (1986) provided an illustration of how a priori probabilities could be used in health care research. Each of three raters was asked to code an item from an interview transcript as belonging to category 1 or category 2. There are eight possible outcomes as listed in Table 3-3. All three raters could agree that the item belonged in category 1 (1-1-1), or they could disagree, for example, with the first rater coding the item as category 1 and the other two coding the item as category 2 (1-2-2). If all of these

---

[1]*Health care researchers who want to draw a random sample avoid having to deal with such details by using a random number table.*

TABLE 3-3

***Probability of Eight Possible Outcomes for Three Raters Coding
an Item Into Dichotomous Categories (1 or 2) by Chance***

Outcome			
Rater #1	*Rater #2*	*Rater #3*	***Probability***
1	1	1	$\frac{1}{8}$
1	1	2	$\frac{1}{8}$
1	2	1	$\frac{1}{8}$
2	1	1	$\frac{1}{8}$
1	2	2	$\frac{1}{8}$
2	1	2	$\frac{1}{8}$
2	2	1	$\frac{1}{8}$
2	2	2	$\frac{1}{8}$

*(Derdiarian, A. K., & Lewis, S. [1986]. The D-L test of agreement: A stronger measure
of interrater reliability.* Nursing Research, 35, *375–378)*

outcomes are equally likely by chance, then each will have a probability of 1 in 8 (see Table 3-3). Derdiarian and Lewis (1986) show how comparing actual results to the tabled probabilities can provide a measure of inter-rater agreement.

Subjective Probability

Another definition for probability is a percentage that expresses our personal, subjective belief that an event will occur. Kotz and Stroup (1983) stress that these judgments are rational assessments, not arbitrary beliefs. In the example of patient X with the suspicious mammogram, what about the health care professional's opinion of the probability of 17.9% that the calcifications are cancer? If the patient were told that the probability was close to zero that the biopsy was malignant, then we would be surprised if it turned out to be cancer. On the other hand, a probability of 17.9% would not be viewed as "close to zero" by most health care professionals. A practitioner would not be very surprised if the calcifications turned out to be cancer, and that is why patient X with five or more calcifications in a cluster was recommended for biopsy.

When testing hypotheses, which is discussed later in this text, researchers focus on probabilities (often called *p* values) that fall at the lower end of the continuum in Figure 3-2. Generally, probabilities that are 5% or less are considered unusual in research. The reasons for this are partly intuitive and partly historical. As part of my statistics classes for many years, I would toss a coin and "arrange" for it to turn up heads all the time. Intuitively, students begin to laugh and be skeptical after seeing four or five heads in a row. The probability of four heads in a row by chance is approximately 6%, and the probability of five heads in a row is approximately 3%. Note that 5% falls between the two.

The historical reasons for the 5% cutoff are partly based on the preference of Sir Ronald Fisher. Moore (1991) quotes Fisher as writing in 1926 that he preferred the 5% point for marking off the probable from the improbable. Because Fisher was an enormously influential statistician, others adopted this rule too. Also, the past inconveniences of calculating have influenced the choice of the 5% mark. Before the computer age, the tables for probabilities for various distributions in textbooks were constructed with handy columns such as 20%, 10%, 5%, and 1%—presumably because we have five fingers, and our number system is based on 10. Today these tables and the use of the 5% level are "almost obsolete" (Freedman, Pisani, Purves, & Adhikari, 1991, p. 494) because the computer can produce an exact probability based on a mathematical equation. Many researchers and editors of journals, however, persist in using the 5% mark as a cutoff for "unusual" simply because it is convenient to have some general standard that is easy to grasp.

Instead of using the 5% criterion, however, researchers often adopt probability cutoffs that are more generous (e.g., 10%) or more strict (e.g., 1%) based on their own intuition or the purposes and design of their research. With regard to intuition, the Nobel physicist, Enrico Fermi, reportedly believed that the 10% level was the cutoff for separating a miracle from a commonplace event. Meininger (1985) used a cutoff of 20% because the purpose of her research was exploratory—testing potential items for a behavior scale; Jacobsen and Lowery (1992) used a cutoff of 1% for statistical reasons—several hypotheses were tested using one dataset.

At the higher end of the probability continuum, probabilities of 95% or more are commonly considered by researchers as evidence for reporting potential events that they are quite confident will occur. The probability of 95% for recovery from skin cancer is empirically derived, and most health care workers would be surprised if recovery did not occur. Additionally, probabilities near the upper end of the probability scale frequently are used to express confidence in a statistic. For example, a poll reported that 38% of a pre-election random sample favored candidate A. The margin of error was given as 3%, with 95% confidence.

Probability Rules

Conditional Probability

The site of malignant breast calcifications can be ductal or lobular. Does the probability of invasive breast cancer vary according to site? The answer to this question can be found in Table 3-4, a crosstabulation of site and invasiveness based on the data in Table 3-2. Given that the site is lobular, what is the probability of invasive cancer? Table 3-4 shows that 11 patients had lobular calcifications, and two of these were invasive. Therefore, the probability of invasive breast cancer, *on the condition* that the site is lobular, is 2 in 11 or 18.2%. What is the probability of invasive cancer, given that the site was ductal? Table 3-4 shows that 34 patients had duct calcifications, and nine of these were invasive. Therefore, the probability of invasive breast cancer, *on the condition* that the site was ductal, is 9 in 34 or 26.5%. Notice that the

TABLE 3-4
*Crosstabulation of Malignant Pathology of X-Ray Calcifications
by Site and by Whether the Cancer Was Invasive*

	Invasive		
Site	*Yes*	*No*	*Totals*
Duct	9	25	34
Lobular	2	9	11

(Based on Table 3-2.)

two probabilities are different, indicating that invasiveness depends, to some extent, on site. A formula for conditional probability is given below:

$$\text{probability of event B, given event A} = \frac{(\text{total number with event A and event B})}{\text{total number with event A}} \times 100$$

In the previous example, relative to the lobular site, the formula would be:

$$\text{probability of invasive, given lobular} = \frac{(\text{total number with lobular invasive})}{\text{total number with lobular cancer}} \times 100$$

The substitutions would be as follows:

$$\text{probability of invasive, given lobular} = \frac{2}{2+9}(100) = \frac{2}{11}(100) = 18.2\%$$

Multiplication Rule

Earlier in this chapter, the idea of independence in choosing a random sample is defined as lack of ability to predict what person will be chosen next. More formally, independence means that given knowledge of event A, the probability of event B does not change. In coin tossing, the a priori probability of a head on a single toss of a fair coin is 1 in 2 (event A). If you are told that a person has obtained a head on the first toss of a coin, what is the probability of a head on the second toss (event B)? Because a fair coin has no memory, the probability of a head on the second toss is still 1 in 2. That is, the probability of a head on the second toss remains the same, in spite of the fact that you have been given information about the first toss. Therefore, successive tosses of a fair coin are independent. In the previous example regarding breast biopsies for calcifications, the probabilities for invasive breast cancer changed according to site; therefore, the variables of site and invasiveness were not independent.

When two events are independent, the probability that both events will occur is equal to the product of their probabilities. What is the probability of tossing two heads in a row? Because each coin toss is independent, the answer may be obtained simply by multiplying the probabilities for two separate coin tosses: $\frac{1}{2} \times \frac{1}{2} = \frac{1}{4}$ or 25%. Thus, when events are independent, one does not have to think about conditional probabilities. The formula for the probability of two events both occurring, *if the two events are independent,* follows:

probability of event A *and* event B = the probability of A times the probability of B

This formula can easily be extended to include more than two events. For the probability of tossing four heads in a row, the substitutions would be:

$$\text{probability of four heads in a row} = 100 \left(\frac{1}{2} \times \frac{1}{2} \times \frac{1}{2} \times \frac{1}{2} \right) = 100 \left(\frac{1}{16} \right) = 6.25\%$$

The ideas of independence and dependence are important in statistics. If the events are dependent, then the formula for conditional probability is used. If they are independent, then the probabilities may be multiplied. It is sometimes difficult to tell in health care situations whether events are independent or not. Indeed, the fundamental aim of many research projects is to learn whether two variables are independent. Also, many statistical procedures require the assumption of independence of events. If a sample is chosen at random or assigned to groups at random, then this assumption of independence is much easier to defend.

Addition Rule

Two events are said to be mutually exclusive when they cannot occur simultaneously; that is, the occurrence of one prevents the other. For instance, in the example of breast biopsies for women with a cluster of five or more calcifications, the site of the clustered calcifications is either ductal or lobular—it cannot be both. If two events are mutually exclusive, the probability that either event will occur is the sum of their probabilities, as given in the following formula:

probability of event A *or* event B = the probability of A + probability of B

In Table 3-2, if we want to compute the probability that a cluster of cancerous calcifications is invasive, the substitutions follow:

$$\text{probability of ductal invasive or lobular invasive} = 100(9/45 + 2/45)$$
$$= 100(11/45) = 24\%$$

As another example, in Table 3-3, the raters can agree perfectly in two ways. All three can assign the interview item to category 1, or all three can assign it to category 2. Thus, the outcomes of 1-1-1 and 2-2-2 are mutually exclusive because the three raters cannot do both simultaneously. Therefore, the probability of perfect agreement by chance is:

$$\text{probability of 1-1-1 or 2-2-2} = 100(\tfrac{1}{8} + \tfrac{1}{8}) = 100(\tfrac{2}{8}) = 25\%$$

In statistics, the probability of two such mutually exclusive events, both located at the extremes of a distribution, is called a "two-tailed probability." If our interest is in only one extreme of a distribution, such as all three raters assigning the interview item to category 1, then the substitutions are:

$$\text{probability of 1-1-1} = 100(\tfrac{1}{8}) = 12.5\%$$

This probability is called "one tailed" and is exactly half of the two-tailed probability.

Some events are not mutually exclusive, such as diabetes and cardiovascular disease. A patient may have both of these diseases simultaneously. The addition rule for such events is somewhat more complicated. This more complex rule is omitted because it is not used in later sections of this text. The interested reader can find the addition rule for nonmutually exclusive events in Freund (1988).

HYPOTHESIS TESTING

Given an underlying theoretical structure, a representative sample, and an appropriate research design, the researcher is able to test hypotheses. We test to see whether the data support our hypothesis. We do not claim to "prove" that our hypothesis is true, because one study can never prove anything. It is always possible that some error has distorted the findings.

Null Hypothesis

The *null hypothesis* is often written H_o. It proposes that there is no difference. The null hypothesis is the basis of the statistical test. If a "significant" difference is found, the null hypothesis is *rejected,* but if no difference is found, the null hypothesis is *accepted.* In older studies, hypotheses were usually stated in null form; however, this is not done as often today. When you hypothesize, you are stating that you believe there is a difference or a relationship. It is clearer if you state what differences or relationships you expect, rather than write a string of null hypotheses. It is important to understand the null hypothesis, however, because without it, there is no significance test. Suppose you stated that there is "no significant difference" between breast- and bottle-fed babies in terms of weight gain. If you really had no idea about this issue, you would not be stating a hypothesis but would simply ask the question: Is there a difference in weight gain between breast- and bottle-fed babies? If you had rationale for a hypothesis, you might state a research hypothesis (H_1), such as breast-fed babies gain more weight in the first week of life than bottle-fed babies.

Types of Error

Types of "error" are defined in terms of the null hypothesis. After analyzing the data, the researcher *accepts* the null hypothesis if there are no significant results or *rejects* the null hypothesis if there are significant results. Rejecting a null hypothesis means that significant differences *have* been found. Because no study is perfect, there is always a chance for error; perhaps this is one of the five chances in 100 ($p < 0.05$) that such an extreme result has happened by chance.

Two potential errors could be made. They are called *type I* and *type II*. Before describing these errors, the possibilities related to decisions about the null hypothesis are presented using the following diagram:

Null Hypothesis

Decision	*True*	*False*
Accept H_o	OK	Type II
Reject H_o	Type I	OK

If a null hypothesis is true and we accept that hypothesis, we have responded correctly. The incorrect response would be to reject a true null hypothesis (type I error). If the null hypothesis is false and we reject it, we have responded correctly. The wrong response would be to accept a false null hypothesis (type II error).

Suppose you compared two groups taught by different methods (A and B) on their knowledge of statistics, and the data indicated that group A scored significantly higher than group B. You would then reject the null hypothesis. Suppose, however, that group A had people with higher math ability in it and that actually the method did not matter at all. Rejecting the null hypothesis is a type I error.

The probability of making a type I error is called alpha (α) and can be *decreased* by altering the level of significance. That is, you could set the p at 0.01, instead of 0.05. Then there is only 1 chance in 100 that the result termed "significant" could occur by chance alone. If you do that, however, you will make it more difficult to find a significant result; that is, you will decrease the *power* of the test and increase the risk of a type II error.

A type II error is accepting a *false* null hypothesis. If the data showed no significant results, the researcher would accept the null hypothesis. If there were significant differences, a type II error would have been made. To avoid a type II error, you could make the level of significance less extreme. There is a greater chance of finding significant results if you are willing to risk 10 chances in 100 that you are wrong ($p = 0.10$) than there is if you are willing to risk only 5 chances in 100 ($p = 0.05$). Other ways to decrease the likelihood of a type II error are to increase the sample size, decrease sources of extraneous variation, and increase the *effect* size. The effect size is the impact made by the independent variable. For example, if group A scored 10 points higher on the statistics final than group B, the effect size would be 10 divided by the SD of the measure (Cohen, 1987). There is a trade-off: Decreasing the likelihood of a type II error increases the chance of a type I error. If decreasing the probability of one type of error increases the probability of the other type, the question arises as to which type of error you are willing to risk. As might be expected, that depends on the study. An example would be a test for a particular genetic defect. If the defect exists and is diagnosed early, it can be successfully treated; however, if it is not diagnosed and treated, the child will become severely retarded. On the other hand, if a child is erroneously diagnosed as having the defect and treated, no physical damage is done.

In terms of the types of errors, a type I error would be diagnosing the defect when it does not exist. In that case, the child would be treated but not harmed by the treatment. A type II error would be declaring the child to be normal when he or she is not. In that case, irreparable damage would be done. In such a situation, it is obvious that you would make every attempt to avoid the type II error.

Suppose a federal study was conducted to determine whether a particular approach to preschool preparation of underprivileged children leads to increased success in school. This approach would cost a great deal of money to implement nationwide. Those responsible for deciding whether or not to implement this approach would certainly want to be sure that a type I error had not been made. They would not want to institute a costly new program if it did not really have any effect on success in school.

Type I and II errors are hard for some people to grasp, so following are a few examples:

It is hypothesized that two groups are equal in their knowledge of statistics. Has an error been made, and if so, what type of error, if the researcher does the following?

1. Accepts the hypothesis when the groups are really equal in statistics knowledge
2. Rejects the hypothesis when the groups are really equal in statistics knowledge
3. Rejects the hypothesis when the groups are really different in terms of their knowledge of statistics
4. Accepts the hypothesis when one group has much more knowledge of statistics than the other

These four examples summarize the possibilities surrounding these errors. First, if we are given a situation in which the null hypothesis is true, that is, there is no difference, we can either accept it and make the correct decision (#1) or reject it and make an incorrect decision, or a type I error (#2). Second, if the null hypothesis is false, we can reject it, making a correct decision (#3) or accept it and make an incorrect decision, or a type II error (#4).

Power of a Test

As previously mentioned, a more *powerful* test is one that is more likely to reject a null hypothesis; that is, it is more likely to indicate a statistically significant result when such a difference exists in the population. The level of significance (probability level) and the power of the test are important factors to consider.

One- and Two-Tailed Tests

The "tails" refer to the ends of the probability curve. When we test for statistical significance, we are asking if the difference or relationship is so extreme, so far out in the tail of the distribution, that it is unlikely to have occurred by chance alone. When we hypothesize the direction of the difference, we are indicating in which tail of the distribution we expect to find the difference.

Although there is some controversy about this, the practice among many researchers is to use a *one-tailed* test of significance when a directional hypothesis is stated and a *two-tailed* test in all other situations. The advantage of using the one-tailed test is that it is more powerful, because the value yielded by the statistical test does not have to be so large to be significant at a given level. To gain this advantage, however, you must have a sound theoretical basis for the directional hypothesis. You cannot base it on a hunch.

The normal curve is used to demonstrate the difference between one- and two-tailed tests (Fig. 3-3). Recall from our discussion of CIs that 95% of the distribution fall between ±1.96 SDs from the mean. Thus, only 5% fall beyond these two points. Two and one-half percent of the distribution fall below a z-score of −1.96, and 2.5% fall above +1.96z. To be so "rare" as to occur only 5% of the time, a z-score would have to be −1.96z or less or +1.96z or greater. Note that we are using both tails of the distribution. Because 99% of the distribution fall between ±2.58 SDs from the mean of the normal curve, a score would have to be −2.58 or less or +2.58 or more to be declared significant at the 0.01 level.

Figure 3-4 shows what occurs when a directional hypothesis is stated. We look at only one tail of the distribution. In this example, we look at the positive side of the distribution. Fifty percent of the distribution fall below the mean, and 45% fall

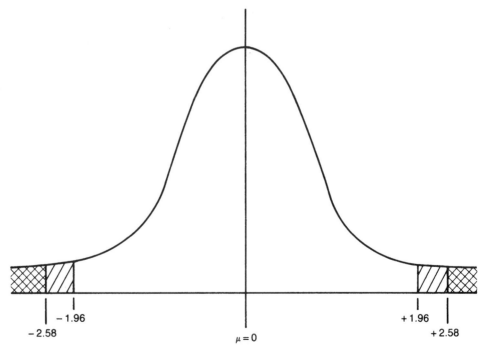

FIGURE 3-3
Two-tailed test of significance using the normal curve.

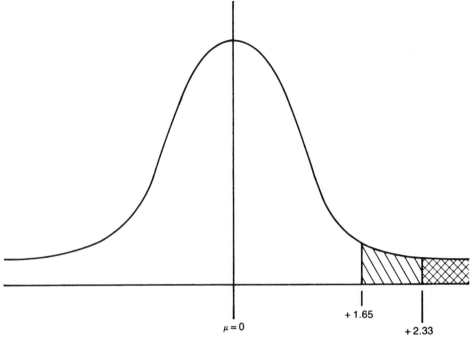

FIGURE 3-4
One-tailed test of significance using the normal curve.

between the mean and a z-score of +1.65 (see Appendix A). Thus, 95% (50 + 45) of the distribution fall below +1.65z. To score in the upper 5% would require a score of +1.65 or greater. Given a one-tailed test of significance, you would need a score of +1.65z to be significant at the 0.05 level, whereas with a two-tailed test, you needed a score of +1.96z. This is an example of the concept of power. With an a priori hypothesis, a lower z-score would be considered significant.

For the 0.01 level of significance and a one-tailed test, a z-score of +2.33 or greater is needed for significance. This is because 49% of the distribution fall between the mean and +2.33, and another 50% fall below the mean.

Degrees of Freedom

The effects of degrees of freedom (*df*) were included in the discussion of the denominator in the computation of the SD. In the sample formula, the denominator is $n - 1$, thus correcting for the possible underestimation of the population parameter. When describing the calculation of various statistics, we discuss dividing by the *df* and looking up levels of significance in tables using *df*s. Because this is sometimes a confusing concept, a simple example of *df* follows.

Degrees of freedom are related to the number of scores, items, or other units in a data set and to the idea of freedom to vary. Given three scores (1, 5, 6), we have three degrees of freedom, one for each independent item. Each score is "free to vary"; that is, before collecting the data we do not know what any of these scores will be. Once we calculate the mean, however, we lose one *df*. The mean of these three scores is four. Once you know the mean and two of the three scores, you can figure out what the third score is. It is no longer free to vary. When calculating the variance or SD, you are calculating how much the scores vary around the sample mean. Because the sample mean is known, one *df* is lost, and the *df*s become $n - 1$, the number of items in the set less one.

STATISTICAL INFERENCE

In statistics, a sample (part) is used to obtain results that represent a target population (whole) to which one wants to generalize. For example, the average birth weight of newborns in a hospital in 1996 (population) can be estimated using observations from a sample of those newborns. Suppose 810 infants were born in the hospital in 1996, and the birth weights of the first 81 newborns (starting January 1) were recorded and averaged. Would the average (mean) birthweight in that sample of 81 be a good estimate of the mean birth weight in the 810 (the population of interest)? It would not be if birth weight depends on time of year or if an effective prenatal nutrition program to improve birth weight had begun in the surrounding community near that time. How can a sample that *is* representative of that population of 810 be selected? One way is by random selection.

A *random sample* is drawn from the population of interest so that every member of the population has the same probability (chance) of being selected in the sample. To make this possible, one must have a list of everyone in the population. A table of random numbers can then be used to select a random sample of any size (Remington & Schork, 1970). Note that samples of convenience or samples drawn in a haphazard manner are *not* random samples. Suppose a 10% random sample was selected from the population of 810. It is extremely unlikely that the resulting random sample would be the first 81 infants born in 1996. Because the process of random sampling does not play favorites, random samples are likely to represent the target population. On the other hand, it is impossible to know that "judgment samples" (such as the first 81 newborns of 1996) are representative of the population of interest. Random samples are unbiased in that the process of random sampling produces samples that represent the population. Most important, the statistical theory on which this book is based assumes random sampling (or random assignment, discussed later).

STATISTICAL ESTIMATES

When an estimate of the population parameter is given as a single number, it is called a *point estimate*. The sample mean is a point estimate. A *CI* is a range or interval of values. Point and CI estimates are types of statistical estimates that allow us to *infer* the true value of an unknown population parameter using information from a *random* sample of that population.

Confidence Intervals

When the means (point estimates) are normally distributed, we can use the standard error of the mean to calculate interval estimates. Typically, the 95% and 99% intervals are used. Recall that 95% of the curve is contained between ±1.96 SDs from the mean and that 99% of the curve is contained between ±2.58 SDs from the mean.

The following formulas are used to calculate the CIs for the population means when the sample size is adequate (generally greater than 30). (For small samples, the *t* distribution may be used to calculate CIs.)

$$95\% = \bar{X} \pm 1.96 \text{ (standard error)}$$
$$99\% = \bar{X} \pm 2.58 \text{ (standard error)}$$

The following hypothetical examples are designed to illustrate point estimates and CI estimates derived from a random sample. Suppose that a random sample of 81 newborns from a hospital in a poor neighborhood during the last year had a mean birth weight of 100 oz with a SD of 27 oz.

1. What is the point estimate for the unknown true value of the average (mean) birth weight of all infants born in that hospital in the last year (called the population parameter)?

   Answer: The mean value of 100 oz (computed from the 81 observations) is the best single number estimate (the point estimate) of the unknown value (parameter) for the population of interest. Another random sample of 81 would have given a sample mean different from 100 oz, so the mean value depends on the particular sample that was taken. The difference between the sample mean of 100 oz and the unknown population mean (which it estimates) is called sampling error. "It is not an error in the sense of a blunder or mistake, but a calculated error we make because we do not collect data on the entire population" (Remington & Schork, 1970).

   Because the point estimate, 100 oz, is a single number, it gives no indication of its sampling error. CIs computed from random samples enable us to measure sampling error in numerical terms.

2. What is the value of the 95% CI estimate for mean birth weight?

   Answer: First, we must calculate the standard error. Remember that the formula is the SD divided by the square root of the sample size:

   $$\frac{\text{standard deviation}}{\sqrt{n}}$$

For our example, this is:

$$= \frac{27}{\sqrt{81}} = \frac{27}{9} = 3$$

Next, we calculate the 95% CI:

$$\bar{X} \pm 1.96 \text{ (standard error)}$$

$$100 \pm (1.96)(3)$$

$$100 \pm 5.88$$

$$94.12 \text{ and } 105.88$$

The 95% CI ranges from 94.12 to 105.88. It is a range or interval of estimates for the unknown true value. Thus, a CI consists of an entire interval of estimates for the population parameter.

3. How do we interpret the 95% CI?

Answer: First, another sample of 81 would almost surely yield a different point estimate. The width of the 95% CI reflects the sampling error resulting from using an estimate based on a random sample of 81 rather than the entire population. In other words, the width of the 95% CI indicates the range of variation for point estimates that may be expected by chance differences from one random sample of the hospital population to another. It is a 95% CI because about 95% of such CIs (obtained from different random samples of that size) will include the true mean value of hospital birth weights. Because that parameter value is usually unknown, we use statistical estimates, the point estimate and the CI estimate, to approximate it. However, if the parameter value (the true mean birth weight for *all* newborns born in that hospital during the last year) were known, approximately 95% of the 95% CIs computed from different random samples of 81 would include that true value.

It is important to understand that the value of the point estimate and the CI estimate depends on the birth weights in the particular sample, and the estimates will vary from sample to sample. Therefore, we may *not* conclude that the probability is 95% that the mean hospital birth weight is between 94 and 106 oz.

Either the parameter (the mean of all birth weights in the hospital during 1991) is between 94 and 106 oz or it is not; we do not know which. "Thus, the 95% refers to the average accuracy of the procedure for constructing the varying CIs, and not to the one interval that is itself presented" (Hahn & Meeker, 1991). However, the width of the CI provides useful information about the sampling error or uncertainty of the point estimate unavailable from the point estimate itself. To interpret the specific CI we computed from our sample (here, 95% CI, 94.12 to 105.88), it is necessary to understand the relationship between CIs and significance tests.

The Relationship Between Confidence Intervals and Significance Tests

To help explain the relationship between CIs and the levels of significance (*p* values) derived from statistical tests, the following four questions might be asked in relation to our sample mean:

1. Is the mean birth weight in this hospital sample (100 oz) statistically significantly different from 88 oz (5.5 lb, the definition of low birth weight)?

2. Is the mean birth weight in this sample statistically significantly different from 106 oz (6.6 lb, the mean birth weight in that city)?
3. Is the mean birth weight in this sample statistically significantly different from a birth weight of 103 oz?
4. Is the mean birth weight in this sample statistically significantly different from 100 oz, the sample estimate itself?

To test the null hypothesis that there is no statistically significant difference between the mean of 100 oz and each of the other values, we apply the t test. The results follow:

Question	Null Hypothesis	Difference Between Values	p Value
1.	88	12 oz	0.0006
2.	106	6 oz	0.0456
3.	103	3 oz	0.3174
4.	100	0 oz	1.0000

For the first question, the null hypothesis is rejected. The observed mean of 100 oz is statistically significantly higher than the hypothesized value of 88 oz; that is, the 12-point difference is a significant difference. The p value indicates that a difference that large would occur by chance alone only 6 in 10,000. The null hypothesis is also rejected for question 2; that is, the hospital mean of 100 oz is statistically significantly lower than the city mean of 106 oz. A difference that large would occur by chance alone only 4½ times in 100 random samples of equal size. For questions 3 and 4, the null hypothesis is not rejected; that is, the observed mean of 100 oz is not statistically significantly different from the values of 103 or 100 oz. In the case of the 3-oz difference (question 3), if there really was no difference between the population means, a difference at least that large could be expected to occur by chance in 32% of the random samples. In question 4, the point estimate and the null hypothesis are numerically indistinguishable (both 100 oz) and statistically indistinguishable ($p = 1$), because the difference between the two values being compared is zero.

From the chart of the p values, you can see that the further a particular null hypothesis is from the point estimate (100 oz), the lower the p value. In other words, hypotheses become less compatible with the mean of the observed values (here 100 oz) the larger the difference between the point estimate and the hypothesized or comparison score becomes.

Figure 3-5 summarizes our results. The null hypotheses are numbered and indicated by H_o. For example, our first null hypothesis compared our mean of 100 with a value of 88. The CI of 94.12 to 105.88 is included in the figure. What can be said about the p values for null hypotheses that fall outside the 95% CI? The two that fall outside of the CI are 88 and 106 from questions 1 and 2, and in both cases, the p

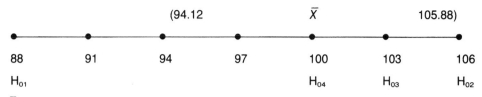

FIGURE 3-5
Relationship of confidence intervals to hypothesis testing.

was $<.05$. Notice that H_o:106 is just outside the 95% CI, and its p value is barely below 0.05. If a null hypothesis falls at either end of a 95% CI, $p = 0.05$.

Because all numbers outside of the CI have p values less than 0.05, we would expect that all numbers within the CI would have p values greater than 0.05. This leads to a characterization of a 95% CI in terms of p values. A 95% CI contains all the (null hypothesis) values for which $p \geq 0.05$. In other words, a 95% CI contains values (hypotheses) that are statistically compatible (will not be rejected at the 0.05 level) with the point estimate (observed value).

Consistency Checks for Evaluating Research Reports

The relationships between point estimates, CI estimates, and significance tests make it possible to uncover inconsistencies in manuscripts. The point estimate cannot be outside of the CI. A value for a null hypothesis within the 95% CI should have a p value greater than 0.05, and one outside of the 95% CI should have a p value less than 0.05.

Value of Confidence Intervals

Levels of significance (p values) ascertain whether a particular hypothesis is statistically compatible with the observed sample value, while 95% CIs specify all the population values that are statistically indistinguishable from the observed sample value. "The CI contains more information (than the p value) because it is equivalent to performing a significance test for all values of the parameter, not just a single value" (Berry, 1986).

A Word of Caution

Statistical tests and statistical estimates assume random sampling. When using either significance tests or CIs, clear-cut conclusions regarding the entire population apply only when the study sample is a random sample of that population. Because study patients are rarely random samples from a population, we should be wary about statistical inferences and ask "From what population might this group constitute a random sample?"(Remington & Schork, 1970, p. 93). If the sample appears to represent some population (but not a random sample), the width of the CI is often conceived of as a lower bound (minimum) for the uncertainty in the point estimate. However, clinical judgment must supplement statistical analysis whenever nonrandom samples are used to generalize to individuals not studied (Riegelman, 1981, p. 205).

When reading a research report, it is essential to determine if there is an explicitly defined population of interest and to ascertain if and how the study sample was selected. Although a representative (nonrandom) sample from an explicitly defined population falls short of a random sample, it is superior to a nonrepresentative sample or to a situation in which the population or the study sample is not clearly defined. When inferences about the population are drawn using statistical tests or CIs in such situations, the reader should beware. Descriptions of the study sample (e.g., using point estimates) provide useful information in all situations. When the population is ill defined, the study sample unrepresentative, or the relation of the study sample to the population unclear, point estimates and other statistics describing the sample may provide the only reliable information.

SAMPLE SIZE

When planning research, the question always arises as to how large a sample is needed. Determination of sample size involves ethical and statistical consideration. If the sample size is too small to detect significant differences or relationships or includes far more subjects than necessary, the cost to subjects and researchers cannot be justified. Sample size is addressed as it relates to the specific statistics covered in this book. Here, we cover only the main determinants of sample size. A major contribution to sample size determination was made by Jacob Cohen (1987). His book provides tables to help determine the appropriate sample size for a particular statistical test.

Sample size is related to power, effect size, and significance level. Power is the likelihood of rejecting the null hypothesis (i.e, avoiding a type II error). An 80% level is generally viewed as an adequate level. As noted, effect size is the difference between the groups or the strength of the relationship. For example, for the t test, which compares the means of two groups, Cohen (1987) defines a small effect as 0.2 of an SD, a moderate effect as 0.5 of an SD, and a large effect as 0.8. In relation to GRE scores with an SD of 100, a small effect would be 20 points (100×0.2); a moderate effect, 50 points; and a large effect, 80 points.

The significance level is the probability of rejecting a true null hypothesis (making a type I error); it is called alpha and is often set at 0.05. Given three of these parameters, the fourth can be determined. Cohen's book has power and sample size tables. If we know the sample size, effect size, and significance level, we can determine the power of the analysis. This can be particularly helpful when critiquing research, because nonsignificant results may be related to an inadequate sample size, and significant results may be related to a very large sample, rather than to a meaningful result. When planning a study, one determines the desired power, acceptable significance level, and expected effect size and uses these three parameters to determine the necessary sample size. In addition to Cohen's book, software programs have been developed to assist with determining sample size. Power relevant to specific statistical tests is discussed in subsequent chapters.

SUMMARY

Topics covered in this chapter are basic to understanding the use of the specific statistical techniques contained in the second section of this book. Please be sure you understand these topics before proceeding.

APPLICATION EXERCISES AND RESULTS

EXERCISES

1. Scores on a particular test are normally distributed with a mean of 80 and a standard deviation of 20. Between what two scores would you expect:

   a. 68% of the scores to fall between: _____ and _____

   b. 96% of the scores to fall between: _____ and _____

2. In a negatively skewed distribution, the "tail" extends toward the _____ (right/left) or _____ (higher/lower) scores of the distribution.

3. When raw scores are converted to standard scores, the resulting distribution has a mean equal to _____ and a standard deviation equal to _____.

4. A distribution of scores has a mean of 70 and a standard deviation of 5. The following four scores were drawn from that distribution: 58, 65, 73, and 82.

   a. Transform the raw scores to standard scores and *T*-scores.

   b. Calculate the percentile for each score.

   c. Use the standard scores that you have calculated for the four scores, and transform them into scores from a distribution with a mean of 100 and a standard deviation of 25.

5. Look at your frequencies for the variables AGE and EDUC. Determine whether or not the variables are significantly skewed. If they are skewed, perform the appropriate transformations and then run descriptives on the new variables to determine whether or not the transformations were successful.

6. At your hospital, there were 1,200 deliveries last year; 288 of the women had cesarean sections. What is the probability of having a cesarean section at your hospital? _____

7. A researcher tests for differences between the mean scores of two groups. She sets the level of significance at 0.05. If the mean difference is so large that it would occur by chance 1% of the time, the researcher should _____ (accept/reject) the *null hypothesis*.

8. When the researcher makes a prediction regarding the direction of mean differences between an experimental and control group, he or she should use a _____ (one-tailed/two-tailed) test of significance.

9. Which is the more powerful test? _____ (one tailed/two-tailed)

10. You hypothesize that there is no significant difference between nurses and social workers in terms of weight. In each of the following, determine whether or not an error has been made and if so, what type of error.

   a. Social workers really weigh significantly more than nurses, and you accept the null hypothesis.

   b. Nurses really weigh more than social workers, and you reject the null hypothesis.

   c. Nurses and social workers really do weigh the same, and you accept the null hypothesis.

   d. Nurses and social workers really do weigh the same, and you reject the null hypothesis.

11. In general, will a nonparametric or parametric test, each designed to accomplish the same analytical function, more frequently reject the null hypothesis?

12. You have measured 120 subjects on a particular scale. The mean is 75 and the standard deviation is 6.

   a. What is the standard error of the mean?

   b. Set up the 95% confidence interval for the mean.

   c. Set up the 99% confidence interval for the mean.

RESULTS

1.

   a. $68\% = \pm 1z$

   80 ± 20

   68% fall between 60 and 100

   b. $96\% = \pm 2z$

   80 ± 40

   96% fall between 40 and 120

2. left, lower

3. 0, 1

4. a. Standard scores and *T*-scores:

Raw Scores	*Standard Scores*	*T-Scores*
	$z = \dfrac{X = \bar{X}}{s}$	$T = 10z + 50$
58	$z = \dfrac{58 - 70}{5} = -2.4$	$T = (10)(-2.4) + 50 = 26$
65	$z = \dfrac{65 - 70}{5} = -1.0$	$T = (10)(-1.0) + 50 = 40$
73	$z = \dfrac{73 - 70}{5} = 0.6$	$T = (10)(.6) + 50 = 56$
82	$z = \dfrac{82 - 70}{5} = 2.4$	$T = (10)(2.4) + 50 = 74$

b. Percentiles: Areas between mean and z-score (see Appendix B)

Raw Score	z-score	Tabled Values	Percentiles
58	−2.4	49.18	50 − 49.18 = .82
65	−1.0	34.13	50 − 34.13 = 15.87
73	.6	22.57	50 + 22.57 = 72.57
82	2.4	49.18	50 + 49.18 = 99.18

c. New distribution:

$$\text{Transformed } z\text{-scores} = (\text{new } s)(z) + (\text{new } \bar{X})$$
$$= 25z + 100$$

z-Scores	Transformed Scores
−2.4	25(−2.4) + 100 = 40
−1.0	25(−1.0) + 100 = 75
.6	25(.6) + 100 = 115
2.4	25(2.4) + 100 = 160

5. Here are the relevant values for the two variables.

Descriptive Statistics

	N	Mean	Std.	Skewness		Kurtosis	
	Statistic	Statistic	Statistic	Statistic	Std. Error	Statistic	Std. Error
Subject's age	170	38.06	12.84	1.281	.186	2.519	.370
Education in years	168	16.15	3.65	-.775	.187	1.191	.373
Valid N (listwise)	165						

To determine the degree of skewness, divide the measure of skewness by its standard error. Values greater than 1.96 are significant at the .05 level, and values greater than 2.58 are significant at the .01 level.

$$\text{AGE: } 1.281/.186 = 6.89$$

$$\text{EDUC: } -.775/.187 = -4.14$$

Because both variables are significantly skewed ($p < .01$), we attempt some transformations. First, we do square root transformations. We must first reverse the scoring of EDUC, because it is negatively skewed. We created two new variables through the following compute statements:

$$\text{AGESQRT} = \text{SQRT (AGE)}$$
$$\text{EDUCSQRT} = \text{SQRT (27−EDUC)}$$

In the first equation, we created a new variable that we named AGESQRT. The new variable consists of the square roots of every subject's age. SQRT is the name SPSS uses for square root.

The second equation creates a new variable that we called EDUCSQRT. Here we have first reverse scored EDUC by subtracting each value from one more than the largest value (the highest years of education recorded was 26). Then the square root of the recoded variable is taken.

After creating the two new variables, we checked to see if the transformations had corrected the skewness.

Descriptive Statistics

	N	Mean	Std.	Skewness		Kurtosis	
	Statistic	Statistic	Statistic	Statistic	Std. Error	Statistic	Std. Error
AGESQRT	170	6.0902	.9899	.714	.186	.956	.370
EDUCSQRT	168	3.2469	.5549	.010	.187	1.390	.373
Valid N (listwise)	165						

$$\text{AGESQRT:} \quad .714/.186 = 3.84$$
$$\text{EDUCSQRT:} \quad .010/.187 = .05$$

Age is still significantly skewed ($p < .01$), but education now has a normal distribution. Remember that we reverse scored education, so when the transformed variable is used, it must be interpreted as scored so that a high score indicates few years of education and vice versa. One might decide to recode education in some other way, such as elementary school, high school, and so forth, rather than doing this data transformation.

We try once more to transform age. We did this by doing a log transformation on AGE. In SPSS, our statement looked like:

$$\text{AGELOG} = \text{LG10 (AGE)}$$

The resulting statistics were:

Descriptive Statistics

	N	Mean	Std.	Skewness		Kurtosis	
	Statistic	Statistic	Statistic	Statistic	Std. Error	Statistic	Std. Error
AGELOG	170	1.5582	.1382	.160	.186	.388	.370
Valid N (listwise)	170						

$$\text{AGELOG:} \quad .160/.186 = .86$$

We could use the log transformation of the age variable, because it results in a normal distribution.

6. 100 times 288/1200 = 24%

7. reject

8. one tailed

9. one tailed

10.

    a. type II

    b. no error

    c. no error

    d. type I

11. parametric

12.

$$s_{\bar{x}} = \frac{s}{\sqrt{n}}$$

    a.
$$= \frac{6}{\sqrt{120}} = 0.55$$

    b.
$$95\% = \bar{X} \pm 1.96 \; s_{\bar{x}}$$
$$= 75 \pm (1.96)(0.55)$$
$$= 75 \pm 1.08$$
$$= 73.92 \text{ to } 76.08$$

    c.
$$99\% = \bar{X} \pm 2.58 \; s_{\bar{x}}$$
$$= 75 \pm (2.58)(0.55)$$
$$= 75 \pm 1.42$$
$$= 73.58 \text{ to } 76.42$$

Confidence Interval Estimates and Significance Tests for Percentages: Examples to Aid Understanding of Statistical Inference

Leonard Braitman

OBJECTIVES FOR CHAPTER 4

After reading this chapter, you should be able to do the following:

1 • Explain the relationships between point estimates, confidence intervals, and probability values.

2 • Distinguish between a random sample and randomization.

3 • Differentiate between statistical significance and clinical significance.

Data are usually collected on a sample of people selected from a larger group (population) to which the researchers want to generalize their findings. The two major approaches to statistical inference from sample to population are significance tests and statistical estimates (point estimates and confidence intervals [CIs]). Point estimates and CIs can address the general question: How large is the difference between groups? This subsumes the question addressed by significance tests, whether there is a nonzero (statistically significant) difference. In this section, statistical estimates, including point estimates and CI estimates of percentages, are discussed through the use of examples.

CONFIDENCE INTERVALS FOR PERCENTAGES

Example 1

None of 20 healthy study subjects younger than 65 years fell during the last year. The point estimate is the percentage, $^0\!/_{20} = 0\%$, of subjects in the study sample who actually fell. If the study sample represents the population of interest, the point estimate, 0%, is the best single number that approximates the unknown true percentage of people who fell during the last year in the population of interest (healthy people younger than 65 years). However, "if nothing goes wrong [in the sample], is everything all right [in the population of interest]?" (Hanley & Lippman-Hand, 1983, p. 1,743). We cannot conclude that no one in the population of interest fell just because no one fell in the sample of 20. We need to know the margin of error of the point estimate (0%) in estimating the unknown true percentage.

A rough idea of the uncertainty in a point estimate is provided using a CI. The 95% CI of the percentage $^0\!/_{20} = 0\%$ ranges from 0% to 17%. The values, 0% to 17% in the 95% CI, provide a range of values that is reasonably compatible with the observed result: 0 out of 20 fell in the study group (sample). The point estimate of 0% and values nearby are most compatible with the observed data. However, we cannot be certain that the true percentage of interest is 0% or even near it. The CI provides a range of plausible estimates. Because repeated samples from the same population usually give different results, the point estimate from that sample (0%) is unlikely to be exactly equal to the unknown population value (parameter). Thus, a range of estimated values is needed.

How is a CI for a single percentage determined? It can be found using a computer program, Confidence Interval Analysis (CIA; available from *Annals of Internal Medicine,* 6th and Race streets, Philadelphia, PA 19106-1657) or read from tables for groups up to size $N = 100$ (Lentner, 1982). However, when the point estimate is 0 (0%), a simple approximate method called the rule of three applies. The rule of three gives an approximate 95% CI from 0 to $^3\!/_N$ when the point estimate is $^0\!/_N$ (Hanley & Lippman-Hand, 1983). For this sample of $N = 20$, the 95% CI ranges from 0 to $^3\!/_{20}$ (from 0%–15%), close to the correct answer of 0% to 17%. The numbers in this 95% CI are the values from the population that are reasonably compatible with the observed sample percentage (0%). Candidates for the unknown population value (parameter) become less compatible with the sample value (0%), the further they are from 0%; those outside the 95% CI are unlikely candidates but still possible.

Example 2

Suppose none of 100 normal subjects younger than 65 years fell during the last year. Find the point estimate and 95% CI for the percentage that fell.

Answer: The point estimate is 0% ($^0\!/_{100} = 0\%$). The rule of three shortcut results in a 95% CI of 0% to 3% ($^3\!/_N = ^3\!/_{100} = 3\%$). (Using the table or the computer program yields 0%–3.6%.) This 4-percentage point interval is much smaller than the 0% to 17% in example 1. Although no one fell in either group, the larger sample of 100 in example 2 has a narrower 95% CI and is a more reliable statistical estimate of the unknown percentage of subjects who fell.

This is because the width of the 95% CI reflects the sampling error resulting from using an estimate based on a random sample rather than using the entire population. In two random samples with the same point estimate (in this case, 0%), the larger sample yields a more reliable estimate (a narrower 95% CI, indicating less sampling error) than the smaller sample. In other words, if other things are equal, a statistical estimate derived from a larger random sample has a smaller margin of error.

Example 3

Of 100 people at least 65 years old, 34 fell in the last year. Find the point estimate and 95% CI for the percent that fell.

Answer: The point estimate is $^{34}/_{100}$ = 34%. The table and computer program both give 95% CI of 25% to 48%. (The rule of three does not apply here because *p* is not 0%.)

Now compare the uncertainty in statistical estimates based on two groups (samples) of the same size that are representative of the population of interest. In examples 2 and 3, groups of 100 people were followed. Despite the same size sample, the 95% CI is much wider in example 3 (48%–25% = 23 percentage points) than in example 2 (3.6 percentage points). This is because in example 2, 0 of 100 fell, so there is no variability in the response (falling or not falling). This extreme uniformity of response facilitates a precise generalization to the population of interest. However, in example 3, there was substantial variability; approximately ⅓ (34%) fell and ⅔ did not. This greater variability results in a more uncertain estimate (of the true but unknown percentage) indicated by the wider 95% CI in example 3. "This difference exemplifies a property of CI for percentages (proportions): For a given sample size, percentages near 50% have wider CIs (more uncertainty) than percentages near either 0% or 100%" (Braitman, 1988). Greater variability of response leads to greater random sampling errors in predictions from sample data to the population of interest.

Example 4

Suppose that in a group of people at least 65 years old and taking benzodiazepines daily, 60% fell during the last year. Find the point estimate and CI estimate for the percent that fell. The point estimate is 60%. However, the CI estimate cannot be determined without knowledge of the size of the group.

ASSUMPTIONS UNDERLYING CONFIDENCE INTERVALS OF SINGLE PERCENTAGES

CIs for percentages depend on underlying assumptions about the process of sampling:

1. Observations within the sample must be independent of one another for a CI to be valid (within-sample independence).
2. The sample must be a random sample of the population of interest.

Example 5

Suppose there were 35 falls in the last year in 50 patients at least 65 years old taking benzodiazepines daily. Find the point estimate and 95% CI for the percentage that fell.

Answer: Note that 35 falls in 50 patients does not mean that 35 of 50 patients fell. We need to know how many times each patient fell because multiple falls by the same person are not independent observations. By using the number of patients who fell (rather than the 35 falls), we would eliminate the multiple falls, which are the nonindependent observations.

Example 6

Suppose there were 35 falls in 50 patients at least 65 years old and taking benzodiazepines daily. One person fell six times, and everyone else fell once during the last year. Find the point estimate and 95% CI.

Answer: The patient, not the fall, is the phenomenon of clinical interest. In addition, patients who fall once are more likely on average to fall again, so falls are not independent observations. Because the patient, not the fall, represents an independent observation, the patient (not the fall) is a proper unit of statistical analysis. One patient fell six times, and each of the remaining 29 falls occurred to a different patient. Thus, $1 + 29 = 30$ patients out of 50 fell at least once during the last year for a point estimate of $30/50 = 60\%$ (not $35/50 = 70\%$). The percentage of patients who fell *one or more times* is 60% (95% CI is 45%–74%). Because 29 patients fell once and one patient fell six times, the percentage of patients who fell *more than once* is $1/50 = 2\%$ (95% CI of 0.5%–14%). Which estimate is appropriate depends on the substantive question being addressed.

Notice that 95% CI of 0.5% to 14% is much narrower (13.5 percentage points wide) than 95% CI of 45% to 74% (approximately 29 percentage points wide) because 1/50 has less variability of response (one fell, 49 did not) than 30/50 (30 fell, 20 did not), despite both percentages being based on groups of 50.

STATISTICAL MISTAKES VERSUS STATISTICAL ERRORS

Example 6 illustrated that unless the assumption of within-sample independence of observations is satisfied, the computed point estimate and associated CI will not be correct. A similar mistake involves using the percentage of serum samples (with nonindependent multiple serum samples for some patients) with a particular characteristic to draw conclusions about the percentage of patients with that characteristic. Another example of a statistical *mistake* is using statistical formulas when the sample size is too small. Such mistakes are avoidable and are completely different from sampling errors and type I and type II errors (see Chapter 3), all of which can be minimized but not entirely avoided. If a result is obviously wrong, for example a probability greater than 1 or a percentage less than 0, we would check our calculations and our assumptions to determine where the error lies. An inconsistency gives us valuable information that leads us to correct our mistakes. However, unrecognized statistical mistakes (e.g., when the answer is incorrect but not inconsistent or otherwise obviously wrong) are common and more dangerous. Many statistical mistakes result from assuming that answers generated by computers are necessarily correct. Most computer programs do not check any assumptions before providing results, and no computer program checks all assumptions. Thus, it is essential to verify all calculations and assumptions underlying statistical tests.

ASSUMPTIONS OF RANDOM SAMPLING AND RANDOMIZATION UNDERLYING CONFIDENCE INTERVALS AND SIGNIFICANCE TESTS

Significance tests and CIs assume random sampling (or random assignment, which is discussed later). The random sampling assumption is an integral part of the interpretation of CIs. The term *random sample* often is used incorrectly to denote a convenience sample of whatever patients are available. In random sampling, a relevant population (from which the sample will be selected) must be carefully listed. Suppose that a sample of 100 was randomly selected from the population of patients receiving a new treatment. That means every sample of 100 has the same chance of being selected from a listing of the population (Wonnacott & Wonnacott, 1985).

The uncertainty that results from making an estimate using a part (sample) rather than the entire population of interest is called sampling error. Such uncertainty in the point estimate depends on the amount of sampling variability (chance variation from sample to sample) expected in random samples of that size. Because we expect more sampling variability in small samples than large samples, we were not surprised that $^0/_{20}$ has a 95% CI of 0% to 17%, approximately five times as wide as the 95% CI of 0% to 3.6% for $^0/_{100}$ in example 2. The margin of error expressed by the width of a CI includes random or chance error (sampling error) that accompanies choosing a random sample rather than the entire population, but does not include observer errors of measurement or classification or any other systematic errors. Such systematic errors often are larger than random (sampling) errors and are difficult to detect. Thus, appropriate measurement and careful study design and study execution remain crucial to control systematic (nonrandom) errors in clinical studies (Rothman, 1986).

RANDOMIZATION AS AN ALTERNATIVE ASSUMPTION TO RANDOM SAMPLING

Randomization is the "allocation of individuals to groups, e.g., to experimental and control regimens, by chance. Within the limits of chance variation, randomization should make the control and experimental groups similar at the start of an investigation and ensure that personal judgement and prejudices of the investigator do not influence allocation. Randomization or random assignment should not be confused with haphazard assignment. The pattern of assignment may appear to be haphazard, but this arises from the haphazard nature with which digits occur in a table of random numbers, and not from the haphazard whim of the investigator in allocating patients" (Last, 1983). Using randomization, chance differences between treatment groups can be measured using probabilities, and nonchance differences are minimized.

Random assignment facilitates fair comparisons. By randomly assigning patients to treatment so that each patient is equally likely to receive either treatment (randomization), treatment groups are formed that differ (before treatment) only by chance, not by human choice. Methods such as keeping subjects and observers unaware of treatment assignments (blinding) and giving placebos to controls are intended to keep other things (besides treatment) equal in the groups during the execution of the study. When carefully performed, such maneuvers make it likely that any observed group differences in response to treatment are due to actual differences between treatments (if sample size is sufficiently large) and not to other differences between the groups.

Randomization (random assignment) also justifies the use of hypothesis tests and CIs. If patients are randomly assigned to treatment and control groups but the entire study group is not a random sample of the population of interest, statistical inferences apply to differences in treatment effects between the study samples but *not* necessarily to the population. This is because such random assignment is equivalent to selecting two random samples from the total study sample (not from the population).

TAILORING THE STATISTICAL ANALYSIS TO THE SUBSTANTIVE PROBLEM

Example

Suppose 15 of 25 patients (60%) responded to a new treatment compared to 7 of 25 (28%) on a standard treatment. Before beginning a study to collect such data, the investigators should decide what specific substantive or clinical questions are to be addressed. At least four separate substantive questions can be addressed using these data:

1. What percent of patients responded to the new treatment?
2. What percent of patients responded to the standard treatment?
3. Is there a statistically significant difference between the percentages that responded to the two treatments?
4. What is the size of the difference between the percentages of patients that responded to the new and the standard treatment?

Possible Approaches to the Four Questions

To address question 1 and question 2, estimate separate percentages responding to the new and standard treatments without comparing them. The percentage that responded to the new treatment was $^{15}/_{25} = 60\%$ (95% CI of 39%–79%). The percentage that responded to the standard treatment was $^{7}/_{25} = 28\%$ (95% CI of 12%–49%).

To address question 3, compare the percentages responding to the new and standard treatments using a statistical test, and report the p value. Because the expected cell sizes in the 2×2 table are all above five, the chi-squared test is used to compare the percentages (Norusis, 1996a). The chi-squared test (discussed in the next chapter) yields $p = 0.046$. Thus, we say that there is a statistically significant (detectable) difference between the percentages.

To address question 4, estimate the difference between those two percentages by determining the point and CI estimates of the difference. The point estimate of the difference is $60\% - 28\% = 32\%$ or 32 percentage points. Because the difference between two percentages is not a percentage but is instead measured in percentage points, we should *not* use the method for the CI of a percentage that was used in the previous examples.

The *CI for the difference between two percentages* is used to find the appropriate 95% CI. The computer program, CIA, gives the 95% CI of 6% to 58% (differences between 6 and 58 percentage points). In sum, 32% (percentage points) is the best single number estimate of the magnitude of the difference in the population of interest, and 95% CI of 6% to 58% provides a range of estimates (interval estimate) that is statistically compatible with the observed difference of 32%.

A common misconception is that statistical significance can be determined by observing whether the individual 95% CIs for the two groups overlap. However, we saw that the two percentages, 60% and 28%, are statistically significantly different despite the overlap in their individual CIs (from 39%–49%). The statistical significance of the difference can be correctly determined from the CI of the difference, 95% CI of 6% to 58%, but not from the two separate CIs found in addressing questions 1 and 2. However, the 95% CI of the difference provides much information in addition to statistical significance. The 95% CI of 6% to 58% provides a set of estimates (indeed, an entire interval) that is statistically compatible with the observed 32-percentage point difference. Thus, it addresses the size of the difference, not just whether there is a statistically significant difference. The four examples in the next section show the advantages of the CI of the difference when the substantive question of interest is the size of the difference between responses to two treatments.

CONFIDENCE INTERVALS OF DIFFERENCES BETWEEN PERCENTAGES

Authors of papers reporting tests of new treatments often address only statistical significance (or p values) and not the question of a real clinical advantage. This section distinguishes clinical (practical) significance from statistical significance and shows how CIs of differences can assess both (Braitman, 1991). Hypothetical examples comparing the percentages of arthritis patients responding to two treatments provide interpretations of p values, point estimates, and CIs.

Example 1

Suppose in a multicenter clinical trial, 156 of 400 patients (39%) responded to a new treatment for arthritis, and 128 of 400 different patients (32%) responded to the standard treatment. Significance tests and statistical estimates address distinct but related questions using these data. A significance test addresses the question, *"How likely was the difference to occur by chance?"* Statistical estimates of differences (point estimates and CIs) address, *"How large is the difference in the population of interest?"* (Wonnacott & Wonnacott, 1985).

Whether a difference in the percentages responding to the two treatments exists in the *population* of arthritis patients is ascertained using a significance level or p value. The null hypothesis, H_o, states that there is really no difference between the percentages responding in the population of interest. The alternative hypothesis is that such a difference (in either direction) exists. The significance test uses the p value to weigh the evidence that there is a real difference (the alternative hypothesis) against the null hypothesis that the observed difference is due to chance variation. The p value, $p = 0.046$, comes from a chi-squared test comparing $156/400$ (39%) with $128/400$ (32%). $p = 0.046$ is the probability of obtaining the observed difference (7% = 39% − 32%) or one larger in the study sample *assuming* H_o: no difference in the percentages responding in the population of interest. A low p value suggests incompatibility between the observed data and H_o. Because $p = 0.046 < 0.05$ (0.05 is the conventional cutoff point), the observed difference is called statistically significant at the $\alpha = 0.05$ level. While this p value indicates a statistically detectable difference between the populations of interest, it provides no information on the size of that difference.

Two statistical measures estimating the size of the unknown population difference are the point estimate and the CI. The point estimate of the difference in this example is the difference between the observed percentages responding in the two groups (samples), 39% − 32% = 7%. Because the observed difference, 7% (7 percentage points), is unlikely to be exactly equal to the unknown true difference between the percentages of all arthritis patients responding to these two treatments (called the parameter), a range or CI estimate is needed. The method for the 95% CI of the difference between percentages (proportions) yields a 95% CI ranging from 0.4% to 14% (see example 1 in Fig. 4-1). A 95% CI means that approximately 95% of such intervals constructed from repeated (random) samples of that size will include the parameter (the unknown true population difference). This definition focuses on the average accuracy (95%) of the CI estimation process but does not help us interpret the single 95% CI of 0.4% to 14% that was computed. Each value in the 95% CI is not statistically significantly different from the observed difference (in this case, 7%).

"Experienced clinicians weigh the side effects, long-term complications and other costs against the benefits of the two treatments to judge the size of the smallest

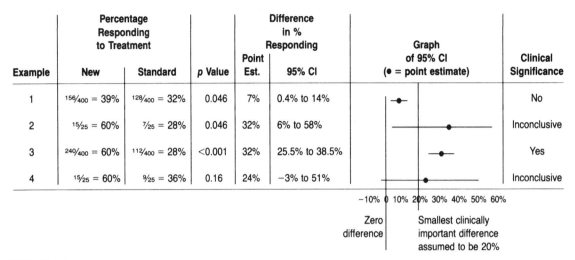

| Example | Percentage Responding to Treatment | | *p* Value | Difference in % Responding | | Graph of 95% CI (● = point estimate) | Clinical Significance |
	New	Standard		Point Est.	95% CI		
1	156/400 = 39%	128/400 = 32%	0.046	7%	0.4% to 14%		No
2	15/25 = 60%	7/25 = 28%	0.046	32%	6% to 58%		Inconclusive
3	240/400 = 60%	112/400 = 28%	<0.001	32%	25.5% to 38.5%		Yes
4	15/25 = 60%	9/25 = 36%	0.16	24%	−3% to 51%		Inconclusive

−10% 0 10% 20% 30% 40% 50% 60%

Zero difference   Smallest clinically important difference assumed to be 20%

FIGURE 4-1
Confidence intervals of differences.

clinically important difference" (Braitman, 1991, p. 515). Assume that the *smallest* clinically important difference is 20% (20 percentage points) in all the examples. Because *every* value in the 95% CI of 0.4% to 14% is below 20% (example 1 in Fig. 4-1), the difference is considered "not clinically significant." Thus, this statistically significant difference is not clinically significant.

Example 2

In a smaller study in which 15 of 25 patients (60%) responded to a new treatment compared with 7 of 25 (28%) on a standard treatment, the *p* value = 0.046. The point estimate of the difference is 60% − 28% = 32% (32 percentage points). Because the same *p* value (0.046) corresponds to highly disparate differences of 32% in example 2 and 7% in example 1 (see Fig. 4-1), the *p* value gives no information on the size of the difference. This point estimate and the 95% CI (6% − 58%) estimate the size of the unknown "true" difference.

How are hypothesis tests and CIs related to one another? When comparing two groups, the usual null hypothesis (H_o) is zero (no) difference between the two groups. If zero is outside the 95% CI of a difference, the observed difference is statistically significantly different from zero ($p < 0.05$). In Figure 4-1 the 95% CIs do not include zero in examples 1 through 3, and the associated *p* values are less than 0.05. In example 4, zero is included in the 95% CI (−3%–51%) and $p = 0.16$. Thus, a 95% CI can be viewed as the set of values hypothesized for the parameter that cannot be rejected at the $\alpha = 0.05$ level (Braitman, 1991). In other words, a 95% CI contains values that are not statistically significantly different ($p \geq 0.05$) from the observed value.

Example 3

Suppose that 240 of 400 patients (60%) responded to a new treatment compared with 112 of 400 (28%) on the standard. In this larger study, the same percentages as in example 2 respond to the new (60%) and standard (28%) treatments, respectively. Using a chi-squared test, $p < 0.001$. Because $p < 0.05$, the difference is statistically significant; however, is it clinically significant? Remember that a p value does not address the size or importance of the difference.

The statistical estimates of the difference, the point estimate and CI estimate, address these issues. A difference is clinically significant when the entire 95% CI is above the predetermined smallest clinically important difference (Braitman, 1991). Because all of the 95% CI of 25.5% to 38.5% is above 20%, the difference is clinically significant. CIs permit readers to assess clinical significance using their own value for the smallest clinically important difference rather than having to depend on the author's interpretation (Berry, 1986).

In example 1, the difference is not clinically significant because the whole 95% CI is below the smallest clinically important difference of 20%. When the smallest clinically important difference is included within the 95% CI, as in example 2, no definitive conclusion about clinical significance is possible. Nevertheless, the point estimate and CI suggest trends in the data. Because in example 2 the point estimate (32%) and more than ⅔ of the 95% CI exceed 20%, these data tend toward clinical significance.

When two groups receive different treatments, a commonly used (but less informative) alternative statistical analysis presents two separate 95% CIs, one for the percentage responding to each treatment. If the relevant question is the percentage that respond to each treatment separately without providing a treatment comparison, these two CIs suffice. However, if they overlap, we cannot conclude whether the difference is statistically significant. The 95% CI of the difference enables us to assess statistical significance and clinical significance. In example 2, the difference of 32 percentage points (95% CI of 6%–58%) is statistically significant and tends toward clinical significance. Thus, only the 95% CI of the difference, not the two single sample 95% CIs, makes the assessment of statistical and clinical significance possible.

INTERPRETATION OF CONFIDENCE INTERVALS

The 95% CI means that approximately 95% of such varying random CIs (one for each random sample), if constructed, would include the population parameter, and 5% would not. The words "95% confidence" refer to the 95% average accuracy of the estimation process and *not* to a probability of 95% for a single computed CI (Wonnacott & Wonnacott, 1985). Either the 95% CI includes the parameter (the unknown true value) or it does not; we cannot tell which. The single 95% CI may be interpreted as the set of hypotheses for parameter values that cannot be rejected at $p \geq 0.05$.

Although 32% is the point estimate for the unknown parameter in examples 2 and 3, its value is more uncertain in the smaller sample. The narrower 95% CI of

25.5% to 38.5% (13 percentage points wide) from the larger sample is more precise than a 95% CI of 6% to 58% (52 percentage points wide). The width of a 95% CI indicates the amount of uncertainty (called sampling variability or sampling error) about the population parameter inherent in examining only a random sample rather than the population. The 95% CI's combined information on the size of the "true" difference and how precisely that size is known (Rothman, 1986) helped us assess clinical and statistical significance.

Although CIs and significance tests can help us assess the impact of sampling or random error, other methods involving the design and analysis of research studies are needed to deal with nonrandom systematic errors. Neither the p value nor the statistical estimates enable us to decide what caused the observed difference in response. A careful analysis of the experimental design and execution of the study is necessary before alternative explanations for the results can be discarded. CIs communicate only the effects of sampling error on the precision of point estimates; they cannot control for systematic (nonsampling) errors, such as unmeasured confounders or measurement error. To limit the effects of systematic errors and biases, careful attention must be given to study design (e.g., randomization) and epidemiologic methods (Rothman, 1986; Wonnacott & Wonnacott, 1985). In the analysis phase, multivariable regression models can address the net effect of treatment on study outcome by controlling statistically for confounding variables (see Chapter 12, Regression).

Although inferences about the population of interest actually presume random (or probability) sampling, point and CI estimates and p values generally are considered to be useful approximations to the extent that the study sample is representative of the population.

INFORMATION CONTENT OF COMMON FORMS OF STATISTICAL PRESENTATIONS

The next example illustrates the relevance of statistical estimates of the difference between treatment response rates even when the difference is not statistically significant. In addition, it demonstrates the different types of information provided by p values, point estimates, and CIs.

Example 4

Suppose a study produced results similar to those in example 2, with 15 of 25 responding to the new treatment but 9 of 25 responding to the standard treatment. In other words, the same number responded to the new treatment, but two additional patients responded to the standard treatment.

Intuitively, we would expect the statistical presentation to lead to an interpretation similar to the one in example 2. However, traditional presentations too often state only that the difference was "significant ($p < 0.05$)" in example 2 and "not significant ($p > 0.05$)" in example 4. Such presentations incorrectly suggest very different conclusions in examples 2 and 4. Although all of examples 1 through 3 contain statistically significant results, the $p < 0.001$ in example 3 provides a much greater weight of evidence against H_o (the hypothesis of zero difference) than $p = 0.046$. Thus, more specific information is provided by an exact p value than by a statement of statistical significance or by $p < 0.05$. However, by themselves, p values yield *no* information on the size of the difference. Indeed, among these examples, the highest p value (0.16) does not correspond to the smallest difference (7%). That shows how a large difference between two small samples can yield a large (nonsignificant) p value.

p values cannot be used to gauge the size of differences because they also depend on sample size. p values address the existence of a real nonzero difference between treatments but not the size of that treatment difference. Thus, they cannot be used to assess clinical (practical) significance. The point estimate of the difference measures the magnitude of differences in the observed samples.

The point estimates in examples 2 through 4 are all large differences (of at least 24 percentage points) contrasted with a small difference of 7 percentage points in example 1. The point estimate *describes* the observed data (the size of the difference between samples) and estimates the unknown difference parameter. Point estimates and CIs of differences estimate the size of the treatment effect. However, being a single number, a point estimate cannot indicate its own sampling error as a CI does. The 95% CI provides two related types of information: the uncertainty in their respective point estimates and the clinical significance of the differences.

The larger group sizes of 400 in examples 1 and 3 yield more precise CI estimates (width approximately 14 percentage points) than the smaller groups of 25 in examples 2 and 4, in which 95% CIs are more than 50 percentage points wide. Assuming that the smallest clinically important difference is 20 percentage points, the observed difference is clinically significant in example 3 and not clinically significant in example 1. In examples 2 and 4 the clinical significance of the differences is inconclusive. However, in example 2, the point estimate, 32%, and almost ¾ of the 95% CI of 6% to 58% are above the smallest clinically important difference (20%), so the difference tends toward clinical significance. Although the difference in example 4 is not statistically significant, it may be real and even clinically important because the point estimate (24%) and more than half of the 95% CI correspond to clinically important differences. Thus, using CIs to evaluate practical significance avoids the common fallacy of "equating non-significance with no [difference]" (Berry, 1986). It is important to include a 95% CI of any substantial difference even if that difference is not statistically significant.

SUMMARY OF ROLES OF POINT ESTIMATES, CONFIDENCE INTERVALS, AND P VALUES

p values, point estimates, and CIs are used to make statistical inferences about a population parameter. Both p values and CIs are defined in terms of the compatibility of hypothesis with the sample difference, while the point estimate is that sample difference. Only the point estimate describes what is actually observed in the sample. Thus, it is a descriptive and an inferential statistic. When there is no random assignment and the sample is neither random nor representative, statistical inference using either the p value or CI is problematic; the point estimate still accurately describes the sample difference. Thus, the point estimate of a difference should be reported because it extracts the most fundamental and consistently meaningful information from a statistical comparison. Point estimates, CIs, and p values extract complementary information from study data and should be reported for major results.

APPLICATION EXERCISES AND RESULTS

This chapter is a series of examples that were designed to help readers understand concepts presented in the first three chapters. It therefore requires no additional exercises.

II

Specific Statistical Techniques

Selected Nonparametric Techniques

Barbara Hazard Munro

OBJECTIVES FOR CHAPTER 5

After reading this chapter, you should be able to do the following:

1 • Identify situations in which the use of nonparametric techniques is appropriate.

2 • Interpret computer printouts containing specified nonparametric analyses.

3 • Relate the results of the analysis to the research question posed.

THE RESEARCH QUESTION

Nonparametric tests can be used to answer research questions ranging from whether or not a relationship exists between two variables to whether or not groups differ on an outcome measure. The focus of this chapter is on comparing groups of subjects on outcome measures. The nonparametric techniques to be covered in this chapter are contained in Table 5-1. This is not intended to be comprehensive, but rather a discussion of the commonly used nonparametrics. The parametric analogs that are covered in later chapters also are included.

THE TYPE OF DATA REQUIRED

Parametric Versus Nonparametric Tests

When we use *parametric* tests of significance, we are estimating at least one population parameter from our sample statistics. To be able to make such an estimation, we must make certain assumptions; the most important one is that the variable we

TABLE 5-1
Nonparametric Tests and Corresponding Parametric Analogs

	Nonparametric Tests		
	Nominal Data	*Ordinal Data*	*Parametric Analog*
One-Group Case	Chi-square goodness of fit	—	—
Two-Group Case	Chi-square	Mann-Whitney U	*t* test
k-Group Case	Chi-square	Kruskal-Wallis H	One-way ANOVA
Dependent Groups (Repeated Measures)	McNemar test for significance of change	Wilcoxon matched-pairs signed rank test	Paired *t* tests
		Friedman Matched samples	Repeated measures ANOVA

have measured in the sample is normally distributed in the population to which we plan to generalize our findings. With *nonparametric* tests, there is no assumption about the distribution of the variable in the population. For that reason, nonparametric tests often are called *distribution free.*

At one time, level of measurement was considered an important element in deciding whether to use parametric or nonparametric tests. It was believed that parametric tests should be reserved for use with interval- and ratio-level data. However, it has been shown that the use of parametric techniques with ordinal data rarely distorts the results.

Parametric techniques have several advantages. Other things being equal, they are more *powerful* and more *flexible* than nonparametric techniques. They not only allow the researcher to study the effect of many independent variables on the dependent variable, but also make possible the study of their interaction. Nonparametric techniques are much easier to calculate by hand than parametric techniques, but that advantage has been eliminated by the use of computers. Small samples and serious distortions of the data should lead one to explore nonparametric techniques.

CHI-SQUARE

The Research Question

Chi-square is the most commonly reported nonparametric statistic. It can be used with one or more groups. It compares the actual number (or frequency) in each group with the "expected" number. The "expected" number can be based on theory, experience, or comparison groups. The question is whether or not the expected number differs significantly from the actual number.

TABLE 5-2
A Comparison of the Rate of Hematoma Formation Between Two Methods of Introducer Care

	Flushed	*Capped*
Present	19 (40%)	20 (40.8%)
Absent	28 (60%)	29 (59.2%)

χ^2 (1 *df*) = 0.0285; p = NS.

(From Craney, J. M., Hart, E. K., & Munro, B. H. [1992]. A comparison of two techniques of care for indwelling arterial introducers after coronary angioplasty. Journal of Cardiovascular Nursing, 7(1), 50–55.)

The Type of Data Required

Chi-square is used when the data are nominal (categorical). Later chapters discuss how the chi-square is used to test the fit of models in techniques such as logistic regression and path analysis.

Craney, Hart, and Munro (1992) compared two techniques of care for indwelling arterial introducers after coronary angioplasty. One outcome measure was hematoma formation. As you can see in Table 5-2, two variables are measured at the nominal level. One is a method of introducer care with two levels, flushed and capped, and the other is hematoma formation with two levels, present and absent. Is there a significant difference in hematoma formation between the two methods of introducer care? There was no significant difference in hematoma formation between the two groups (p = ns). The rate of hematoma formation was 40% in the flushed group and 40.8% in the capped group. Although in this table, the actual p value is not reported, it is better practice to report the actual value, rather than just indicate that it was not significant.

Assumptions Underlying Chi-Square

1. Frequency data
2. Adequate sample size
3. Measures independent of each other
4. Theoretical basis for the categorization of the variables

The first assumption is that the data are frequency data, that is, a count of the number of subjects in each condition under analysis. The chi-square cannot be used to analyze the difference between scores or their means. If data are not categorical, they must be categorized before being used. Whether or not to categorize depends on the data and the question to be answered.

If the data are not normally distributed and violate the assumptions underlying the appropriate parametric technique, then categorization might be appropriate. The categories developed must adequately represent the data and be based on sound rationale. If you had the ages of subjects, you could categorize them as 20 to 29, 30 to 39, and 40 to 49. However, you have treated all people within one of your three categories as being equal in age. Does a 29 year old belong in the same group as a 20 year old, or is he or she more like the 30 year old? Specificity and variability are decreased through this categorization, and as a result, the analysis will be less powerful.

The question addressed affects the categorization of subjects. Suppose the researcher was interested in whether or not being in school affects some categorical outcome measure. Then grouping the children as preschool and in school would make sense, rather than using their actual ages. When categories have clinical relevance, statistical analyses that preserve these categories are more likely to provide useful interpretations. They are less likely to provide "differences that do not make a difference."

The second assumption is that the sample size is adequate. Expected frequencies of less than five in 2 × 2 tables present problems. In larger tables, a cell with an expected frequency of less than five is less of a problem, but when more than 20% of the cells have less than five or if one of the cells has no frequencies, the researcher is advised to reduce the number of cells in the analysis by grouping the subjects into a smaller number of categories (Hinkle, Wiersma, & Jurs, 1994).

The third assumption is that the measures are independent of each other. This means that the categories created are mutually exclusive; that is, no subject can be in more than one cell in the design, and no subject can be used more than once. It also means that the response of one subject cannot influence the response of another. This seems relatively straightforward, but difficulties arise in clinical research situations when data are collected for a period of time. If you are testing subjects in a hospital, you must be sure that a person who is readmitted does not get enrolled in the study for a second time. You also must be sure that subjects in one condition are not communicating with subjects in their own or different conditions in such a way that responses are "contaminated."

The fourth assumption is that there is some theoretical reason for the categories. This ensures that the analysis will be meaningful and prevents "fishing expeditions." The latter would occur if the researcher kept recategorizing subjects, hoping to find some relationship between the variables. Research questions and methods for analysis are established prior to data collection. While these may be modified to suit the data obtained, the basic theoretical structure remains.

Power

Power must be considered when planning sample size. If you have 40 subjects, 10 in each of the four cells in a 2 × 2 design, set your probability level at 0.05, and expect a moderate effect—your power is only 0.47 (Cohen, 1987, p. 235). You have less than a 50% chance of finding a significant relationship between the two variables. Under the same conditions, a sample of 80 results in a power of 76 and a sample of 90 in a power of 81. Following the description of the computer printout, an example of power is given.

TREATMENT GROUP

WTLOSS		*Drug Therapy*	*Behavior Mod*	*Row Total*
	Yes	35	30	65
	No	11	24	35
	Column Total	46	54	100

FIGURE 5-1
Data for chi-square analysis.

Example for Computer Analysis

Suppose we were testing two methods of weight loss, drug therapy and behavior modification. We randomly assign subjects to one of the two therapies. Figure 5-1 contains the fictional results. By looking at the column totals, we can see that the final sample contains 46 people in the drug therapy group and 54 people in the behavior modification group for a total sample of 100 subjects.

The null hypothesis is that there is no difference between the two therapies in the effect on weight loss. Because the numbers of subjects in the two groups are not equal, adding percentages to the table is helpful in clarifying the results (Fig. 5-2). Now you can see that 76.1% of the subjects in the drug therapy group lost weight, compared to 55.6% in the behavior modification group. The statistical question is whether or not a difference this large is likely to have occurred by chance. If there are less than five chances in 100 that the difference occurred by chance alone, the difference is significant at the 0.05 level. The row totals show that 65 of the subjects in the entire sample (65%) were successful in losing weight. If the rates of weight loss are the same between the two therapies, then we would expect that 65% of the drug therapy group and 65% of the behavior modification group would lose weight. These "expectations" become the expected frequencies in the calculation of the chi-square. For the drug therapy group, the expected frequencies would equal 29.9

TREATMENT GROUP

WTLOSS	*Count Col Pct*	*Drug Therapy*	*Behavior Mod*	*Row Total*
	Yes	35	30	65
		76.1	55.6	65.0
	No	11	24	35
		23.9	44.4	35.0
	Column Total	46	54	100
		46.0	54.0	100.0

FIGURE 5-2
Percentage of subjects within each group who did or did not lose weight.

TREATMENT GROUP

WTLOSS

Count Exp Val	Drug Therapy	Behavior Mod	Row Total
Yes	35	30	65
	29.9	35.1	65.0%
No	11	24	35
	16.1	18.9	35.0%
Column Total	46	54	100
	46.0%	54.0%	100.0%

FIGURE 5-3
Actual and expected frequencies.

$(.65 \times 46 = 29.9)$, and for the behavior modification group, they would equal 35.1 $(.65 \times 54)$. Figure 5-3 contains the actual and expected frequencies.

Computer Output for Chi-Square Analysis

Figure 5-4 contains the computer printout of this analysis. The output was produced by SPSS for Windows. It was edited slightly, and comments have been added in lighter print. The table titled Weight Loss * STUDY GROUP Crosstabulation, contains the number and percent of subjects in each cell and the row and column totals.

CROSSTABS

Weight Loss * STUDY GROUP Crosstabulation

			STUDY GROUP		
			Drug Therapy	Behavior Modification	Total
Weight Loss	Yes	Count	35	30	65
		% of STUDY GROUP	76.1%	55.6%	65.0%
	No	Count	11	24	35
		% of STUDY GROUP	23.9%	44.4%	35.0%
Total		Count	46	54	100
		% of STUDY GROUP	100.0%	100.0%	100.0%

FIGURE 5-4
Computer output of chi-square analysis. (*continued*)

Chi-Square Tests

	Value	df	Asymp. Sig. (2-tailed)	Exact Sig. (2-tailed)	Exact Sig. (1-tailed)
Pearson Chi-Square	4.603[b]	1	.032		
Continuity Correction[a]	3.744	1	.053		
Likelihood Ratio	4.691	1	.030		
Fisher's Exact Test[a]				.037	.026
Linear-by-Linear Association	4.557	1	.033		
N of Valid Cases	100				

a. Computed only for a 2x2 table

b. 0 cells (.0%) have expected count less than 5. The minimum expected count is 16.10.

The Pearson value is the usual chi-square value. The other values are described in the text.

Symmetric Measures

		Value	Approx. Sig.
Nominal Measures	Phi	.215	.032
	Cramer's V	.215	.032
N of Valid Cases		100	

Phi is a shortcut method of calculating a correlation coefficient that can be used when both variables are dichotomous (have only two levels). It is only appropriate when chi-square is significant.

Cramer's V is a modified version of Phi that can be used with larger tables.

FIGURE 5-4 (CONTINUED)

Under Chi-Square Tests, we see four different values, with their degrees of freedom (*df*) and significance levels. The *Pearson value* is what you would get if you did this by hand using the usual formula. It is based on the differences between the observed and expected frequencies. For example, the actual (or observed) number of subjects in the drug therapy group who lost weight is 35, but the expected number (based on an overall rate of 65%) is 29.9. The difference between these two values is 5.1. The chi-square value based on the differences between observed and expected frequencies in each of the four cells in our design is 4.603. There is 1 *df,* and the significance level is 0.032. Therefore, we would say that the null hypothesis of no difference between the two treatment groups has been rejected. There is a significant difference between the two groups in percentage of subjects who lost weight. The drug therapy group had a significantly higher (76.1%) rate of weight loss than the behavior modification group (55.6%).

In Chapter 3, *df* is defined as the extent to which values are free to vary given a specific number of subjects and a total score. In chi-square analysis, however, frequencies are used rather than scores. The number of cells that are free to vary depends on the number of cells found in the table. How many cell frequencies would we need to know to derive the others? The answer to that question is equal to the *df.* Given the row and column totals, we only need to know one cell value in a 2 × 2 table to be able to calculate the rest by simple subtraction. Therefore, only one cell is free to vary; the others are dependent on that value. The *df* for a 2 × 2 chi-square analysis is always 1, regardless of sample size. The formula for calculating the *df* for any size table in a chi-square analysis follows:

$$df = (r - 1)(c - 1)$$

For our 2 × 2 table, this becomes $df = (2 - 1)(2 - 1) = 1$.

The *continuity correction* is often called the Yates' correction. Although nominal data are used to calculate a chi-square, chi-square values have a distribution (see Appendix B). The distribution is continuous, but when the expected frequency in any of the cells in a 2 × 2 table is less than 5, the sampling distribution of chi-square for that analysis may depart substantially from normal (Hinkle et al., 1994). In these cases, the continuity correction is recommended. The correction consists of subtracting 0.5 from the difference between each pair of observed and expected frequencies. In our example, the difference of 5.1 would be reduced to 4.6 by subtracting 0.5. This results in an overall lower chi-square value. On the output, we see that the Pearson value is 4.603, but with the continuity correction, this drops to 3.7444. Thus, applying the correction reduces the power of the analysis. In our example, the *minimum expected count* is 16.10 (see "b" under the Chi-Square Tests); therefore, we would report the Pearson result. If the minimum expected count (or frequency) had been less than 5, the continuity correction value or Fisher's exact test should have been reported.

The *likelihood ratio* chi-square is based on maximum likelihood theory (Norusis, 1996a) and is of more interest when we discuss the fitting of models, such as with structural equation models. When the sample is large, the likelihood ratio is similar to the Pearson, which is evident in our example.

Fisher's exact test is an alternative to Pearson's chi-square for the 2 × 2 table. It assumes that the marginal counts remain fixed at the observed values and calculates exact probabilities of obtaining the observed results if the two variables are independent (Norusis, 1996). It is most useful when sample sizes and expected frequencies are small. If the minimum expected value is less than 5 in a 2 × 2 table, Fisher's exact is more appropriate that Pearson's chi-square.

The *linear-by-linear association chi-square* is the "square of the usual Pearson correlation multiplied by the sample size minus one" (Norusis, 1996, p. 84). Although printed when chi-square is requested, it is not always appropriate, because it is based on the relationship between the two variables as measured by the Pearson correlation coefficient. The Pearson correlation coefficient assumes normally distributed data, and this is not usually the case with nominal data, especially with two dichotomous variables as in a 2 × 2 table.

Two measures are listed in the table titled Symmetric Measures. They are Phi and Cramer's V.

Phi is a shortcut method of calculating a correlation coefficient that can be used when both variables are dichotomous (have only two levels). It is only appropriate when the chi-square value is significant. It is interpreted as a measure of association; that is, in this example, the correlation between these two variables is .215. It allows us to interpret the strength of the relationship. It is most useful with 2 × 2 tables in which the values of phi range from 0 to 1. In tables with more cells, the value can be greater than 1, decreasing its usefulness. It is complementary to chi-square because it is less sensitive to sample size. It could be used to compare the strength of the relationship across studies.

Cramer's V is a slightly modified version that can be used with larger tables. Phi is adjusted for the number of rows and columns. Thus, given a significant chi-square, report phi for 2 × 2 tables and Cramer's V for larger tables.

An Example of Power Analysis

Cohen (1987) defines the effect sizes related to the chi-square as follows:

Small = .1
Moderate = .3
Large = .5

Using our example, what does this mean? Table 5-3 demonstrates these effect sizes for our example. The null hypothesis in our example is based on the fact that 65% of the entire sample lost weight. Thus, if the null hypothesis is true, 65% of each group should lose weight. By Cohen's definition, a small effect would be a 10% difference between the two groups, such as 70% of the drug therapy group losing weight versus 60% of the behavior modification group. A moderate effect would be a 30% difference between the two groups, and a large effect would be a 50% difference.

TABLE 5-3
An Example of Cohen's (1987) Definition of Effect Sizes

	Drug Therapy	*Behavior Modification*	*Difference Between Groups*
Null Hypothesis	65%	65%	0%
Small Effect	70%	60%	10%
Moderate Effect	80%	50%	30%
Large Effect	90%	40%	50%

Example From the Literature

Sulzbach, Munro, and Hirshfeld (1995), in a randomized clinical trial of the effect of bed position after percutaneous transluminal coronary angioplasty, compared two groups of patients on the number of packages of 4 × 4's used (Table 5-4). There are two nominal level variables. The first is group membership, which has two levels, experimental and control. The experimental group was allowed to use their bed controls as desired. The control group was not allowed to use the bed controls. Their heads were elevated no more than 30 degrees, and the affected leg was kept straight and immobilized. The second variable was bleeding as measured by the number of 4 × 4's used. There were three levels: none used, 1 to 6 used, and 7 to 20 used. The null hypothesis was that there would be no significant difference in bleeding between the two groups; the null hypothesis was supported ($p = .56$). Nineteen percent of the control group (5/26) and 21% of the experimental group (6/28) required seven or more packages of 4 × 4's.

Calculation of Chi-Square

When calculating chi-square, the expected and observed frequencies in each cell are compared. Using the expected and observed frequencies in Figure 5-3, we demonstrate the use of the chi-square formula. Note that in each cell, the expected frequency is subtracted from the observed frequency; that result is squared and then divided by the expected frequency. The sum of these calculations is the chi-square.

Chi-Square Formula

$$\Sigma\ \frac{(35 - 29.9)^2}{29.9} + \frac{(30 - 35.1)^2}{35.1} + \frac{(11 - 16.1)^2}{16.1} + \frac{(24 - 18.9)^2}{18.9} = 4.60264$$

TABLE 5-4
Number of Packages of 4×4's Required for Bleeding at Catheter Insertion Site

Packages of 4×4's	Control Group Frequency	Experimental Group Frequency
0	10	14
1–6	11	8
7–20	5	6

$\chi^2 = 1.16$, $df = 2$, $p = .56$

(From Sulzbach, L. M., Munro, B. H. & Hirshfeld, Jr., J. W. [1995]. A randomized clinical trial of the effect of bed position after PTCA. American Journal of Critical Care, 4(3), 221–226.)

SUMMARY FOR CHI-SQUARE

Chi-square is the appropriate technique when variables are measured at the nominal level. It may be used with one or more groups. In the *one-group* case comparison, data may be provided from a theoretical perspective, norms, or past experience. Suppose a hospital had a cesarean section rate of 30%. This percentage could be compared with reported rates (locally, regionally, or nationally) through the use of chi-square.

Although only a 2 × 2 design has been used as an example, this *two-group* case with two levels in each group can be extended to larger designs. The groups in a chi-square analysis must be mutually exclusive; however, an adaptation of chi-square is the McNemar test for use with repeated measures at the nominal level.

NOMINAL-LEVEL DATA, DEPENDENT MEASURES

The *McNemar test* can be used with two dichotomous measures on the same subjects. It is used to measure change. Figure 5-5 contains an example of a computer printout produced by SPSS for Windows.

We are interested in whether or not satisfaction with weight varies over time. Subjects are asked to rate their satisfaction with their weight when they were 18 years old and currently. One indicates dissatisfaction, and two indicates satisfaction. The cells show that 122 people did not change their rating, 47 were dissatisfied at both times, and 75 were satisfied at both times. Among those who changed, 38 who were satisfied with their weight at age 18 are dissatisfied with their current weight, and 13 people who were dissatisfied with their weight at age 18 are satisfied with their current weight. The significance of .001 indicates that more people became dissatisfied with their weight over time.

SUMMARY FOR MCNEMAR

The McNemar test uses an adaptation of the chi-square formula to test the direction of change. Only the two cells that include changes are included in the analysis; therefore, the *df* = 1.

ORDINAL DATA, INDEPENDENT GROUPS

Two commonly used techniques are the *Mann-Whitney U*, which is used to compare two groups and is thus analogous to the *t* test, and *Kruskal-Wallis*, which is used to compare two or more groups and is thus analogous to the parametric technique analysis of variance. An example of these techniques comes from analysis of data collected from three groups in a program grant supported by the National Institute for Nursing Research (Jacobsen, Munro, & Brooten, 1996). The Multiple Af-

Test Statistics[a]

	SATISCUR & Satisfaction with weight at age 18
N	173
Chi-Square[b]	11.294
Asymp. Sig.	.001

a. McNemar Test

b. Continuity Corrected

SATISCUR & Satisfaction with weight at age 18

	Satisfaction with weight at age 18	
SATISCUR	1	2
1	47	38
2	13	75

Row totals—Satisfaction with current weight
   85 people (47 + 38) dissatisfied
   88 people (13 + 75) satisfied

Column totals—Satisfaction with weight at age 18
   60 people (47 + 13) dissatisfied
   113 people (38 + 75) satisfied

Cells
   Reflecting no change
      47 people dissatisfied both times
      75 people satisfied both times
   Reflecting change
      38 people who are dissatisfied currently, were satisfied at age 18
      13 people who are currently satisfied, were dissatisfied at age 18

FIGURE 5-5
Computer output of McNemar test.

fect Adjective Checklist Revised was used to collect data from three groups of subjects: cesarean section mothers, diabetic pregnant women, and hysterectomy patients. In our preliminary check of the data, we found that the measure of anxiety seriously violated the assumptions underlying the use of parametric techniques. We elected, therefore, to compare the three groups through the use of the nonparametric technique, the Kruskal-Wallis one-way analysis of variance (ANOVA). In this technique, scores for subjects are converted into ranks, and the analysis compares the mean rank in each group. Figure 5-6 contains the computer printout.

With 277 subjects, rankings can go from 1 to 277. The actual scores on the anxiety scale ranged from 0 to 10. Two chi-square values are given; one is corrected for ties in rankings. Because 56% of our subjects scored 0 or 1 on this measure, the correction for ties is important. With a significance of 0.0026, we know that the three groups differ, but further analysis must be done to determine which pairs of groups differ.

We used the Mann-Whitney U for the post-hoc comparisons. It does not require

```
                        SPSS/PC+

NPAR TESTS /KRUSKAL-WALLIS ANXIETY BY GROUP (1,3).


- - - - - Kruskal-Wallis 1-way ANOVA

       ANXIETY
  by GROUP


     Mean Rank    Cases
        128.73       121   GROUP = 1   CESAREAN
        135.88       112   GROUP = 2   HYSTERECTOMY
        175.19        44   GROUP = 3   DIABETIC
                     ---
                     277   Total

                                          Corrected for Ties
        CASES    Chi-Square  Significance   Chi-Square  Significance
         277       11.1416         .0038      11.8730         .0026
```

FIGURE 5-6

Kruskal-Wallis test. (Data collected in program grant funded by the National Center for Nursing Research, PO1-NR1859. P. I., D. Brooten, *Early Hospital Discharge and Nurse Specialist Followup.*)

normally distributed data but is sensitive to the central tendency and the distribution of the scores. To protect against a type I error, we used a *Bonferroni correction*. We divided the level of significance by the number of comparisons we would make (0.05/3 = 0.0167). For a comparison to be considered significant, it must have a significance level of 0.0167, not 0.05. Figure 5-7 contains the three analyses.

As with the Kruskal-Wallis analysis, ranks are assigned and compared. U is a measure of how often ranks in one group are lower than ranks in the other group. U is calculated for each group, and the printout contains the smaller of the two U's. W is the sum of the ranks for the group with the smaller number of subjects. The significance level is obtained by transforming the score into a standard score, Z (Norusis, 1996a).

The first analysis compares the cesarean and hysterectomy groups. They did not differ significantly on their anxiety scores ($p = .4680$).

The second analysis compares the cesarean and diabetic groups. The diabetic group scored significantly higher (mean rank = 103.10) than the cesarean group (mean rank = 75.69), $p = 0.0007$.

In the third analysis, the hysterectomy and diabetic groups are compared, and we see that the diabetic group scored significantly higher than the hysterectomy group.

To summarize, the post-hoc tests demonstrated that the diabetic pregnant women had significantly higher anxiety scores than the cesarean or hysterectomy patients. The latter two groups did not differ significantly from each other.

NPAR TESTS /MANN-WHITNEY ANXIETY BY GROUP (1,2).

- - - - - Mann-Whitney U - Wilcoxon Rank Sum W Test

    ANXIETY
by GROUP

Mean Rank	Cases			
114.04	121	GROUP = 1	CESAREAN
120.20	112	GROUP = 2	HYSTERECTOMY

	233	Total	

		Corrected for Ties	
U	W	Z	2-tailed P
6417.5	13462.5	-.7258	.4680

NPAR TESTS /MANN-WHITNEY ANXIETY BY GROUP (1,3).

- - - - - Mann-Whitney U - Wilcoxon Rank Sum W Test

    ANXIETY
by GROUP

Mean Rank	Cases			
75.69	121	GROUP = 1	CESAREAN
103.10	44	GROUP = 3	DIABETIC

	165	Total	

		Corrected for Ties	
U	W	Z	2-tailed P
1777.5	4536.5	-3.3717	.0007

NPAR TESTS /MANN-WHITNEY ANXIETY BY GROUP (2,3).

- - - - - Mann-Whitney U - Wilcoxon Rank Sum W Test

    ANXIETY
by GROUP

Mean Rank	Cases			
72.18	112	GROUP = 2	HYSTERECTOMY
94.59	44	GROUP = 3	DIABETIC

	156	Total	

		Corrected for Ties	
U	W	Z	2-tailed P
1756.0	4162.0	-2.8604	.0042

FIGURE 5-7

Mann-Whitney. (Data collected in program grant funded by the National Center for Nursing Research, PO1-NR1859. P. I. D. Brooten, *Early Hospital Discharge and Nurse Specialist Followup.*)

TABLE 5-5
Mann Whitney U *Comparison of Antiemetic Consumption in Milligrams Between PCAE and NCAE Groups at Hour 1, Hour 12, and Hour 24 Following Chemotherapy*

	Mean	*SD*	*Range*	*Mann-Whitney* U	p
Benadryl					
Hour 1					
PCAE	5.6	.88	5–8		
NCAE	12.5	.00	13–13	0	<.001
Hour 12					
PCAE	3.8	7.7	0–24		
NCAE	35.2	7.5	13–38	1	<.001
Hour 24					
PCAE	1.1	2.7	0–8		
NCAE	12.5	.00	13–13	0	<.001

PCAE = patient-controlled analgesia; NCAE = nurse-administered analgesia.

(From Edwards, J. N., Herman, J., Wallace, B. K., Pavy M. D., & Harrison-Pavy, J. [1991]. Comparison of patient-controlled and nurse-controlled antiemetic therapy in patients receiving chemotherapy. Research in Nursing & Health, *14(4), 249–257.)*

Example From the Literature

Edwards, Herman, Wallace, Pavy, and Harrison-Pavy (1991), compared patient-controlled and nurse-controlled antiemetic therapy in patients receiving chemotherapy. One of the outcome measures was antiemetic consumption in milligrams (Table 5-5). The independent variable is a type of antiemetic therapy with two levels, patient controlled and nurse controlled. The outcome measure of milligrams of diphenhydramine (Benadryl) consumed was measured at three points. A separate Mann Whitney U was used to compare the two study groups at each of the three times. At all three times, the patient-controlled group consumed significantly less diphenhydramine than the nurse-controlled group ($p <$ .001).

Summary of Kruskal-Wallis and Mann-Whitney U

Kruskal-Wallis is the nonparametric analogue for the Oneway Analysis of Variance and Mann-Whitney U is the nonparametric analogue for the *t* test. They may be used when the data violate the assumptions underlying the parametric tests, especially when the data are not normally distributed.

ORDINAL DATA, DEPENDENT GROUPS

The last two nonparametric techniques to be presented are the *Wilcoxon matched-pairs signed rank test* and the *Friedman matched samples*. The Wilcoxon matched-pairs is analogous to the parametric paired *t* test, and the Friedman matched samples is analogous to a repeated measures analysis of variance. We start with the Friedman to demonstrate how initial analysis and post-hoc tests might be done using non-parametric techniques.

This is a fictitious example of a repeated measures design in which subjects are their own controls. Each subject is exposed to each treatment. The order of their exposure to the three treatments is random, and adequate time is allowed between treatments to prevent carryover effects. The subjects are elderly with limited mobility. The outcome measure is the distance they are able to walk in 5 minutes, measured in yards. This outcome measure is not normally distributed. The three treatments are listening with an earphone while walking to a tape that gives encouragement on walking, watching a video prior to walking that shows good walking technique and explains the value of walking, and simply being asked to walk as far as they can in 5 minutes (control). Figure 5-8 contains the computer output.

Each subject has a score on each of these variables representing his or her distance walked. The question is whether or not the subjects' distance differed across the three treatments. The mean ranks for the three conditions are given first, and the ranks vary from a high of 2.82 for the earphone group to a low of 1.18 for the control group.

The chi-square has a significance level of .0000. Because the initial analysis is significant, we conduct comparisons of each pair of ranks. The Wilcoxon matched-pairs is used for the three comparisons, and the Bonferroni correction is 0.05/3 or 0.0167. Figure 5-9 contains the results.

In the first comparison, ranks in the earphone condition are compared with ranks in the video condition. In 20 cases, the subject's distance was greater with the earphone than in the video condition. In three cases, the subject walked farther after watching the video than with the earphone. There were two ties (i.e., the subject did equally well under both conditions). The p value of .002 is less than our level of sig-

Ranks

	Mean Rank
EARPHONE	2.82
VIDEO	2.00
CONTROL	1.18

Test Statistics[a]

N	25
Chi-Square	35.766
df	2
Asymp. Sig.	.000

a. Friedman Test

FIGURE 5-8
Computer output, Friedman.

Ranks

		N	Mean Rank	Sum of Ranks
EARPHONE - VIDEO	Negative Ranks	20[a]	12.05	241.00
	Positive Ranks	3[b]	11.67	35.00
	Ties	2[c]		
	Total	25		

a. EARPHONE > VIDEO

b. EARPHONE < VIDEO

c. EARPHONE = VIDEO

Test Statistics[a]

	EARPHONE - VIDEO
Z	-3.139[b]
Asymp. Sig. (2-tailed)	.002

a. Wilcoxon Signed Ranks Test

b. Based on positive ranks.

Ranks

		N	Mean Rank	Sum of Ranks
EARPHONE - CONTROL	Negative Ranks	24[a]	12.50	300.00
	Positive Ranks	0[b]	.00	.00
	Ties	1[c]		
	Total	25		

a. EARPHONE > CONTROL

b. EARPHONE < CONTROL

c. EARPHONE = CONTROL

Test Statistics[a]

	EARPHONE - CONTROL
Z	-4.292[b]
Asymp. Sig. (2-tailed)	.000

a. Wilcoxon Signed Ranks Test

b. Based on positive ranks.

Ranks

		N	Mean Rank	Sum of Ranks
VIDEO - CONTROL	Negative Ranks	20[a]	13.30	266.00
	Positive Ranks	3[b]	3.33	10.00
	Ties	2[c]		
	Total	25		

a. VIDEO > CONTROL

b. VIDEO < CONTROL

c. VIDEO = CONTROL

Test Statistics[a]

	VIDEO - CONTROL
Z	-3.899[b]
Asymp. Sig. (2-tailed)	.000

a. Wilcoxon Signed Ranks Test

b. Based on positive ranks.

FIGURE 5-9

Computer output, Wilcoxon.

nificance of 0.0167, so subjects walked significantly farther while listening to the tape than after watching the video.

In the second comparison, the control condition is compared with the earphone. Twenty-four subjects walked farther with the earphone than in the control condition. No subjects walked farther in the control condition, and there was one tie. Thus, with a p value of .000, subjects walked significantly farther with the earphone than in the control condition.

The control and video conditions are compared next. Twenty subjects walked farther after watching the video than in the control condition. Three subjects walked farther in the control than the video, and there were two ties.

After reviewing the three analyses, we can say that subjects walked significantly farther with the earphone than with the video or in the control condition. Subjects walked significantly farther with the video than in the control condition.

Example From the Literature

McCain (1992) used Friedman's and Wilcoxon in a study designed to test efficacy of three different interventions to facilitate optimal feeding states in preterm infants (Table 5-6). Inactive awake behavioral states have been associated with more successful feeding. Twenty preterm infants served as their own controls by being exposed to each of four conditions in a random order. The conditions were non-nutritive sucking, non-nutritive sucking plus rocking, stroking, and a control condition. There were significantly more inactive awake states with the non-nutritive sucking and non-nutritive sucking plus rocking interventions than with the stroking or control conditions.

TABLE 5-6
Intervention Heart Rates and Post Hoc Comparisons: Tukey's Test of Differences Among Means (N = 20)

| Intervention | M | Range | Differences among Means | | | |
			Control	NNS	NNS/R	Stroking
Control	161.5	138–192	—	9.4	6.15	11.4*
NNS	152.1	131–173		—	3.25	20.6**
NNS/Rocking	155.5	124–179			—	17.35**
Stroking	172.7	140–212				—

*$p < .05$; **$p < .01$

(From McCain, G. C. [1992]. Facilitating inactive awake states in preterm infants: A study of three interventions. Nursing Research, 41(3), 157–160.)

Summary of Friedman's and Wilcoxon

These techniques are the nonparametric analogues of the repeated measures analysis of variance and the paired t test.

SUMMARY

A few of the more commonly reported nonparametric techniques have been presented. Investigators must examine their data prior to analysis to determine which techniques are appropriate.

APPLICATION EXERCISES AND RESULTS

EXERCISES

In the exercises below, conduct the appropriate nonparametric analysis to answer the research question. Write a description of your results as it might appear in a manuscript.

1. Do men and women differ in their political affiliation?

2. Does current quality of life differ significantly from quality of life at age 18? To answer this question, first use the recode procedure to create two *new* variables. Recode both QOL-CUR and QOL18 into **new** variables where the values of $1 - 4 = 1$, and $5 - 6 = 2$. This will create two dichotomous variables with the sample fairly evenly divided between the two values. Conduct your analysis on the dichotomous variables.

3. Does smoking status affect overall state of health?

4. Do ratings of satisfaction with current weight, overall state of health, and quality of life in the past month differ significantly?

RESULTS

1. Exercise Figure 5-1 contains the results of this analysis. We would report that chi-square was used to answer the research question. Men and women differed significantly in their political affiliation ($p = .038$). More men (34.5%) registered as republicans than women (17.4%), and more women (33.9%) registered as democrats than men (24.1%).

2. Exercise Figure 5-2 contains the results. McNemar was used to answer the research question. There is no significant difference between ratings of quality of life currently and at age 18 ($p = .193$). On the dichotomized variables, of the 173 individuals included in the analysis, 114 reported the same level of quality of life at both times. Of those who changed their ratings, 24 reported a lower level currently than at age 18, and 35 reported a lower level at age 18.

3. Exercise Figure 5-3 contains the results of the analysis. Kruskal-Wallis was used to answer the research question. Smoking status is significantly related to overall state of health ($p = .010$). To test pairwise differences, Mann-Whitney U was used. Subjects who never smoked rated their health significantly higher than those who were still smoking ($p = .002$). There were

(text continues on page 121)

Political Affiliation * Gender cross-tabulation

			Gender		
			Male	Female	Total
Political Affiliation	Republican	Count	20	20	40
		% of gender	34.5%	17.4%	23.1%
	Democrat	Count	14	39	53
		% of gender	24.1%	33.9%	30.6%
	Independent	Count	24	56	80
		% of gender	41.4%	48.7%	46.2%
Total		Count	58	115	173
		% of gender	100.0%	100.0%	100.0%

Chi-Square Tests

	Value	df	Asymp. Sig. (2-tailed)
Pearson Chi-Square	6.520[a]	2	.038
Likelihood Ratio	6.304	2	.043
Linear-by-Linear Association	3.567	1	.059
N of Valid Cases	173		

[a] 0 cells (.0%) have expected count less than 5. The minimum expected count is 13.41.

EXERCISE FIGURE 5-1. Results for Exercise 1, chi-square.

Current QOL, Dichotomous & QOL at 18, Dichotomous

Current QOL, Dichotomous	QOL at 18, Dichotomous	
	1	2
1	58	24
2	35	56

Test Statistics[a]

	Current QOL, Dichotomous & QOL at 18, Dichotomous
N	173
Chi-Square[b]	1.695
Asymp. Sig.	.193

a. McNemar Test

b. Continuity Corrected

EXERCISE FIGURE 5-2. Results for Exercise 2, McNemar.

Ranks

	Smoking History	N	Mean Rank
Overall state of health	Never smoked	109	93.97
	Quit smoking	42	85.95
	Still smoking	23	59.65
	Total	174	

Test Statistics[a,b]

	Overall state of health
Chi-Square	9.156
df	2
Asymp. Sig.	.010

a. Kruskal Wallis Test

b. Grouping Variable: Smoking History

Ranks

	Smoking History	N	Mean Rank	Sum of Ranks
Overall state of health	Never smoked	109	77.77	8477.00
	Quit smoking	42	71.40	2999.00
	Total	151		

Test Statistics[a]

	Overall state of health
Mann-Whitney U	2096.000
Wilcoxon W	2999.000
Z	-.817
Asymp. Sig. (two-tailed)	.414

a. Grouping Variable: Smoking History

Ranks

	Smoking History	N	Mean Rank	Sum of Ranks
Overall state of health	Never smoked	109	71.20	7761.00
	Still smoking	23	44.22	1017.00
	Total	132		

Test Statistics[a]

	overall state of health
Mann-Whitney U	741.000
Wilcoxon W	1017.000
Z	-3.126
Asymp. Sig. (2-tailed)	.002

a. Grouping Variable: Smoking History

Ranks

	Smoking History	N	Mean Rank	Sum of Ranks
Overall state of health	Quit smoking	42	36.05	1514.00
	Still smoking	23	27.43	631.00
	Total	65		

Test Statistics[a]

	overall state of health
Mann-Whitney U	355.000
Wilcoxon W	631.000
Z	-1.782
Asymp. Sig. (2-tailed)	.075

a. Grouping Variable: Smoking History

EXERCISE FIGURE 5-3. Exercise 3, Kruskal-Wallis and Mann-Whitney U.

Ranks

	Mean Rank
Satisfaction with current weight	1.99
Overall state of health	2.66
Quality of life in past month	1.35

Test Statistics[a]

N	174
Chi-Square	165.513
df	2
Asymp. Sig.	.000

a. Fr

Ranks

		N	Mean Rank	Sum of Ranks
Satisfaction with current weight – overall state of health	Negative Ranks	30[a]	47.33	1420.00
	Positive Ranks	106[b]	74.49	7896.00
	Ties	39[c]		
	Total	175		
Overall state of health – quality of life in past month	Negative Ranks	157[d]	81.87	12853.00
	Positive Ranks	3[e]	9.00	27.00
	Ties	15[f]		
	Total	175		

a. satisfaction with current weight > overall state of health

b. satisfaction with current weight < overall state of health

c. satisfaction with current weight = overall state of health

d. overall state of health > quality of life in past month

e. overall state of health < quality of life in past month

f. overall state of health = quality of life in past month

Test Statistics[a]

	Satisfaction With Current Weight- Overall State of Health	Overall State of Health- Quality of Life in Past Month
Z	-7.088[b]	-10.980[c]
Asymp. Sig. (2-tailed)	.000	.000

a. Wilcoxon Signed Ranks Test

b. Based on negative ranks.

c. Based on positive ranks.

Test Statistics[a]

	Satisfaction With Current Weight- Quality of Life in Past Month
Z	-7.217[b]
Asymp. Sig. (2-tailed)	.000

a. Wilcoxon Signed Ranks Test

b. Based on positive ranks.

Ranks

		N	Mean Rank	Sum of Ranks
Satisfaction with current weight – quality of life in past month	Negative Ranks	114[a]	89.32	10182.00
	Positive Ranks	42[b]	49.14	2064.00
	Ties	18[c]		
	Total	174		

a. satisfaction with current weight > quality of life in past month

b. satisfaction with current weight < quality of life in past month

c. satisfaction with current weight = quality of life in past month

EXERCISE FIGURE 5-4. Results of Exercise 4, Friedman and Wilcoxon.

no significant differences between those who never smoked and those who quit smoking or between those who quit and those who were still smoking.

4. Exercise Figure 5-4 contains the results. Friedman was used to answer the main question. There was an overall significant result ($p = .000$) in the comparison of the following ratings: satisfaction with current weight, overall state of health, and quality of life in the past month. Wilcoxon tests were conducted to test the pairwise comparisons. Subjects rated their overall state of health significantly higher than their satisfaction with their current weight ($p = .000$) and significantly higher than their quality of life ($p = .000$). They also rated their satisfaction with their current weight significantly higher than their quality of life in the past month ($p = .000$).

t *Tests: Measuring the Differences Between Group Means*

BARBARA HAZARD MUNRO

OBJECTIVES FOR CHAPTER 6

After reading this chapter, you should be able to do the following:

1 • Determine when the *t* test is appropriate to use.

2 • Discuss how mean difference, group variability, and sample size are related to the statistical significance of the *t* statistic.

3 • Discuss how the results of the homogeneity of variance test are related to choice of *t* test formula.

4 • Select the appropriate *t* test formula (separate, pooled, or correlated) for a given situation.

5 • Interpret computer printouts of *t* test analyses.

Many research projects are designed to test the differences between two groups. The t-test involves an evaluation of means and distributions of each group. The *t* test, or Student's *t* test, is named after its inventor, William Gosset, who published under the pseudonym of Student. Gosset invented the *t* test as a more precise method of comparing groups. He described a set of distributions of *means* of randomly drawn samples from a normally distributed population. These distributions are the *t* distributions.

The shape of the distributions varies depending on the size of the samples drawn from the populations. However, all the *t* distributions have a normal distribution with a mean equal to the mean of the population. Unlike the *z* distributions, which are based on the normal curve and estimate the theoretical population parameters, the *t* distributions are based on sample size and vary according to the degrees of freedom (*df*). Theoretically, when an infinite number of samples of equal size is drawn from a normally distributed population, the mean of the sampling distribution will equal the mean of the population. If the sample sizes were large enough, the shape of the sampling distribution would approximate the normal curve.

THE RESEARCH QUESTION

When we compare two groups on a particular characteristic, we are asking whether the groups are different. The statistical question asks *how different* the groups are; that is, is the difference we find greater than that which could occur by chance alone? The null hypothesis for the *t* test states that any difference that occurs between the means of two groups is a difference in the sampling distribution. The means are different not because the groups are drawn from two different theoretical populations, but because of different random distributions of the samples from such a population. The null hypothesis is represented by the *t* distributions constructed by the random sampling of one population. When we use the *t* test to interpret the significance of the difference between groups, we are asking the statistical question, "What is the probability of getting a difference of this magnitude in groups this size if we were comparing random samples drawn from the same population?" That is, *"What is the probability of getting a difference this large by chance alone?"*

An example of the *t* test used to compare two groups is the study of Youngblut, Loveland-Cherry, and Horan (1994) who investigated the effects of maternal employment on families with preterm infants (Table 6-1). The investigators tested whether the mother's employment status affected family functioning by comparing employed and nonemployed mother's groups on the Feetham Family Functioning survey, where a lower score indicates a higher level of functioning. The nonemployed mothers rated their family functioning as significantly higher (mean = 18.5) than did the employed mothers (mean = 26.3). The husbands of the nonemployed

TABLE 6-1
Significant Comparisons of Family Functioning Between Employment Status Groups and Attitude/Behavior Consistency Groups

Feetham Family Functioning Survey	Employed Mother Group	Nonemployed Mother Group	t value
Mothers	26.3 (13.8)	18.5 (9.2)	2.78*
Fathers	25.8 (13.8)	16.3 (8.1)	3.43*

*$p < 0.01$

(From Youngblut, J. M., Loveland-Cherry, C. J., & Horan, M. [1994]. Maternal employment effects on families and preterm infants at 18 months. Nursing Research, *43(6), 331–337.)*

mothers also rated their family functioning significantly higher than did the husbands of the employed mothers.

To answer research questions through use of the *t* test, we compare the difference we obtained between our means with the sampling distribution of such differences. In general, the larger the *difference* between our two means, the more likely it is that the *t* test will be significant. However, two other factors are taken into account: the variability and the sample size. An increase in variability leads to an increase in error, and an increase in sample size leads to a decrease in error.

Given the same mean difference, groups with less variability will be more likely to be significantly different than groups with wide variability. This is because in groups with more variability, the error term will be larger. If the groups have scores that vary widely, there is likely to be considerable overlap between the two groups; thus, it will be difficult to ascertain whether a difference exists. Groups with less variability and a real mean difference will have distributions more clearly distinct from each other; that is, there will be less overlap between their respective distributions. With *more* variability (thus, larger error), we need a larger difference to be reasonably "sure" that a real difference exists.

TYPE OF DATA REQUIRED

For the *t* test, we need one nominal-level variable, with two levels as the independent variable. A simpler way to say this is that we must have two groups. The dependent variable should be "continuous."

Some people have criticized the use of the term continuous, rather than specifying the level of measurement of the variable (ordinal, interval, ratio). However, even when data are measured at the ordinal level, they may be appropriate for use in parametric analyses if they approximate the data required to meet the assumptions of a given analysis. Nunnally and Bernstein (1994) consider any measure that can assume 11 or more dichotomous levels as continuous and state that with multi-category items, "somewhat fewer items are needed to qualify" (p. 570). Scales with less items are considered discrete. For ease of expression, we use the term continuous to describe scale scores.

The *t* test has been commonly used to compare two groups. The mathematics involved are simpler than those required for analysis of variance, which is discussed in Chapter 7. However, when comparing two groups, it does not matter whether one uses a *t* test or a one-way analysis of variance. The results will be mathematically identical. The *t* statistic (derived from the *t* test formula) is equal to the square root of the *F* statistic (derived from the one-way analysis of variance). Symbolically then, $t = \sqrt{F}$ and $F = t^2$.

With the use of the computer, ease of calculation is not an issue, so some people use analysis of variance to compare two groups. Either way is correct. The typical *t* test table has the advantage of clearly presenting the means being compared in the analysis.

ASSUMPTIONS

The three assumptions underlying the *t* test concern the type of data used in the test and the characteristics of the distribution of the variables:

1. The independent variable is categorical and contains two levels; that is, you have two mutually exclusive groups of subjects. Mutually exclusive means that a subject can contribute just one score to one of the two groups. This is the assumption of independence. When this assumption is violated, as when subjects are measured twice, a correlated or paired *t* test may be appropriate.
2. The distribution of the dependent variable is normal. If the distribution is seriously skewed, the *t* test may be invalid.
3. The variances of the dependent variable for the two groups are similar. This is related to the assumption implied by the null hypothesis that the groups are from a single population. This assumption is called the requirement of *homogeneity of variance.*

Meeting this last assumption protects against type II errors—incorrectly accepting the null hypothesis. When the variances are unequal, that is, when the variation in one sample is significantly greater than the variation in the other, we are less likely to find a significant *t* value. Therefore, we might incorrectly conclude that the groups were drawn from the same population when they were not.

What if the variances are significantly different? Occasionally, groups that we want to compare do not have equal variances. Fortunately, a statistical method approximates the *t* test and can be interpreted in the same way using a different calculation for the standard error.

Actually, three different formulas based on the *t* distribution can be used to compare two groups:

1. The basic formula, sometimes called the *pooled formula*, is used to compare two groups when the three assumptions for the *t* test are met.
2. When the variances are *unequal*, the *separate formula* is used. This takes into account the fact that the variances are not alike. It is a more conservative measure.
3. When the two sets of scores are not independent (assumption 1), that is, there is correlation between the data taken from the two groups, adjustment must be made for that relationship. That formula often is called the *correlated t test* or the *t* test for *paired comparisons.* Comparing a group of subjects on their pretest and posttest scores is an example of when this technique would be used. Because these are not two independent groups, but rather one group measured twice, the scores will most likely be correlated. Another example is when the two groups consist of matched pairs. If the pairs are carefully matched, their scores will correlate, and the standard *t* test would not be appropriate.

When checking the assumptions, the first step is to be sure that each subject contributes only one score to one of the groups. In a randomized clinical trial with angioplasty patients (Sulzbach, Munro, & Hirshfeld, 1995), some patients who had been enrolled in our study in one of the two groups returned to the hospital for a second angioplasty. They could not be reentered into the study without violating the principles underlying the notion of mutual exclusivity.

Next, examine the frequency distribution of the dependent variable. Is it normally distributed? Remember that you divide the skewness by the standard error of the skewness to make this determination. Values that are greater or less than 1.96 are considered skewed. Alternatives for dealing with skewed data include data transformations, categorizing the variable, or using a nonparametric (distribution free) test. If data transformation is selected and successful, then the t test can still be used. If the variable is categorized, then a chi-square would be appropriate. The Mann-Whitney U is an appropriate nonparametric test.

For the test of homogeneity of variance, one runs the analysis and examines the results. The computer produces a test of the assumption, the results of two t tests, the pooled or equal variance formula, and the separate or unequal variance formula. An example is given following the discussion of sample size considerations.

SAMPLE SIZE CONSIDERATIONS AND POWER

How many subjects do you need for a t test? Cohen (1987) provides tables for determining sample size based on power and effect size determinations. To enter the tables, we must first decide whether we will be conducting a one- or two-tailed test and what our alpha or probability level will be. If there is sufficient theoretical rationale and we are able to hypothesize that one group will score significantly higher than the other, we will be using a one-tailed test. If we simply will answer a question such as, "Is there a difference between the experimental and control groups on the outcome measure?" then we will use a two-tailed test. When planning a study, you set the sample size based on the planned analysis that will require the highest number of subjects. If you were going to run three t tests and one would be two tailed, you would base your sample on that, because it requires more subjects than the other two one-tailed tests.

The power of the test of the null hypothesis is "the probability that it will lead to the rejection of the null hypothesis" (Cohen, 1987, p.4). A power of .80 means, therefore, that there is an 80% chance of rejecting the null hypothesis. The higher the desired power, the more subjects required. Cohen (1987) suggests that for the behavioral scientist, a power of .80 is reasonable, given no other basis for selecting the desired level.

The effect size should be based on previous work, if it exists, rather than simply picking a "moderate" effect from the Cohen (1987) tables. The effect size for the t test is simply the difference between the means of the two groups divided by the standard deviation for the measure. Cohen's moderate effect size is set at .5, which means ½ of a standard deviation unit. As an example, the graduate record examinations (GRE) have a mean of 500 and a standard deviation of 100. One-half of a standard deviation unit on that measure would be 50 (100/2). Thus, a moderate effect would be a difference of 50 points on the GRE between two groups. In a test of the model of transitional nursing care (Brooten et al., 1995), we used the LaMonica-Oberst Patient Satisfaction Scale. We found a 17-point difference between the experimental and control groups. The standard deviation on the scale was 24. If we were going to use that scale again in a similar experiment, what would our expected effect size be?

Answer: Dividing the difference between the means of 17 by the standard deviation of 24 (17/24), we calculate an effect size of .71. Look at Table 6-2 for a section of Cohen's tables.

TABLE 6-2
n *to Detect d by* t *Test*

$a_2 = .05 \ (a_1 = .025)$										
Power	*.10*	*.20*	*.30*	*.40*	*.50*	*.60*	*.70*	*.80*	*1.00*	*1.20*	*1.40*
.25	332	84	38	22	14	10	8	6	5	4	3
.50	769	193	86	49	32	22	17	13	9	7	5
.60	981	246	110	62	40	28	21	16	11	8	6
2/3	1144	287	128	73	47	33	24	19	12	9	7
,70	1235	310	138	78	50	35	26	20	13	10	7
.75	1389	348	155	88	57	40	29	23	15	11	8
.80	1571	393	175	99	64	45	33	26	17	12	9
.85	1797	450	201	113	73	51	38	29	19	14	10
.90	2102	526	234	132	85	59	44	34	22	16	12
.95	2600	651	290	163	105	73	54	42	27	19	14
.99	3675	920	409	231	148	103	76	58	38	27	20

$a_1 = .05 \ (a_2 = .10)$										
					d						
Power	*.10*	*.20*	*.30*	*.40*	*.50*	*.60*	*.70*	*.80*	*1.00*	*1.20*	*1.40*
.25	189	48	21	12	8	6	5	4	3	2	2
.50	542	136	61	35	22	16	12	9	6	5	4
.60	721	181	81	46	30	21	15	12	8	6	5
2/3	862	216	96	55	35	25	18	14	9	7	5
.70	942	236	105	60	38	27	20	15	10	7	6
.75	1076	270	120	68	44	31	23	18	11	8	6
.80	1237	310	138	78	50	35	26	20	13	9	7
.85	1438	360	160	91	58	41	30	23	15	11	8
.90	1713	429	191	108	69	48	36	27	18	13	10
.95	2165	542	241	136	87	61	45	35	22	16	12
.99	3155	789	351	198	127	88	65	50	32	23	17

(From Cohen, J. [1987]. Statistical power analysis for the behavioral sciences (Rev. ed.) Hillsdale, NJ: Lawrence Erlbaum Assn.)

The top section has the table for a two-tailed test (a_2) at the .05 level (or a one-tailed test at the .025 level). Given an effect size of .70 (numbers across top of table) and a power of .80 (numbers down the left side of the table), we would need 33 subjects in each of our groups. If we had used the moderate effect as defined by Cohen as .50, we would need 64 subjects in each of our groups at the same power level. The larger effect size indicates a larger difference between the mean scores and can be detected by less subjects.

Now look at the lower section, which includes a one-tailed test at the .05 level (a_1 = .05). Given an effect size of .70 and a power of .80, we would need 26 subjects per group. Thus, we can see that a one-tailed test is more powerful; that is, we need less subjects to detect a significant difference.

To summarize, for sample size with the *t* test, you must determine the following:

- One tailed versus two tailed
- Alpha level
- Effect size
- Power

One must also estimate how many subjects will be "lost" during data collection and oversample to be sure of having the appropriate numbers for analysis.

COMPUTER ANALYSIS

Figure 6-1 was produced by SPSS for Windows. The first table contains the group statistics. In all three analyses, there were 35 men and 59 women. The second table contains the analyses. In the first comparison, males and females are being compared on a variable, life satisfaction (scored from 1–7).

Levene's Test for Equality of Variances is not significant (p = .274), indicating that the variances are equal. The computer produces the equal (pooled) variance formula and the nonequal (separate) variance formula. Always look first at Levene's Test. If the significance level is greater than .05, report the equal variance (pooled) results, and if the significance level is less than .05 report the nonequal (separate) variance results. In the first analysis, $t = -.656$, $df = 92$, and $p = .513$. Because the p value is

Group Statistics

	GENDER	N	Mean	Std. Deviation	Std. Error Mean
Life Satisfaction	MALE	35	5.3109	.9690	.1638
	FEMALE	59	5.4316	.7936	.1033
Confidence	MALE	35	5.0002	.9027	.1526
	FEMALE	59	4.8001	.6945	9.0E-02
Spirituality	MALE	35	2.5005	.8472	.1432
	FEMALE	59	2.8520	.7614	9.9E-02

FIGURE 6-1

Computer output, independent *t* tests. (CONTINUED)

Independent Samples Test

		Levene's Test for Equality of Variances		t-test for Equality of Means					95% Confidence Interval of the Mean	
		F	Sig.	t	df	Sig. (2-tailed)	Mean Difference	Std. Error Difference	Lower	Upper
Life Satisfaction	Equal variances assumed	1.211	.274	-.656	92	.513	-.1207	.1840	-.4863	.2448
	Equal variances not assumed			-.623	60.797	.535	-.1207	.1937	-.5080	.2666
Confidence	Equal variances assumed	4.468	.037	1.205	92	.231	.2000	.1660	-.1296	.5297
	Equal variances not assumed			1.128	57.887	.264	.2000	.1774	-.1550	.5551
Spirituality	Equal variances assumed	1.595	.210	-2.074	92	.041	-.3515	.1695	-.6880	-1.E-02
	Equal variances not assumed			-2.018	65.564	.048	-.3515	.1742	-.6993	-4.E-03

Levene's test for the assumption of homogeneity of variance is used to determine which t test to report. If the significance level is greater than .05, the assumption is met, and the equal variance (pooled) formula should be reported. If the significance level is less than .05, the assumption has not been met, and the unequal variance (separate) formula should be reported.

FIGURE 6-1 (CONTINUED)

TABLE 6-3
Comparisons of Males and Females

	Males n = 35 Mean (SD)	Females n = 59 Mean (SD)	t	df	p[a]
Spirituality	2.50 (.85)	2.85 (.76)	−2.07[b]	92	.041
Life Satisfaction	5.31 (.97)	5.43 (.79)	−.66[b]	92	.513
Self-Confidence	5.00 (.90)	4.80 (.70)	1.13[c]	57.89	.264

[a]*Two-tailed significance*
[b]*Equal variance formula*
[c]*Unequal variance formula*

greater than .05, the null hypothesis of no statistical difference between the means is supported. We would report that males (mean = 5.3109) and females (mean = 5.4316) did not differ significantly on the variable life satisfaction. The computer printed out the two-tailed significance. For a one-tailed significance, simply divide the *p* value by 2. In this example, the one-tailed *p* valued would equal .513/2 or .2565.

In the second example, we see that males and females are being compared on a variable called confidence (scored 1–7). This time the mean difference between the two groups is .2000. The assumption of homogeneity of variance has not been met. The *p* of .037 for the Levene's Test indicates that the null hypothesis of no difference between the variances should be rejected. Because there is a significant difference between the variances, the unequal variance *t* test should be used. The appropriate results to report are: *t* = 1.128, *df* = 57.887, *p* = .264 (one tailed = .132). We would report that males and females do not differ significantly on the variable confidence.

In the third example, males and females are compared on spirituality (scored 1–4). Check the assumption, determine which *t* test to report, and state the results.

The assumption of homogeneity of variance was met. The equal variance formula is reported, and we would state that females scored significantly higher (mean = 2.8520) on spirituality than did males (mean = 2.5005).

A report of these three comparisons might read as:

t tests were used to compare males and females on life satisfaction, self-confidence, and spirituality. See Table 6-3 for the results. Males and females differed significantly on spirituality, with women (mean = 2.85) scoring significantly higher than men (mean = 2.50). Males and females did not differ significantly in either life satisfaction or self-confidence.

EXAMPLE FROM A PUBLISHED STUDY

Broom (1994), in a study of the extent to which marital quality affects parental sensitivity, compared the first-time parents' responses for study instruments (Table 6-4). She reported that "mothers and fathers had relatively high levels of marital quality, psychological well-being, and parental sensitivity" (p. 141). The only significant dif-

TABLE 6-4
First-Time Parents' Responses for Study Instruments

Instrument	Mother (n = 71)		Father (n = 71)		t
	M	(SD)	M	(SD)	
Quality marriage index	40.6	(3.9)	38.6	(5.5)	2.54*
Revised spouse checklist					
Pleasing	106.7	(46.5)	124.7	(70.2)	−1.80
Displeasing	9.5	(11.4)	10.9	(13.8)	−.66
Interaction/participation	114.4	(40.7)	104.2	(41.5)	1.48
Affect balance scale	30.6	(4.6)	31.2	(4.0)	−1.38
Nursing child assessment					
Teaching scale (total)	30.3	(3.2)	30.1	(3.5)	.50
Sensitivity to cues	9.7	(1.5)	9.5	(1.6)	.81
Response to distress	10.4	(1.1)	10.6	(1.1)	−.61
Socioemotional growth fostering	10.2	(1.2)	10.0	(1.4)	.83

*p < .01

(From Broom, B. L. [1994]. Impact of marital quality and psychological well-being on parental sensitivity. Nursing Research, 43(3), 138–143.)

ference between spouses was that mothers rated their marital quality higher than did fathers.

CORRELATED OR PAIRED t TEST

If the two groups being compared are matched or paired on some basis, the scores are likely to be similar. The chance differences between the two groups will not be as large as when they are drawn independently. In the correlated *t* test, a correction is made that has the effect of increasing *t*, thus making it more likely to find a significant difference if one exists.

Figure 6-2 contains a computer printout produced by SPSS for Windows. We asked subjects how satisfied they were with their current weight and how satisfied they were with their weight at age 18. The rating scale for both measures went from 1, very dissatisfied, to 10, very satisfied. There were 91 respondents. The mean score for satisfaction with current weight was 5.25, and the mean score for satisfaction with weight at age 18 was 6.91. The correlation between the two scores, presented in the second table, was .314, significant at the .002 level. The Paired Samples Test table shows that the means differed by −1.66. The *t* value of −4.846 with 90 *dfs*, has a two-tailed significance of .000 (at least less than .001). There is a significant difference between the two satisfaction scores. Specifically, respondents were significantly more satisfied with their weight at age 18 (mean = 6.91) than with their current weight (mean = 5.25).

The correlated *t* test uses the pooled estimate of variance, so we do not have to decide whether to use a separate or pooled formula.

Paired Samples Statistics

		Mean	N	Std. Deviation	Std. Error Mean
Pair 1	SATISFACTION WITH CURRENT WEIGHT	5.25	91	2.75	.29
	SATISFACTION WITH WEIGHT AT 18	6.91	91	2.83	.30

Paired Samples Correlations

		N	Correlation	Sig.
Pair 1	SATISFACTION WITH CURRENT WEIGHT — SATISFACTION WITH WEIGHT AT 18	91	.314	.002

Paired Samples Test

		Paired Differences					t	df	Sig. (2-tailed)
		Mean	Std. Deviation	Std. Error Mean	95% Confidence Interval of the Difference				
					Lower	Upper			
Pair 1	SATISFACTION WITH CURRENT WEIGHT — SATISFACTION WITH WEIGHT AT 18	-1.66	3.27	.34	-2.34	-.98	-4.846	90	.000

FIGURE 6-2
Computer output, paired t test.

CALCULATING THE BASIC (POOLED) t TEST

The *t* test formula consists of dividing the difference between the two means by the standard error. The standard error is an estimate of the standard deviation in the population from which our subjects are drawn. It represents the "pooled" variance of both groups and is appropriate when the variances of the two groups are equal. An example of the calculation is provided in Table 6-5.

TABLE 6-5
Calculation of Pooled t Test

Group 1 Experimental		Group 2 Control	
X_1	X_1^2	X_2	X_2^2
8	64	15	225
5	25	13	169
7	49	12	144
9	81	8	64
7	49	11	121
6	36	14	196
5	25	9	81
3	9	10	100
4	16	9	81
4	16	10	100
58	*370*	*111*	*1281*

Group 1	Group 2
$\bar{X} = 5.8$	$\bar{X} = 11.1$
$n = 10$	$n = 10$

$$\text{sum of squares } (\Sigma x_1)^2 = 370 - \frac{(58)^2}{10}$$

$$= 33.6$$

$$\text{sum of squares } (\Sigma x_2)^2 = 1281 - \frac{(111)^2}{10}$$

$$= 48.9$$

$$t = \frac{(\bar{X}_1 - \bar{X}_2)}{\sqrt{\left(\dfrac{\Sigma x_1^2 + \Sigma x_2^2}{n_1 + n_2 - 2}\right)\left(\dfrac{1}{n_1} + \dfrac{1}{n_2}\right)}}$$

$$t = \frac{5.8 - 11.1}{\sqrt{\left(\dfrac{33.6 + 48.9}{10 + 10 - 2}\right)\left(\dfrac{1}{10} + \dfrac{1}{10}\right)}}$$

$$t = -5.54$$

Using the table in Appendix C, we find that a *t* value of −5.54 with 18 *df* has a probability level of 0.001 for the two-tailed test and 0.0005 for the one-tailed test.

CALCULATING THE "SEPARATE" t TEST

If the variances for the two groups were not the same, we would use a more conservative formula, because it would be an error to "pool" different variances. The formula for this *t* test is:

$$t = \frac{\bar{X}_1 - \bar{X}_2}{\sqrt{\dfrac{s_1^2}{n_1} + \dfrac{s_2^2}{n_2}}}$$

where s_1^2 = variance for group 1
       s_2^2 = variance for group 2

CALCULATING THE CORRELATED OR PAIRED t-TEST

The formula for calculating the correlated or paired *t* test follows:

$$t = \frac{\bar{X}_1 - \bar{X}_2}{\sqrt{\dfrac{s_1^2}{n_1} + \dfrac{s_2^2}{n_2} - 2r\left(\dfrac{s_1}{\sqrt{n_1}}\right)\left(\dfrac{s_2}{\sqrt{n_2}}\right)}}$$

where s_1^2 = variance for group 1
       s_2^2 = variance for group 2
       s_1 = standard deviation for group 1
       s_2 = standard deviation for group 2

SUMMARY

The *t* test is a statistical method for comparing differences between two groups. The *t* statistic is similar to the *z* statistic. It uses an estimate of the population parameters and thereby is substituted for the *z* statistic when these parameters are unknown. The test requires a continuous dependent variable on which the groups are being compared. The test assumes that the variable is normally distributed in the populations from which the samples are drawn and that the samples have equivalent variances. The *t* test is particularly useful in experimental and quasiexperimental designs in which an experimental and control group are compared.

APPLICATION EXERCISES AND RESULTS

EXERCISES

Answer the following research questions by running the appropriate *t* tests and writing up the results.

1. Do individuals who have never smoked differ significantly from individuals who are still smoking on measures of confidence during stressful situations and life purpose and satisfaction?

2. Do current ratings of quality of life differ significantly from ratings of quality of life at age 18?

RESULTS

1. An independent *t* test should be used to answer this question. On the SMOKE variable, only two groups are selected, those who never smoked (0) and those who are still smoking (2). Exercise Figure 6-1 contains the results.

   For the comparison of the two smoking groups on confidence (CONFID), which *t* test should be reported? Because Levene's test for equality of variances is not significant ($p = .150$), the equal variance (pooled) formula should be reported. We would report that people who never smoked scored significantly higher ($p = .027$) on the measure of confidence (mean = 63.36) than did those who are still smoking (mean = 55.4). Also, there was a large difference in the size of the two groups.

   For life purpose and satisfaction (LIFE), we would report the unequal variances (separate) formula, because the Levene's test was significant ($p = .008$). Subjects who never smoked (mean = 92.84) rated their life purpose and satisfaction significantly higher ($p = .002$) than did subjects who are still smoking (mean = 73.91).

2. There was no significant difference ($p = .670$) between the rating of quality of life in the past month (mean = 4.38) and at age 18 (mean = 4.33). The correlation between the two measures was .248 ($p = .001$). Exercise Figure 6-2 contains the printout.

(See over for figures.)

Group Statistics

	Smoking History	N	Mean	Std. Deviation	Std. Error Mean
Confidence during stressful situations	Never smoked	110	63.3636	14.7024	1.4018
	Still smoking	23	55.3913	18.9922	3.9601
Life purpose and satisfaction	Never smoked	108	92.8426	16.2142	1.5602
	Still smoking	23	73.9130	25.8824	5.3969

Independent Samples Test

		Levene's Test for Equality of Variances		*t* test for Equality of Means					95% Confidence Interval of the Mean	
		F	Sig.	t	df	Sig. (2 tailed)	Mean Difference	Std. Error Difference	Lower	Upper
Confidence during stressful situations	Equal variances assumed	2.094	.150	2.242	131	.027	7.9723	3.5552	.9393	15.0054
	Equal variances not assumed			1.898	27.771	.068	7.9723	4.2009	-.6361	16.5808
Life purpose and satisfaction	Equal variances assumed	7.254	.008	4.522	129	.000	18.9295	4.1863	10.6468	27.2123
	Equal variances not assumed			3.370	25.794	.002	18.9295	5.6179	7.3774	30.4817

EXERCISE FIGURE 6-1. Results of Exercise 1, independent samples *t* test.

Paired Samples Statistics

		Mean	N	Std. Deviation	Std. Error Mean
Pair 1	Quality of life in past month	4.38	173	1.17	8.92E-02
	quality of life at age 18	4.33	173	1.15	8.76E-02

Paired Samples Correlations

		N	Correlation	Sig.
Pair 1	Quality of life in past month & quality of life at age 18	173	.248	.001

Paired Samples Test

		Paired Differences					t	df	Sig. (2 tailed)
					95% Confidence Interval of the Difference				
		Mean	Std. Deviation	Std. Error Mean	Lower	Upper			
Pair 1	Quality of life in past month - quality of life at age 18	4.62E-02	1.43	.11	-.17	.26	.427	172	.670

EXERCISE FIGURE 6-2. Results of Exercise 2, paired samples t test.

Differences Among Group Means: One-Way Analysis of Variance

Barbara Hazard Munro

OBJECTIVES FOR CHAPTER 7

After reading this chapter, you should be able to do the following:

1 • Determine when analysis of variance is appropriate to use.

2 • Interpret a computer printout of a one-way analysis of variance.

3 • Describe between-group, within-group, and total variance.

4 • Explain the use of post-hoc tests and a priori comparisons.

5 • Report the results of one-way analysis of variance in a summary table.

Many times, a clinical research question involves a comparison of several groups on a particular measure. In Chapter 6, we discuss the *t* test as a method for examining the difference between *two* groups. The basic *t* test compares two means in relation to the distribution of the differences between pairs of means drawn from a random sample. When we have more than two groups and are interested in the differences among the set of groups, we are dealing with different combinations of pairs of means. If we choose to analyze the differences by *t* test analysis, we would need to do a number of *t* tests. Suppose that we had four different groups—A, B, C, and D—that we wanted to compare on a particular variable. If we were interested in the differences among the four groups, we would need to do a *t* test for each of the possible pairs that exist in the four groups. We would have A versus B, A versus C, A versus D, B versus C, B versus D, and C versus D. In all, we would have six separate comparisons, each requiring a separate analysis.

The problem with conducting such multiple group comparisons relates to the underlying concept of statistical analysis. Each test is based on the probability that the null hypothesis is *true*. Therefore, each time we conduct a test, we are running the risk of a type I error. The probability level we set as the point at which we reject the null hypothesis also is the level of risk with which we are comfortable. If that level is 0.05, we are accepting the risk that 5 of 100 times, our rejection of the null hypothesis will be in error.

However, when we calculate multiple *t* tests on independent samples that are being measured on the same variable, the rate of error increases exponentially by the number of tests conducted. For example, with our four-group problem, the error rate increases to 18 of 100 times, a substantial increase.[1]

Instead of using a series of individual comparisons, we examine the differences among the groups through an analysis that considers the variation across all groups at once. This test is the analysis of variance (ANOVA).

THE STATISTICAL QUESTION IN ANALYSIS OF VARIANCE

The statistical question using ANOVA is based on the null hypothesis: the assumption that all groups are equal and drawn from the same population. Any difference comes from a random sampling difference. The question answered by the ANOVA test is whether group means differ from each other.

TYPE OF DATA REQUIRED

With ANOVA, the independent variable(s) are at the nominal level. A one-way ANOVA means that there is only *one* independent variable (often called *factor*). That independent variable has two or more levels. Gender would be a variable with two levels, whereas race, religion, and so forth may have varying numbers of levels depending on how the variable is defined. Two-way ANOVA indicates two independent variables, and *n*-way ANOVA indicates that the number of independent variables is defined by *n*. The dependent variable must be continuous.

For example, Williams, Oberst, and Bjorklund (1994) used one-way ANOVA to compare outcomes after hip fracture in three groups of women: those discharged home from the hospital, those discharged to a nursing home and staying there 1 month or more, and those discharged to a nursing home but staying there less than

---

[1]*The calculation of the rate of type I errors is determined by the following formula:*

$$1 - (1 - \alpha)^t$$

where α = *the level of significance for the tests*

t = *the number of test comparisons used*

In our example, the calculation would give us $1 - (1 - 0.05)^4 = 0.18$.

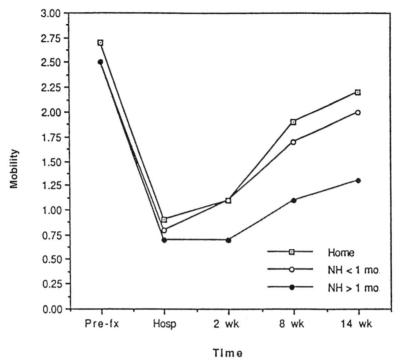

FIGURE 7-1

Trend over time in regaining mobility after hip fracture among women discharged home and to nursing homes. (From Williams, M. A., Oberst, M. T., & Bjorklund, B. C. [1994]. Early outcomes after hip surgery among women discharged home and to nursing homes. *Research in Nursing & Health, 17*(3), 175–183.)

1 month. They reported that women who stayed in the nursing home more than 1 month had significantly lower mobility scores than did the home group or the short-stay nursing home group (Fig. 7-1).

ASSUMPTIONS

ANOVA has been shown to be fairly "robust." This means that even if the researchers do not rigidly adhere to the assumptions, the results may still be close to the truth.

The assumptions for ANOVA are the same as those for the *t* test; that is, the dependent variable should be a continuous variable that is normally distributed, the groups should be mutually exclusive (independent of each other), and the groups should have equal variances (homogeneity of variance requirement).

TABLE 7-1
Sample Size Determination

| | | | | | | u = 4 | | | | | | |
| | | | | | | f | | | | | | |
Power	.05	.10	.15	.20	.25	.30	.35	.40	.50	.60	.70	.80
.10	74	19	9	6	4	3	2	2	—	—	—	—
.50	514	129	58	33	21	15	11	9	6	5	4	3
.70	776	195	87	49	32	22	17	13	9	6	5	4
.80	956	240	107	61	39	27	20	16	10	8	6	5
.90	1231	309	138	78	50	35	26	20	13	10	7	6
.95	1486	372	166	94	60	42	31	24	16	11	9	7
.99	2021	506	225	127	82	57	42	33	21	15	11	9

(From Cohen, J. [1987]. Statistical power analysis for the behavioral sciences [Rev. ed.]. Hillsdale, NJ: Lawrence Erlbaum Assoc.)

SAMPLE SIZE CONSIDERATIONS AND POWER

The principles relating to considerations of sample size and power are based on those outlined in Chapter 6, where two means were compared through use of the *t* test. Using means and standard deviations from previous work, we can calculate expected effect sizes, either by using the formulas provided in Cohen (1987) or by one of the software programs available. Given an expected effect size, desired power, and alpha level, we can determine sample size. For example, Table 7-1 contains an excerpt from Cohen's Table 8.44 (p. 384). It is used to determine appropriate sample size when alpha is .05 and the degrees of freedom (*df;* u) equal 4. Because the *df* is one less than the number of groups, this table is used when there are five groups. The effect sizes are indicated by f across the top of the table, and the power values are listed down the left side. Suppose we calculated an effect size of .30. (Cohen defines a moderate effect size as .25, which with two groups is still half of a standard deviation unit.) If we desired a power of .80, how many subjects would we need in each group, and how many would we need overall?

We would need 27 subjects in each group, and because there are five groups, we would need a total of 135 subjects.

SOURCE OF VARIANCE

According to the null hypothesis, all groups are from the same population, and each of their scores comes from the same population of measures. Any variability of scores can be seen in two ways: First, the scores vary from each other in their own group;

second, the groups vary from each other. The first variation is called *within-group variation;* the second variation is called *between-group variation.* Together the two types of variation add up to the *total variation.*

Students often are confused when we say that ANOVA tells us whether or not the means of groups differ significantly and then proceed to talk about analyzing variance. The *t* test was clearly a test of mean difference, because the difference between the two means was contained in the numerator of the *t* test formula. It is important to understand how analyzing the variability of groups on some measure can tell us whether their measures of central tendency (means) differ.

With ANOVA, the variance of each group is measured separately; all the subjects are then lumped together, and the variance of the total group is computed. If the variance of the total group (total variation) is about the same as the average of the variances of the separate groups (within-group variation), the *means* of the separate groups are not different. This is because if total variation is the sum of within-group variation and between-group variation and if within-group variation and total variation are equal, there is no between-group variation. This should become more clear in the diagrams that follow. However, if the variance of the total group is much larger than the average variation within the separate groups, a significant mean difference exists between at least two of the subgroups. In that case, the within-group variation does not equal total variation. The difference between them must equal the between-group variation.

To visualize the difference in the types of variation, consider three groups exposed to three different experimental conditions. Suppose that the three conditions yielded such widely different scores that there was no overlap among the three

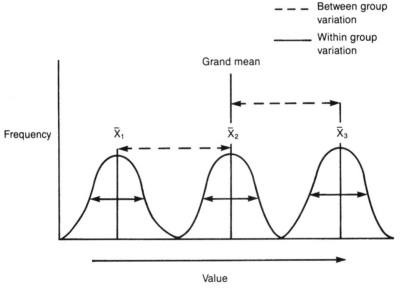

FIGURE 7-2
Between-group and within-group variation: the case of no overlap.

groups in terms of the outcome measure (Fig. 7-2). We could then represent our three groups in terms of their relationship to each other and in terms of a *total group.* Each group would then have its own mean and its own distribution around its mean. At the same time, there would be a *grand mean,* which is a mean for all the groups combined. As shown in Figure 7-2, we can look at the variation *within* the groups and *between* the groups. The combination of the within-group and between-group variation equals the *total* variation.

The ANOVA test examines the variation and tests whether the between-group variation is greater than the within-group variation. When the between-group variance is greater (statistically greater) than the within-group variance, the means of the groups must be different. However, when the within-group variance is approximately the same as the between-group variance, the groups' means are not importantly dif-

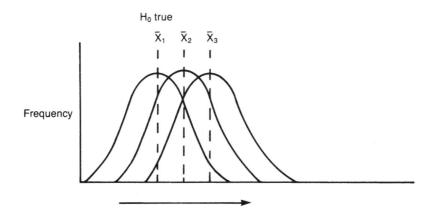

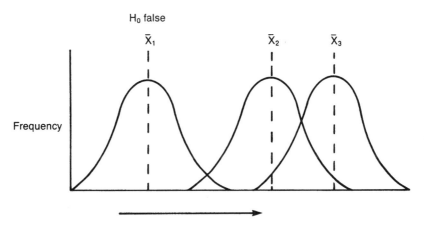

FIGURE 7-3
Relationship of variation to null hypothesis.

ferent. This relationship between the difference among groups and the different types of variance is shown in Figure 7-3.

When the null hypothesis is true, the groups overlap to a large extent, and the within-group variation is greater than the between-group variation. When the null hypothesis is false, the groups show little overlapping, and the distance between groups is greater.

As we can infer from Figure 7-3, the group variation and the deviation between group means determine the likelihood that the null hypothesis is true. More explicitly, when the variation within a group or groups is great, the difference between the groups must be greater than when the distribution within groups is narrow to reject the null hypothesis (Fig. 7-4). In the same way, when the group distributions are nar-

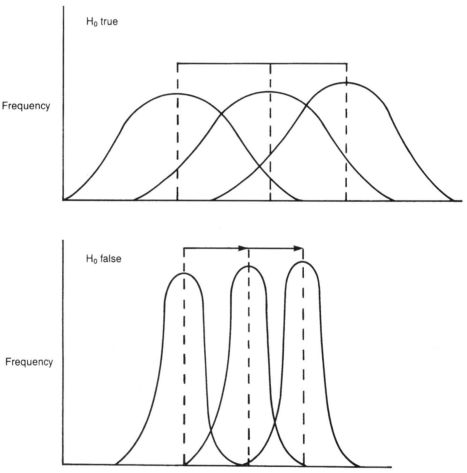

FIGURE 7-4
Effect of within-group variation on null hypothesis.

row (low within-group variance), relatively small between-group differences will be significant.

THE MEASURE OF VARIANCE: SUMS OF SQUARES

The kinds of variation of scores within groups has an intuitive and a statistical meaning. We have discussed the intuitive meaning as the extent to which the scores within a group vary from each other and the extent to which the groups vary from each other. The statistical concept of this variation involves a quantification of the amount of variation of scores around the mean. We have already defined and used this concept with the term *sum of squares*.

The *sum of squares* is the sum of the squared deviations of each of the scores around a respective mean. In ANOVA, the sum of squares is used to measure the total variation, between-group variation, and within-group variation. Table 7-2 contains an example of the calculation of the sums of squares using the formulas based on the deviations of the scores from their respective means. The data consist of four scores in each of three groups. The means for the three groups are 2, 4, and 6, respectively.

The Sum of Squares for Total Variation

The total sum of squares is equal to the sum of the squared deviations of each score in all groups from the grand mean. In our example, the grand mean (mean of the nine scores) is 4. The sum of the deviations around the mean equals zero, and the sum of the squared deviations equals 42. This total sum of squares represents the basis of the null hypothesis that all the subjects belong to one population, which is described by the grand mean.

The Sum of Squares for Within-Group Variation

The within-group variation is the total of the variation that occurs in each subgroup. It is calculated by finding the sum of squares for each group separately and then summing the results. The sums of the squared deviations for the three groups are 2, 2, and 6, and the sum across the three groups is 10.

The Sum of Squares for Between-Group Variation

The between-group variation examines how each of the groups varies from the grand mean. For this calculation, we use group means as representative of the individual groups. The between-group variation examines the variation of the group means from the grand mean. In Table 7-2, the mean for group 1 is two less than the grand mean. The sum of the deviations around the grand mean is (as always) zero, and the squared deviations are 4, 0, and 4, respectively. Because the weight of the difference

TABLE 7-2
Calculation of Sum of Squares

	Group 1	Group 2	Group 3
	1	4	6
	2	5	8
	3	3	5
	2	4	5
$\bar{X}_s$	2	4	6

TOTAL SUM OF SQUARES

Raw Scores	Deviations From Grand Mean	Squared Deviation
1	$1 - 4 = -3$	9
2	$2 - 4 = -2$	4
3	$3 - 4 = -1$	1
2	$2 - 4 = -2$	4
4	$4 - 4 = 0$	0
5	$6 - 4 = 1$	1
3	$3 - 4 = -1$	1
4	$4 - 4 = 0$	0
6	$6 - 4 = 2$	4
8	$8 - 4 = 4$	16
5	$5 - 4 = 1$	1
5	$5 - 4 = 1$	1
Grand Mean = 4	Sum = 0	42

Total sum of squares = 42.

WITHIN SUM OF SQUARES

Group 1

Raw Scores	Deviations From Group Mean	Squared Deviations
1	$1 - 2 = -1$	1
2	$2 - 2 = 0$	0
3	$3 - 2 = 1$	1
2	$2 - 2 = 0$	0
$\bar{X} = 2$	Sum = 0	Sum = 2

(continued)

TABLE 7-2 (CONTINUED)

Group 2

Raw Scores	Deviations From Group Mean	Squared Deviations
4	4 − 4 = 0	0
5	5 − 4 = 1	1
3	3 − 4 = −1	1
4	4 − 4 = 0	0
$\bar{X} = 4$	Sum = 0	Sum = 2

Group 3

6	6 − 6 = 0	0
8	8 − 6 = 2	4
5	5 − 6 = −1	1
5	5 − 6 = −1	1
$\bar{X} = 6$	Sum = 0	Sum = 6

Within sum of squares = 2 + 2 + 6 = 10

BETWEEN SUM OF SQUARES

Deviations of Group Means From Grand Mean	Squared Deviations	Number in Group
Group 1 2 − 4 = −2	4	4
Group 2 4 − 4 = 0	0	4
Group 3 6 − 4 = 2	4	4

Between sum of squares = (4)(4) + (4)(0) + (4)(4) = 32

SUMMARY TABLE

Source of Variance	SS	df	MS	F	p
Between group	32	2	16	14.41	<.01
Within group	10	9	1.11		
Total	42	11			

of any mean from the grand mean is influenced by the number of the scores in the group, we weight the squared deviations by the number in the group. The weighted squared deviations are then summed to provide the between sum of squares (32).

In summary, these three sums of squares define the three different kinds of variation that exist when subjects are members of different groups and measured on a single variable. They include the *total variation* of each of the scores around the grand mean, the variation of scores *within* their respective groups, and the deviation *between* groups measured by the deviation of group means from the grand mean.

DISPLAYING THE RESULTS: THE SUMMARY OF ANALYSIS OF VARIANCE

The results of the calculations leading to the *F* ratio are summarized in table form that is standard for presenting ANOVA results. This presentation of the results is called the *summary of ANOVA* table.

In Table 7-2, *SS* stands for sum of squares, *df* for degrees of freedom, *MS* for mean square, *F* for the statistic generated, and *p* for the probability level.

Degrees of Freedom

The *df* for the between-group variance is equal to the number of groups minus one. In our example, this is $3 - 1 = 2$. The *df* for the within-group variance is equal to the total number of subjects minus the number of groups, or $12 - 3 = 9$. The df for the total variance is equal to the number of subjects minus one ($12 - 1 = 11$). The mean square is the sum of squares divided by its *df*. Thus, the between-group sum of squares, 32, divided by 2 results in a mean square of 16.

Testing the Difference Among Groups: The F Ratio

To determine whether the between-group difference is great enough to reject the null hypothesis, we compare it statistically to the within-group variance. The *F* represents the ratio of between to within variance and is calculated as the between mean square divided by the within mean square, or $16/1.11 = 14.41$. The *F* value is compared to the values obtained when the null hypothesis is true, and the scores are randomly selected from one population. To make the interpretation, we use the table that presents the *F* distributions (Appendix D). We locate the critical values for comparison by using the *df* for the between and within mean squares.

In the example, the between *df* was 2, and the within *df* was 9. We locate the between *df* on the row across the top of the table, and we locate the within *df* on the column on the left side of the table. With these points as coordinates, we locate two critical values for *F*.

The top value (in light print) is 4.26. This is the value required to reject the null hypothesis at a probability level of 0.05 (given a one-tailed test). The value below (in bold print) is 8.02, the value required to reject the null hypothesis at the 0.01 level.

The value of 14.41 is greater than the value required to reach an alpha of 0.01. Therefore, we can reject the null hypothesis at the 0.01 level. We say we have reached a probability level of "less than 0.01." In summary, we obtained an *F* value of 14.41. We therefore rejected the null hypothesis that there were no differences between the groups, and we concluded that the groups were different. In other standard presentations of ANOVA summary tables, the within variance is sometimes called the *error variance* or *error term*. This terminology reflects the assumption of the ANOVA: The within difference is sampling error or random difference.

In addition to the summary table, often it is helpful to include a table in your results section that shows the means and standard deviations for the scores of each group. One can then see which group scored higher and by how much. Without further analysis, however, we do not know which pairs of means differ significantly. A post-hoc analysis would allow us to compare group 1 with group 2, group 1 with group 3, and group 2 with group 3. Before discussing such contrasts in detail, however, we first present another example with a computer analysis of the data.

ONE-WAY ANALYSIS OF VARIANCE

We have one independent categorical variable with *n* levels and one continuous dependent variable. To demonstrate, we use the example in Table 7-3. Suppose we are interested in the effect of advanced practice nurses (APNs) on the functional status of elderly people. We randomly assign clients to a control group, where they receive usual care from their providers; an experimental group where they receive monthly telephone calls from an APN, whom they can call at other times; or to a second experimental group where they are visited monthly by an APN, who is also available to them by telephone.

The question is whether the groups score differently on the functional status

TABLE 7-3
Scores on Functional Status Across Groups

Control	APN Telephone	APN Visits and Telephone
1	7	5
3	4	8
2	2	6
2	3	9
3	9	7
5	4	9
7	4	10
4	8	8
2	6	7
1	5	10
$\bar{X} = 3.0$	$\bar{X} = 5.2$	$\bar{X} = 7.9$
$s = 1.89$	$s = 2.25$	$s = 1.66$

measure; a higher score indicates better functional status. If the groups differ in their scores, the question is, "Which groups are different from which other groups?"

COMPUTER ANALYSIS

To answer the research question, the data were submitted to analysis by the ONEWAY program in SPSS for Windows+. This program handles one-way ANOVA (one independent variable) and post-hoc tests necessary to compare pairs of means. Figure 7-5 contains the computer output. Comments have been added in light print.

The dependent variable is a score on functional status, and the independent variable is a group with three levels, control, APN telephone, and APN visits and telephone. The group statistics are given first. There were 10 subjects in each group, and group means, standard deviations, and standard errors are listed. Based on the standard errors, 95% confidence intervals (CI) also are listed. For the control group, the 95% CI is 1.6511 to 4.3489. The minimum and maximum scores for each group also are listed.

The assumption of homogeneity of variance is met ($p = .520$). The ANOVA summary table is typical of what is reported in the literature. The variance is reported as between groups, within groups, and total. "Between groups" indicates the differences among the three groups, "within groups" is the error term, and "total" is the total variance in the dependent variable.

Sums of squares are reported first. Because there are three groups, the $df = 2$ (number of groups minus one). Dividing the sum of squares by its associated df gives the mean square value. For example, for between groups, $120.467/2 = 60.233$. The F is the ratio of between to within variance, or $60.233/3.796 = 15.866$. This number is significant at the 0.000 (or <0.001) level.

Because the overall F is significant, we want to know which pairs of means are significantly different. The Scheffé procedure was requested. The asterisks indicate that the control group differed significantly from the visit plus phone group, the telephone group differed significantly from the visit plus phone group, and the visit plus phone group differed significantly from the other two groups. By examining the means, we see that the visit plus telephone group had significantly higher functional status scores (mean = 7.9) than did the other two groups (means of 3.0 and 5.2). The final table contains the homogeneous subsets. In this case, because the control group and telephone groups did not differ from each other, they are in the one homogeneous subset.

MULTIPLE GROUP COMPARISONS

Two types of comparisons can be made among group means. The most commonly reported are post-hoc (after the fact) comparisons and a priori (planned) comparisons, based on hypotheses stated prior to the analysis.

Descriptives

		N	Mean	Std. Deviation	Std. Error	95% Confidence Interval for Mean		Minimum	Maximum
						Lower Bound	Upper Bound		
SCORE GROUP	Control	10	3.0000	1.8856	.5963	1.6511	4.3489	1.00	7.00
	Telephone	10	5.2000	2.2509	.7118	3.5898	6.8102	2.00	9.00
	Visit + phone	10	7.9000	1.6633	.5260	6.7101	9.0899	5.00	10.00
	Total	30	5.3667	2.7728	.5062	4.3313	6.4021	1.00	10.00

Test of Homogeneity of Variances

	Levene Statistic	df1	df2	Sig.
SCORE	.669	2	27	.520

The assumption of homogeneity of variance has been met.

ANOVA

		Sum of Squares	df	Mean Square	F	Sig.
SCORE	Between Groups	120.467	2	60.233	15.866	.000
	Within Groups	102.500	27	3.796		
	Total	222.967	29			

The overall analysis is significant ($p = .000$).

FIGURE 7-5

Computer output of oneway analysis of variance with post-hoc comparisons. *(continued)*

Multiple Comparisons

Dependent Variable: SCORE

Scheffe

(I) GROUP	(J) GROUP	Mean Difference (I-J)	Std. Error	Sig.	95% Confidence Interval	
					Lower Bound	Upper Bound
Control	Telephone	-2.2000	.871	.057	-4.4568	5.7E-02
	Visit + phone	-4.9000*	.871	.000	-7.1568	-2.6432
Telephone	Control	2.2000	.871	.057	-6.E-02	4.4568
	Visit + phone	-2.7000*	.871	.016	-4.9568	-.4432
Visit + phone	Control	4.9000*	.871	.000	2.6432	7.1568
	Telephone	2.7000*	.871	.016	.4432	4.9568

* The mean difference is significant at the .05 level.

The control group scored significantly lower than the visit plus phone group.
The telephone group scored significantly lower than the visit plus phone group.
The visit plus phone group scored significantly higher than the other two groups.

FIGURE 7-5

SCORE

Scheffe[a]

GROUP	N	Subset for alpha = .05
		1
Control	10	3.0000
Telephone	10	5.2000
Visit + phone	10	
Sig.		.057

Means for groups in homogeneous subsets are displayed.

a. Uses Harmonic Mean Sample Size = 10.000

The table above shows that the control and telephone groups did not differ from each other.

Post-Hoc Tests

When a significant F test is obtained, the null hypothesis that all the groups are from the same population or that all the populations are equal is rejected; that is, we are able to state that there is a difference among the groups. However, when more than two groups are being compared, we cannot determine from the F test alone which groups differ from each other. In other words, a significant F test does not mean that every group in the analysis is different from every other group. Many patterns of difference are possible. Some of the groups may be similar, forming a cluster that is different from another select group; depending on the number of groups being compared, there may be wide deviation between each pair of the groups.

To determine where the significant differences lie, further analysis is required. Therefore, we must compare group means. However, if we decide to use the standard t test, we are confronted with the possibility of an increased rate of type I errors. To prevent this, secondary analyses following the computation of the F ratio are available to pinpoint the source of the difference.

Many techniques exist. For example, SPSS for Windows+ has seven available. A complete discussion of each is beyond the scope of this book, but the aim of all is to decrease the likelihood of making a type I error when making multiple comparisons. For more detail on post-hoc tests following ANOVA, we suggest Holm and Christman (1985), Klockars and Sax (1986), and Toothaker, (1993).

The *Scheffé test* is reported frequently. The formula is based on the usual formula for the calculation of a t test or F ratio. The critical value used for determining whether the resulting F statistic is significant is different. In other words, the F associated with comparing the two means is the same as if they had been compared in the usual ANOVA, but the critical value is changed based on the number of comparisons. The new critical value is simply the usual value multiplied by the number of groups being compared minus one. In our example in Figure 7-5, the critical value at the 0.05 level with 2 and 27 df is 3.35 (see Appendix D). Multiplying that by 2 (the number of groups minus one) results in a critical value of 6.7. Thus, the critical value is twice as stringent when making all possible comparisons among three groups than it was for the overall analysis. The Scheffé test is quite stringent, but it can be used with groups of equal and unequal size F.

Bonferroni has been explained previously. The desired alpha is divided by the number of comparisons. For example, with an alpha of .05 and 4 comparisons, the significance level would have to be equal to or less than .0125 for the paired comparison to be "significant."

The *Least Significant Difference Test* is equivalent to multiple t tests. The modification is that a pooled estimate of variance is used rather than variance common to groups being compared.

Tukey's Honestly Significant Difference (HSD) is the most conservative comparison test, and as such, is the least powerful. The critical values for Tukey remain the same for each comparison, regardless of the total number of means to be compared.

Student Newman-Keuls is similar to Tukey's HSD, but the critical values do not stay the same. They reflect the variables being compared.

Tukey's Wholly Significant Difference uses critical values that are the average of those used in Tukey's HSD and Newman-Keuls. It is therefore intermediate in conservatism between those two measures.

Planned Comparisons

Planned comparisons, or a priori contrasts, are based on hypotheses stated before data are collected. When you hypothesize ahead of time, you are able to use more powerful statistical tests. One way to do this is through the development of pre-specified contrasts that are orthogonal to each other. *Orthogonal* means that the hypothesis tests are unrelated to each other; that is, knowing one result tells you nothing about the other. For an overview of planned comparisons versus omnibus tests, you can refer to a *Nursing Research* "Methodology Corner" by Wu and Slakter (1990).

Here we demonstrate how orthogonal contrasts can be developed and analyzed in SPSS for Windows+. To have comparisons that are independent, only $n - 1$ comparisons can be made. In our three-group example, therefore, there could only be two orthogonal contrasts. In our example, we might want to test the hypothesis that the two experimental groups will score significantly higher on functional status than the control group and that the group receiving APN visits and telephone calls will score significantly higher on functional status than the group that receives APN telephone calls only. Table 7-4 contains the vectors necessary to code such a contrast. On vector 1 (V1) subjects in both experimental groups receive a -1, and the control group subjects receive 2. This contrast tests the difference between the functional status mean score for all the experimental subjects and the mean for the control group subjects. The second contrast is given in vector 2. The two experimental groups are compared. The control group is not considered in the second contrast.

To ensure that hypothesized contrasts are orthogonal, three tests must be applied:

There must be only $n - 1$ contrasts.
The sum of each vector must equal zero. In the example, the sum of V1 is $2 + (-1) + (-1) = 0$, and the sum of V2 is $0 + (-1) + 1 = 0$.
The sum of the cross-products must equal zero. In the example, $(2 \times 0) + (-1 \times -1) + (-1 \times 1) = 0$.

Table 7-5 provides other examples of possible contrasts, given three groups. Are they all orthogonal? The vectors $X1$ and $X2$ reflect an orthogonal contrast, as do the vectors $Y1$ and $Y2$. Vectors $Z1$ and $Z2$ do not reflect an orthogonal contrast; group 1 is compared to group 2 and to group 3. The sum of the cross-products does not equal zero $(-1 \times 1) + (0 \times -1) + (1 \times 0) = -1$.

We now demonstrate the use of the contrasts specified in Table 7-4 in a computer analysis of these data. See Figure 7-6 for the computer output of the contrasts.

TABLE 7-4
Orthogonal Coding

	Vectors	
Groups	V1	V2
Control	2	0
APN telephone	−1	−1
APN visits and telephone	−1	1

Because this is the same analysis contained in Figure 7-5, we will not repeat the ANOVA table. In the first analysis (Fig. 7-5), we requested a post-hoc test and determined that the APN visit and telephone group scored significantly higher than the other two groups.

In the analysis in Figure 7-6, we are testing a priori orthogonal contrasts. This is a more powerful analysis, that is, it is more likely to find a significant difference among groups. This is because the contrasts are stated a priori (before the fact) and are restricted to orthogonal contrasts. In the case of post-hoc tests, the overall F value must be significant before we can test pairwise comparisons. When using orthogonal contrasts, these contrasts can be examined even when the overall F is not significant.

The first contrast compares the means of the two experimental groups with the control group. The second contrast compares the two experimental groups.

The pooled variance estimate is appropriate, because the assumption of homogeneity of variance has been met (Levene Test, $p = .520$). Both contrasts are significant. The two experimental groups scored significantly higher on functional status than the control group, and the APN visit plus phone group scored significantly higher than the APN telephone group. Thus, given a priori contrasts, the difference between the two experimental groups is significant, whereas with a post-hoc test, the difference was not significant.

A priori contrasts must be based on firm theoretical grounds.

TABLE 7-5
Contrasts

	Pairs of Vectors					
Groups	X1	X2	Y1	Y2	Z1	Z2
1	2	0	−1	1	−1	1
2	−1	1	2	0	0	−1
3	−1	−1	−1	−1	1	0

Contrast Coefficients

	GROUP		
Contrast	Control	Telephone	Visit + phone
1	2	−1	−1
2	0	−1	1

The first contrast tests the difference between the two experimental groups (each given a coefficient of −1) and the control group (coefficient = 2).

The second contrast tests the difference between the two experimental groups.

Contrast Tests

		Contrast	Value of Contrast	Std. Error	t	df	Sig. (2-tailed)
SCORE	Assume equal variances	1	−7.1000	1.5092	−4.704	27	.000
		2	2.7000	.8714	3.099	27	.005
	Does not assume equal variances	1	−7.1000	1.4851	−4.781	18.583	.000
		2	2.7000	.8851	3.051	16.571	.007

Because the homogeneity of variance assumption was met, the equal variance contrasts are appropriate. Both contrasts are significant.

FIGURE 7-6

Computer output containing a priori contrasts.

TABLE 7-6
A Priori Contrasts for Observer-Rated Proficiency and Sensitivity

	Observer Rated Proficiency t value (df = 294)	Sensitivity t value (df = 295)
Control versus belief	1.02	.68
Control versus procedural	6.24*	5.03*
Control versus procedural/belief	6.18*	7.40*
Procedural versus procedural/belief	.02	2.35*
Belief versus procedural/belief	5.10*	7.98*

*$p \leq .01$.

(From Champion, V., & Scott, C. [1993]. Effects of a procedural/belief intervention on breast self-examination performance, Research in Nursing & Health, 16(3), 163–170.)

EXAMPLE FROM THE LITERATURE

Table 7-6 contains a table from a study by Champion and Scott (1993) on the effects of a theoretically based nurse-delivered intervention on the performance of breast self-examination (BSE). Their study included four groups: control, belief intervention, procedural intervention, and procedural/belief intervention. They hypothesized that there would be significant differences between the experimental groups taken together and the control group in frequency and proficiency of BSE. They also hypothesized that the group that received belief and procedural interventions would perform better than the groups that received only one of these interventions.

The authors report the use of a priori contrast to test for hypothesized differences. The control group, as hypothesized, demonstrated significantly lower proficiency and sensitivity than either the procedural or procedural/belief group but did not score lower than the belief group. The procedural/belief group scored significantly higher on sensitivity but not on proficiency than the procedure only group. The procedural/belief group scored significantly higher on proficiency and sensitivity than did the belief only group.

SUMMARY

One-way ANOVA is used to compare the means of two or more groups. When the overall *F* is significant and more than two groups are being compared, post-hoc tests are necessary to determine which pairs of means differ from each other. Additionally, when directional hypotheses are appropriate, a priori contrasts may be specified and tested.

APPLICATION EXERCISES AND RESULTS

EXERCISES

Run the appropriate analyses to answer the question and test the hypotheses. Write a description of the results.

1. Do the three smoking groups differ significantly in their quality of life during the past month?

2. Test the following hypotheses:

   a. The smoking group will score significantly lower on quality of life during the past month than the other two groups.

   b. There will be no significant difference in quality of life between the group that quit smoking and the group that never smoked.

RESULTS

1. To answer this question, a one-way analysis of variance (ANOVA) was run, and the Scheffé post-hoc test was requested. Exercise Figure 7-1 contains the output.

   Looking at the descriptives, we see that the group that is still smoking had the lowest mean score (3.55) on the six-point scale that ranged from a low of 1 (very dissatisfied, unhappy most of the time) to a high of 6 (extremely happy, could not be more pleased). The other two groups had fairly similar scores (4.5 and 4.4). The assumption of homogeneity of variance has been met ($p = .625$). The overall F is significant ($p = .002$).

   The Scheffé tests indicate that the smoking group reported significantly lower quality of life during the past month than did either of the nonsmoking groups. The two nonsmoking groups did not differ significantly from each other ($p = .908$).

2. One-way ANOVA with a priori contrasts was used to test the two hypotheses. Exercise Figure 7-2 contains the output. Only the contrasts have been included, because the ANOVA results are the same as in Exercise 1. The first contrast tests whether or not the still smoking group differs significantly from the other two groups. The second contrast tests whether or not the two nonsmoking groups differ from each other.

   Because the homogeneity of variance assumption has been met, we use the equal variances contrasts. We would report that the first hypothesis was supported ($p = .001$). The group that is still smoking scored significantly lower on their quality of life score than the other two groups combined. The second hypothesis was also supported ($p = .661$). There was no significant difference between the two nonsmoking groups on their reported quality of life.

Descriptives

		N	Mean	Std. Deviation	Std. Error	95% Confidence Interval for Mean		Minimum	Maximum
						Lower Bound	Upper Bound		
Quality of life in past month	Smoking History Never Smoked	109	4.50	1.17	.11	4.27	4.72	1	6
	Quit Smoking	42	4.40	1.11	.17	4.06	4.75	1	6
	Still Smoking	22	3.55	1.01	.22	3.10	3.99	1	5
	Total	173	4.35	1.17	8.90E-02	4.18	4.53	1	6

Test of Homogeneity of Variances

	Levene Statistic	df1	df2	Sig.
Quality of life in past month	.472	2	170	.625

ANOVA

		Sum of Squares	df	Mean Square	F	Sig.
Quality of life in past month	Between Groups	16.670	2	8.335	6.475	.002
	Within Groups	218.821	170	1.287		
	Total	235.491	172			

EXERCISE FIGURE 7-1. One-way analysis of variance with post-hoc test, Exercise 1. *(continued)*

Multiple Comparisons

Dependent Variable: quality of life in past month

Scheffe

(I) Smoking History	(J) Smoking History	Mean Difference (I-J)	Std. Error	Sig.	95% Confidence Interval Lower Bound	95% Confidence Interval Upper Bound
Never smoked	Quit smoking	9.07E-02	.206	.908	-.42	.60
	Still smoking	.95*	.265	.002	.30	1.60
Quit smoking	Never smoked	-9.07E-02	.206	.908	-.60	.42
	Still smoking	.86*	.299	.018	.12	1.60
Still smoking	Never smoked	-.95*	.265	.002	-1.60	-.30
	Quit smoking	-.86*	.299	.018	-1.60	-.12

* The mean difference is significant at the .05 level.

Scheffe[a]

Smoking History	N	Subset for Alpha = .05 — 1
Still smoking	22	4.40
Quit smoking	42	4.50
Never smoked	109	
Sig.		.941

Means for groups in homogeneous subsets are displayed.

a. Uses Harmonic Mean Sample Size = 38.247

EXERCISE FIGURE 7-1. (END)

Contrast Coefficients

Contrast	Smoking History		
	Never Smoked	Quit Smoking	Still Smoking
1	−1	−1	2
2	−1	−1	0

Contrast Tests

		Contrast	Value of Contrast	Std. Error	t	df	Sig. (2 tailed)
Quality of life in past month	Assume equal variances	1	−1.81	.53	−3.441	170	.001
		2	9.07E-02	.21	.440	170	.661
	Does not assume equal variances	1	−1.81	.48	−3.794	31.045	.001
		2	9.07E-02	.20	.444	78.321	.658

EXERCISE FIGURE 7-2. One-way analysis of variance with a priori contrasts, Exercise 2.

Differences Among Group Means: Multifactorial Analysis of Variance

Barbara Hazard Munro

OBJECTIVES FOR CHAPTER 8

After reading this chapter, you should be able to do the following:

1 ● Discuss the advantages of testing for interactions.

2 ● Interpret computer output from a two-way analysis of variance.

3 ● Determine when it is appropriate to use a multivariate analysis of variance.

TWO-WAY ANALYSIS OF VARIANCE

The Research Question

We have discussed the use of analysis of variance (ANOVA) with one categorical independent variable (with two or more levels) and one continuous dependent variable. This chapter discusses the use of ANOVA with more than one independent variable. We then extend the discussion into an analysis that includes more than one dependent variable. Such an analysis usually is called multivariate analysis of variance (MANOVA) and allows the researcher to look for relationships among dependent and independent variables.

There are great advantages in having more than one independent variable in an ANOVA. One advantage is economy: Many hypotheses can be tested for almost the same cost. The other is the ability to test for *interactions*. Although it is interesting and valuable to learn whether one approach works better than another, it may be even more important to find out whether the effect of an approach varies depending on the group of subjects. Testing for an interaction allows us to answer the ques-

TABLE 8-1
Example of an Interaction (Numbers Represent Group Means)

	Information		
	Yes	No	Row Means
Information Style			
Information seeker	100	50	75
Information avoider	50	100	75
Column means	75	75	
Diagonals: Seek/yes and avoid/no	**Mean = 100**		
Seek/no and avoid/yes	**Mean = 50**		

(From Munro, B. H. [1990]. Testing for interactions: The analysis of variance model. Clinical Nurse Specialist, 4(3), 128–129.)

tion of whether or not the results of a treatment vary depending on the groups or conditions in which it is applied.

Table 8-1 illustrates this with a contrived example, first published in *Clinical Nurse Specialist* (Munro, 1990). This is an example of a 2 × 2 design, often called a 2 × 2 factorial design. Each of the two independent variables (or factors) has two levels. The first between-subject factor is information, with two groups, one that received information (yes) and one that did not receive information (no). The second factor (independent variable) is information style, with two groups (information seekers and information avoiders). If we analyzed each independent variable separately, we would not derive the information that is provided by studying the interaction effect in the two-way ANOVA. If we compared those who received information with those who did not, there would be no difference between the groups, because the mean of each group (column means) is 75. Similarly, if we compared information seekers with information avoiders, we would find no difference (row means). Looking at the cells in the table, however, we can see that those whose information style fit with the information provided did much better (means of 100) than those whose style did not fit (means of 50). The test of the interaction is the statistical comparison of the diagonal means, 100 versus 50.

In the example provided, three research questions (or hypotheses) can be addressed:

1. Is there a significant difference between those who receive information and those who do not?
2. Is there a significant difference between those who seek information and those who avoid it?
3. Is there a significant interaction between information provided and the information-seeking style of the subject?

Testing of the interaction provides information about whether or not effects are altered by other factors. This allows us to investigate differences among groups of subjects in relation to an outcome measure.

The Type of Data Required

This is simply an extension of the one-way ANOVA. The independent variables are nominal (categorical), and the dependent variable is continuous. For example, Yoder (1994) was interested in comparing learning outcomes between two methods of technology-assisted instruction: linear video (a video program with no interruptions) and computer-assisted interactive video instruction (CAIVI). She hypothesized that learning style would affect learning; specifically, that learners with reflective observing styles would learn better with linear video. She used a two-way ANOVA in which one main effect was learning style with two levels, active experimenter and reflective observer, and the second main effect was treatment, with two levels, linear video and CAIVI. The results are contained in Table 8-2. There is a significant main effect for treatment ($p = .001$), and a significant interaction effect ($p = .003$). When there is a significant interaction effect, that should be studied first. Figure 8-1 contains a graph of the interaction. Yoder's hypothesis was supported: Reflective observers did better with linear video, and the active experimenters did better with CAIVI. The significant effect for treatment resulted because taken together, the mean for the CAIVI group was higher than the mean for the linear video group.

Assumptions

The assumptions are the same as those for the one-way ANOVA. The independent variables must be made up of mutually exclusive groups. The dependent variable must be normally distributed and demonstrate homogeneity of variance across groups.

TABLE 8-2
Two-way ANOVA Post-test by Learning Style and Treatment Group

Source	SS	MS	F	Significance
Main Effects	25.82	6.46	4.51	.003
Learning Style	3.83	1.28	.89	.451
Treatment	16.94	16.94	11.84	.001
Interaction	13.44	13.44	9.40	.003
Residual	80.10	1.43		

(From Yoder, M. E. [1994]. Preferred learning style and educational technology. Nursing & Health Care, 15(3), 128–132.)

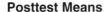

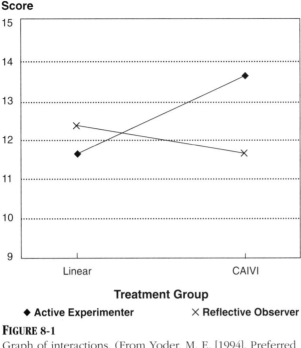

FIGURE 8-1

Graph of interactions. (From Yoder, M. E. [1994]. Preferred learning style and educational technology. *Nursing & Health Care, 15*(3), 128–132.)

Power

We have described the relationships among alpha level, effect size, power, and sample size for the *t* test and the one-way ANOVA. To test for an interaction, you must calculate the expected effect size for the interaction and for the independent variables to determine the appropriate sample size. You can request effect and power calculations as part of the output in ANOVA programs.

Example of a Computer Printout of a Two-Way Analysis of Variance

Figure 8-2, produced by SPSS for Windows, contains data drawn from a program grant funded by National Institute for Nursing Research (NINR), which included three randomized clinical trials. The purpose of the three studies was to test a model of nurse specialist transitional care (Brooten et al., 1989). Patient satisfaction, as measured by the La Monica-Oberst Patient Satisfaction Scale, was one of the outcome variables.

The descriptive statistics are presented first. In this analysis, we have two main effects, one labeled research study, and the other labeled study group. Research study

(text continues on page 168)

Descriptive Statistics

	RESEARCH STUDY	STUDY GROUP	Mean	Std. Deviation	N
PATIENT SATISFACTION	CESAREAN	EARLY DISCHARGE	187.2222	16.8888	54
		ROUTINE DISCHARGE	163.4464	24.8230	56
		Total	175.1182	24.3347	110
	DIABETIC	EARLY DISCHARGE	179.4474	20.3665	38
		ROUTINE DISCHARGE	167.6757	25.8307	37
		Total	173.6400	23.8138	75
	HYSTERECTOMY	EARLY DISCHARGE	181.7600	19.2646	50
		ROUTINE DISCHARGE	168.7143	25.1228	56
		Total	174.8679	23.3797	106
	Total	EARLY DISCHARGE	183.2183	18.8616	142
		ROUTINE DISCHARGE	166.4765	25.1309	149
		Total	174.6460	23.7815	291

Levene's Test of Equality of Error Variances

	F	df1	df2	Sig.
PATIENT SATISFACTION	1.336	5	285	.249

Tests the null hypothesis that the error variance of the dependent variable is equal across groups.

a. Design: Intercept+STUDY+GROUP+STUDY * GROUP

166

Tests of Between-Subjects Effects

Dependent Variable: PATIENT SATISFACTION

Source	Type III Sum of Squares	df	Mean Square	F	Sig.	Eta Squared	Noncent. Parameter	Observed Power[a]
Corrected Model	22739.3[b]	5	4547.864	9.175	.000	.139	45.874	1.000
Intercept	8613413	1	8613413	17376.4	.000	.984	17376.420	1.000
STUDY	166.101	2	83.050	.168	.846	.001	.335	.076
GROUP	18509.0	1	18509.0	37.339	.000	.116	37.339	1.000
STUDY * GROUP	2184.016	2	1092.008	2.203	.112	.015	4.406	.448
Error	141273	285	495.696					
Total	9039874	291						
Corrected Total	164013	290						

a. Computed using alpha = .05

b. R Squared = .139 (Adjusted R Squared = .124)

Grand Mean

Dependent Variable: PATIENT SATISFACTION

Mean	Std. Error
174.7110	1.325

RESEARCH STUDY

Dependent Variable: PATIENT SATISFACTION

RESEARCH	Mean	Std. Error
CESAREAN	175.3343	2.123
DIABETIC	173.5615	2.571
HYSTERECTOMY	175.2371	2.166

STUDY GROUP

Dependent Variable: PATIENT SATISFACTION

STUDY	Mean	Std. Error
EARLY DISCHARGE	182.8099	1.890
ROUTINE DISCHARGE	166.6121	1.859

FIGURE 8-2
TWO-WAY ANOVA.

has three levels, one for each of the three studies: unplanned cesarean birth mothers, childbearing diabetics, and nononcologic hysterectomy patients. The second main effect, study group, has two levels: early discharge and routine discharge. The early discharge group received the services of an advanced practice nurse who prepared them for discharge, made home visits after discharge, and was available by telephone.

Looking at the means, we see that within each study, the early discharge group had a higher mean score on patient satisfaction than did the routine discharge group.

With these two independent variables, three questions can be addressed:

1. Do the three research study groups differ on satisfaction with nursing care?
2. Do the two experimental groups differ on satisfaction with care?
3. Is there an interaction between research study group and experimental group in relation to satisfaction?

The assumption of homogeneity of variance has been met; Levene's test indicates $p = .249$. Looking at the ANOVA table, which is labeled Tests of Between-Subjects Effects, we see that there were 291 subjects in the analysis. The three study groups did not differ on satisfaction with care ($p = .846$). The two experimental groups do differ from each other ($p = .000$). There is no interaction between research study and experimental group in relation to satisfaction with nursing care. Before discussing the power estimates, look at the tables of means. The means for the research study groups are similar (173.6–175.3). In the experimental groups, the early discharge group rated their satisfaction significantly higher (mean = 182.8) than did the routine discharge group (mean = 166.6). Some people would prefer to see all the means in one table, rather than in three as provided by this output. Table 8-3 contains all the means associated with this analysis.

Now, look back at the ANOVA table at the measures of effect size and power. Power is related to the effect size and the sample size. SPSS for Windows provides an eta-squared statistic as a measure of effect size. Eta-squared is used to describe the proportion of variance explained by the differences among groups. It is the ra-

TABLE 8-3
Row, Column, and Cell Means From Figure 8-2

Discharge Group	Cesarean	Diabetic	Hysterectomy	Row Means
		Study		
Early	187.22	179.45	181.76	182.81
Routine	163.45	167.68	168.71	166.61
Column Means	175.33	173.56	175.24	

tio of the between-groups sum of squares and the total sum of squares (Norusis, 1996b). The observed power reflects the fact that there was very little difference between the means of the three study groups but a large difference (effect) between the two experimental groups. Because it was not the intent of the program grant to seek significant differences between the study groups, the lack of power is not a problem. The intent was to have enough subjects to compare early and routine discharge groups within each study. We planned to include 128 subjects in each study, 64 in each of the two groups within a study, for a power of .80, alpha of .05, and a moderate effect size. The difference in satisfaction between experimental and control groups was so large that the resulting power was 1.00, rather than the planned .80.

MULTIVARIATE ANALYSIS OF VARIANCE

The Type of Data Required

Often we are interested in more than one outcome. For example, Watters and Kristiansen (1995) compared the effects of combined mother-infant postnatal nursing care (where one nurse cares for both mother and infant) with traditional, separate postpartum and newborn care. Given the number of outcomes measured, they chose to use MANOVA. Mothers in the mother-infant care group rated themselves significantly higher in competence with infant care and satisfaction with parent education, nurse–client relationship, and parent–infant contact than did the traditional care group.

Although MANOVA techniques were developed in the 1930s and 1940s, not until the computer software became readily available were they reported in the social science literature. Today, MANOVA can be performed on a personal computer. Because in health professions we are usually interested in more than one outcome, MANOVA is being reported with increasing frequency in research publications.

Advantages of Multivariate Analysis of Variance

Health care outcomes measures, including physiological, psychological, and sociological, often are correlated. MANOVA includes the inter-relation among the outcome measures, whereas separate ANOVAs (one for each dependent variable) do not. Goodwin (1984) cites three general advantages of a multivariate, rather than several univariate analyses, to test hypotheses: to keep alpha at a known level; to increase power; and for ease in computation and interpretation. Conducting one overall analysis protects against type I errors. An alternative would be to use a Bonferroni correction, but that would ignore any relationship among the dependent variables. MANOVA is more powerful than separate ANOVAs, and the interpretation of the results may be improved by considering the outcome measures simultaneously (Bray & Maxwell, 1985). If the outcome measures are not correlated, however, there is no advantage to conducting a MANOVA.

Assumptions of Multivariate Analysis of Variance

For ANOVA, the assumptions include random sample, normal distribution, and equal variances across the groups on the dependent variable. When this is extended to MANOVA, not only should the univariate assumptions hold, but the dependent variable should have a "multivariate normal distribution with the same variance covariance matrix in each group" (Norusis, 1990b, p. B-64). To meet the assumption of multivariate normal distribution, each dependent variable must have a normal distribution, but this does not ensure that the overall measure of the dependent variables taken together will be normally distributed. Thus, the multivariate assumption needs to be tested. The requirement that each group will have the same variance–covariance matrix means that the homogeneity of variance assumption is met for each dependent variable, and the correlation between any two dependent variables must be the same in all groups (Bray & Maxwell, 1985).

Box's M is a measure of the multivariate test for homogeneity of variance and can be requested as part of the MANOVA program in SPSS for Windows. However, that Box's M, although widely used, is sensitive to departures from normality (Olson, 1974). Therefore, data must be submitted to preliminary checks for meeting the underlying assumptions for outliers and so forth before the analysis is conducted.

Statistical Power

It is difficult to ascertain the power when planning a MANOVA study because of the number of parameters to be estimated. Increasing the number of dependent variables requires an increase in sample size to maintain a given level of power. For example, for two groups with an alpha of 0.05, power of 0.80, and moderate effect size, 64 subjects in each group are required when there is one dependent variable. With two dependent variables, 80 subjects are required in each group (Lauter, Lauter, & Schmidtke, 1978). Because it is now possible to request power and effect measurements as part of the output from statistical analyses, prior work should be used for estimates on which to base sample size determinations.

Results of Multivariate Analysis of Variance

The first step in assessing the results is to look at the overall MANOVA. This is similar to looking at the F in the ANOVA. It tells whether there is an overall significant result. If there is, it indicates that there is a difference in at least one of the dependent variables. There is only one outcome measure for ANOVA, F, but there are four outcome measures for MANOVA:

1. Wilks' lambda
2. Pillai-Bartlett trace
3. Roy's greatest characteristic root
4. Hotelling-Lawley trace

Wilks' lambda is also explained in the sections on canonical correlation and discriminant analysis. It represents the product of the unexplained variances, that is, the error variance. Thus, a small value indicates significance.

Pillai-Bartlett trace represents the sum of the explained variances; therefore, a large value indicates significance.

Roy's greatest characteristic root is based on the first discriminant variate (see the section on discriminant function analysis for further detail).

Hotelling-Lawley trace is the sum of the ratio of the between and within sums of squares for each of the discriminant variates.

Any of these statistics might be used to test the overall multivariate hypothesis. According to Bray and Maxwell (1985), choosing the appropriate test involves a complex consideration of robustness and statistical power; Wilks' lambda is historically the most widely used, and Pillai-Bartlett trace has been found to be the most robust.

If the overall MANOVA is significant, you want to determine where the differences lie. Do the groups differ on all the dependent variables or only one? Generally, investigators have conducted univariate analyses following a multivariate significant result; that is, they conduct an ANOVA for each dependent variable. The danger of type I error is "protected" by the overall significant MANOVA. This has been called the least significant difference test or the protected *F* (Bray & Maxwell, 1985). This approach has been criticized, however, because it does not control for the number of comparisons made and does not adequately analyze the multivariate nature of the analysis. According to Bray and Maxwell (1985) the most general method of analyzing a significant MANOVA is to use Roy-Bose simultaneous confidence intervals. "This is a completely multivariate approach in which any linear combination of the classification or criterion variables can be investigated" (Bray & Maxwell, p. 53). In our computer example, we use the univariate analysis following the significant multivariate result, which is what is provided by SPSS for Windows.

Computer Output of a Multivariate Analysis of Variance

To demonstrate a MANOVA analysis, we use data collected by doctoral students at Boston College for use in their course on statistical analysis. For this example, we assume that all variables have been checked for departures from normality, the assumption of homogeneity of variance has been met, and that Box's M (the measure of equality of covariance matrices) is not significant.

Figure 8-3 contains the output. There are two independent variables, smoking history and experience of depression, and there are two dependent variables, life satisfaction and confidence. Smoking status contains three levels: never smoked, quit smoking, and still smoking. Experience of depression contains two levels: rarely depressed and sometimes to frequently depressed. The outcome measures are taken from the Inventory of Positive Psychological Attitudes (Kass et al., 1991). The life purpose and satisfaction scale contains 17 items and has a potential range of 17 to 119. The self-confidence during stressful situations scale contains 13 items, with a potential range of scores of 13 to 91.

The cell means are presented first. The multivariate tests determine where the differences lie. Remember that rather than one statistic (F in ANOVA), we get four multivariate tests.

The multivariate tests of the main effect smoking status are all significant ($p = 0.010–0.019$). The multivariate tests of the main effect experience of depression are given next. They are significant at the 0.000 level. The multivariate tests of the interaction are significant with the p values ranging from .005 to .028.

The univariate results are contained in the next table. There are two dependent variables, life satisfaction and confidence. The univariate results tell us whether the significant multivariate results apply to both dependent variables.

Although the multivariate results for the smoking groups were significant, the univariate results indicate that the three smoking groups did not differ significantly on either life satisfaction or confidence. The depressed groups differ significantly on both outcome measures. The interaction is significant on confidence ($p = .042$) but not on life satisfaction.

Using the cell means from the descriptive statistics table and the means from the smoking history and depressed tables, we have created Table 8-4 to assist with the interpretation of these results. The significant results are summarized:

1. Although there was a multivariate significant result for smoking status, neither of the univariate tests was significant
2. Significant main effects for the experience of depression on life satisfaction and confidence
3. A significant interaction between smoking status and experience of depression on confidence

Look at the column means for the effect of smoking group on outcome measures. On life satisfaction, we see that the group that is still smoking scored the lowest, but the difference is not statistically significant ($p = .108$). On the confidence outcome measure, the mean scores are similar across the three smoking groups as reflected by the p value of .235.

Examine the row means for both outcome variables to explain the main effects for experience of depression. On both outcome measures, the rarely depressed group scored significantly higher than the sometimes to routinely depressed group.

Look at Table 8-4, and determine why there was a significant interaction on the outcome confidence. Looking at the cell means, we can see that among people who are rarely depressed, those who quit smoking report the lowest confidence score (mean = 68.842). For the sometimes to frequently depressed group, those who quit smoking report the highest confidence score (mean = 59.864).

The power of the analysis is reported in the Multivariate Tests table. The power for the main effects ranges from .789 to 1.000. For the interaction, the power ranges from .757 to .845.

(text continues on page 179)

Descriptive Statistics

	Smoking History	Depressed	Mean	Std. Deviation	N
Life Satisfaction	Never Smoked	Rarely	99.9571	11.5976	70
		Sometimes to routinely	81.0526	18.1137	38
		Total	93.3056	16.8065	108
	Quit Smoking	Rarely	101.3684	12.8548	19
		Sometimes to routinely	83.4545	14.5593	22
		Total	91.7561	16.3536	41
	Still Smoking	Rarely	94.0000	13.2665	4
		Sometimes to routinely	69.6842	26.0940	19
		Total	73.9130	25.8824	23
	Total	Rarely	99.9892	11.8702	93
		Sometimes to routinely	78.9873	19.9657	79
		Total	90.3430	19.1786	172
Confidence	Never Smoked	Rarely	70.5857	10.0715	70
		Sometimes to routinely	50.5000	13.1370	38
		Total	63.5185	14.7632	108
	Quit Smoking	Rarely	68.8421	11.0517	19
		Sometimes to routinely	59.8636	9.0412	22
		Total	64.0244	10.8823	41
	Still Smoking	Rarely	72.2500	14.3846	4
		Sometimes to routinely	51.8421	18.1636	19
		Total	55.3913	18.9922	23
	Total	Rarely	70.3011	10.3628	93
		Sometimes to routinely	53.4304	14.0171	79
		Total	62.5523	14.7816	172

FIGURE 8-3

Multivariate analysis of variance (MANOVA). *(continued)*

Multivariate Tests[a]

Effect		Value	F	Hypothesis df	Error df	Sig.	Eta Squared	Noncent. Parameter	Observed Power[b]
Intercept	Pillai's Trace	.944	1394.871[c]	2.000	165.000	.000	.944	2789.741	1.000
	Wilks' Lambda	.056	1394.871[c]	2.000	165.000	.000	.944	2789.741	1.000
	Hotelling's Trace	16.908	1394.871[c]	2.000	165.000	.000	.944	2789.741	1.000
	Roy's Largest Root	16.908	1394.871[c]	2.000	165.000	.000	.944	2789.741	1.000
SMOKE5	Pillai's Trace	.069	2.988	4.000	332.000	.019	.035	11.951	.794
	Wilks' Lambda	.931	2.988[c]	4.000	330.000	.019	.035	11.951	.794
	Hotelling's Trace	.073	2.987	4.000	328.000	.019	.035	11.949	.794
	Roy's Largest Root	.058	4.783	2.000	166.000	.010	.054	9.566	.789

174

		Value	F	Hypothesis df	Error df	Sig.	Partial Eta Squared	Noncent. Parameter	Observed Power
DEPRESS	Pillai's Trace	.205	21.295[c]	2.000	165.000	.000	.205	42.589	1.000
	Wilks' Lambda	.795	21.295[c]	2.000	165.000	.000	.205	42.589	1.000
	Hotelling's Trace	.258	21.295[c]	2.000	165.000	.000	.205	42.589	1.000
	Roy's Largest Root	.258	21.295[c]	2.000	165.000	.000	.205	42.589	1.000
SMOKE5 * DEPRESS	Pillai's Trace	.064	2.761	4.000	332.000	.028	.032	11.043	.757
	Wilks' Lambda	.936	2.785[c]	4.000	330.000	.027	.033	11.139	.761
	Hotelling's Trace	.068	2.808	4.000	328.000	.026	.033	11.234	.765
	Roy's Largest Root	.066	5.494	2.000	166.000	.005	.062	10.988	.845

a. Design: Intercept+SMOKE5+DEPRESS+SMOKE5 * DEPRESS

b. Computed using alpha = .05

c. Exact statistic

FIGURE 8-3 (CONTINUED)

175

Tests of Between-Subjects Effects

Source	Dependent Variable	Type III Sum of Squares	df	Mean Square	F	Sig.	Eta Squared	Noncent. Parameter	Observed Power[a]
Corrected Model	Life Satisfaction	21266.0[b]	5	4253.203	16.959	.000	.338	84.797	1.000
	Confidence	13503.6[c]	5	2700.730	18.791	.000	.361	93.953	1.000
Intercept	Life Satisfaction	635341	1	635341	2533.383	.000	.939	2533.383	1.000
	Confidence	316752	1	316752	2203.829	.000	.930	2203.829	1.000
SMOKE5	Life Satisfaction	1131.271	2	565.635	2.255	.108	.026	4.511	.454
	Confidence	420.489	2	210.244	1.463	.235	.017	2.926	.309
DEPRESS	Life Satisfaction	8468.672	1	8468.672	33.768	.000	.169	33.768	1.000
	Confidence	5545.842	1	5545.842	38.586	.000	.189	38.586	1.000
SMOKE5 * DEPRESS	Life Satisfaction	105.175	2	52.587	.210	.811	.003	-.419	.082
	Confidence	928.107	2	464.054	3.229	.042	.037	6.457	.609
Error	Life Satisfaction	41630.7	166	250.788					
	Confidence	23858.9	166	143.728					
Total	Life Satisfaction	1466737	172						
	Confidence	710363	172						
Corrected Total	Life Satisfaction	62896.8	171						
	Confidence	37362.5	171						

a. Computed using alpha = .05

b. R Squared = .338 (Adjusted R Squared = .318)

c. R Squared = .361 (Adjusted R Squared = .342)

Smoking History

Dependent	Smoking	Mean	Std. Error
Life Satisfaction	Never Smoked	90.5049	1.595
	Quit Smoking	92.4115	2.480
	Still Smoking	81.8421	4.356
Confidence	Never Smoked	60.5429	1.208
	Quit Smoking	64.3529	1.877
	Still Smoking	62.0461	3.298

Depressed

Dependent	Depressed	Mean	Std. Error
Life Satisfaction	Rarely	98.4419	2.972
	Sometimes to routinely	78.0638	1.862
Confidence	Rarely	70.5593	2.250
	Sometimes to routinely	54.0686	1.409

FIGURE 8-3 (END)

TABLE 8-4
Row, Column, and Cell Means From Figure 8-3

Dependent Variable—Life Satisfaction

| | **Smoking Status** | | | |
Depressed	*Never*	*Quit*	*Still Smoking*	**Row Means**
Rarely	99.957	101.368	94.000	98.442
Sometimes to frequently	81.053	83.455	69.684	78.064
Column means	*90.505*	*92.411*	*81.842*	

Dependent Variable—Confidence

| | **Smoking Status** | | | |
Depressed	*Never*	*Quit*	*Still Smoking*	**Row Means**
Rarely	70.586	68.842	72.250	70.559
Sometimes to frequently	50.500	59.864	51.842	54.069
Column means	*60.543*	*64.353*	*62.046*	

TABLE 8-5
Effects of Type of Care on Mothers' Hospital and Mail Scores in Study I

| | | **Traditional** | | **Mother-Infant** | | **Care Effects** | |
| | **Max** | **(n = 121 − 147)*** | | **(n = 142 − 152)*** | | | |
Outcome	**Score**	M	SD	M	SD	F	df
1. Competence							
Self-care	12	9.5	1.7	9.6	1.5	1.31	(1,295)
Infant care	20	15.9	2.5	16.5	2.4	7.21[†]	(1,295)
2. Satisfaction							
Parent education	16	11.7	2.7	13.0	2.1	18.18[‡]	(1,259)
Nurse–client relationship	16	13.0	2.1	13.8	1.9	7.15[†]	(1,259)
Parent–infant contact	8	5.8	1.9	6.4	1.5	8.01[†]	(1,259)
Overall rating	10	8.2	1.2	8.5	1.2	6.13**	(1,259)

*Sample sizes vary due to missing data.   **$p < .02$.   [†]$p < .01$.   [‡]$p < .001$.
(From Watters, N. E., & Kristiansen, C. M. [1995]. Two evaluations of combined mother-infant versus separate postnatal nursing care. Research in Nursing & Health, 18, *20.)*

EXAMPLE FROM THE PUBLISHED LITERATURE

Table 8-5 contains a slightly edited version of the results from the study by Watters and Kristiansen (1995) on evaluations of combined mother-infant versus separate postnatal care. They are comparing traditional care in which different nurses care for mothers and babies with a system in which the same nurse cares for both mother and baby. They compared the two groups on two measures of competence and four measures of satisfaction. On five of these outcome measures, the mother-infant group scored significantly higher than the traditional group.

SUMMARY

ANOVA is a powerful, robust test that allows us to test for relationships between categorical independent variables and a continuous (measured at the interval or ratio level) dependent variable. Testing for interactions between the independent variables is particularly useful when we want to determine whether or not the effects of some intervention will be the same for all types of people or conditions. ANOVA may be extended to the use of more than one dependent variable in a given analysis. This analysis is usually called MANOVA and allows the researcher to look for relationships among dependent and many independent variables.

APPLICATION EXERCISES AND RESULTS

EXERCISES

1. Run the appropriate analysis to answer the following questions, and write up the results:
   a. Do the three political groups differ significantly in reported quality of life during the past month?
   b. Do men and women differ significantly in reported quality of life during the past month?
   c. Is there an interaction between political affiliation and gender in relation to reported quality of life?

2. Add a second dependent variable, years of education, to the analysis in Exercise 1. Run the analysis, and write up the results.

RESULTS

1. A two-way analysis of variance was used to answer the questions. Exercise Figure 8-1 contains the output. The two independent variables were political affiliation with three levels, republican, democrat, and independent, and gender with two levels, male and female. The dependent variable was quality of life during the past month, which was measured on a six-point scale in which 1 = very dissatisfied, unhappy most of the time, and 6 = extremely happy, could not be more pleased.

   The assumption of homogeneity of variance was met ($p = .573$). The three political groups do differ significantly in reported quality of life ($p = .040$). Looking at the means,

Between-Subjects Factors

		Value Label
Political affiliation	1	Republican
	2	Democrat
	3	Independent
Gender	0	male
	1	female

Levene's Test of Equality of Error Variances[a]

	F	df1	df2	Sig.
Quality of life in past month	.769	5	165	.573

Tests the null hypothesis that the error variance of the dependent variable is equal across groups.

a. Design: Intercept+POLAFF+GENDER+POLAFF * GENDER

Tests of Between-Subjects Effects

Dependent Variable: quality of life in past month

Source	Type III Sum of Squares	df	Mean Square	F	Sig.	Eta Squared	Noncent. Parameter	Observed Power[a]
Corrected model	18.349[b]	5	3.670	2.796	.019	.078	13.978	.824
Intercept	2581.646	1	2581.646	1966.644	.000	.923	1966.644	1.000
POLAFF	8.593	2	4.296	3.273	.040	.038	6.546	.616
GENDER	2.784	1	2.784	2.121	.147	.013	2.121	.305
POLAFF * GENDER	7.820	2	3.910	2.978	.054	.035	5.957	.573
Error	216.598	165	1.313					
total	3472.000	171						
Corrected Total	234.947	170						

a. Computed using alpha = .05

b. R Squared = .078 (Adjusted R Squared = .050)

Political Affiliation

Grand Mean

Dependent Variable: quality of life in past month

Mean	Std. Error
4.32	.097

Dependent Variable: quality of life in past month

Political	Mean	Std. Error
Republican	4.31	.184
Democrat	4.61	.179
Independent	4.03	.140

Gender

Dependent Variable: quality of life in past month

Gender	Mean	Std. Error
Male	4.18	.154
Female	4.46	.119

EXERCISE FIGURE 8-1. Two-way analysis of variance, Exercise 1. (CONTINUED)

Multiple Comparisons

Dependent Variable: quality of life in past month

Scheffe

(I) Political Affiliation	(J) Political Affiliation	Mean Difference (I-J)	Std. Error	Sig.	95% Confidence Interval	
					Lower Bound	Upper Bound
Republican	Democrat	−.29	.243	.495	−.89	.31
	Independent	9.52E-02	.224	.914	−.46	.65
Democrat	Republican	.29	.243	.495	−.31	.89
	Independent	.38	.204	.174	−.12	.89
Independent	Republican	−9.52E-02	.224	.914	−.65	.46
	Democrat	−.38	.204	.174	−.89	.12

Quality of Life in Past Month

Scheffe[a,b]

Political Affiliation	N	Subset
		1
Independent	80	4.21
Republican	39	4.31
Democrat	52	4.60
Sig.		.234

Means for groups in homogeneous subsets are displayed.
Based on Type III Sum of Squares

a. Uses Harmonic Mean Sample Size = 52.291.

b. Alpha = .05.

EXERCISE FIGURE 8-1. (CONTINUED)

we see that independents had the lowest mean score (4.03), and democrats the highest (4.61). Although the overall F for the comparison was significant, none of the pairwise comparisons using the Scheffé test were significant.

Men and women did not differ significantly on reported quality of life ($p = .147$). There was no interaction between political affiliation and gender in relation to quality of life ($p = .054$).

2. A multivariate analysis of variance was used for this analysis. Exercise Figure 8-2 contains the output. There were two independent variables, political affiliation and gender, and two dependent variables, quality of life in the past month and years of education.

(text continues on page 187)

Box's Test of Equality of Covariance Matrices[a]

Box's M	16.698
F	1.068
df1	15
df2	37120
Sig.	.380

Tests the null hypothesis that the observed covariance matrices of the dependent variables are equal across groups.

a. Design: Intercept+POLAFF+GENDER+POLAFF * GENDER

Between-Subjects Factors

		Value Label
Political Affiliation	1	Republican
	2	Democrat
	3	Independent
Gender	0	Male
	1	Female

Levene's Test of Equality of Error Variances[a]

	F	df1	df2	Sig.
Quality of life in past month	.926	5	156	.466
Education in years	1.755	5	156	.125

Tests the null hypothesis that the error variance of the dependent variable is equal across groups.

a. Design: Intercept+POLAFF+GENDER+POLAFF * GENDER

Multivariate Tests[a]

Effect		Value	F	Hypothesis df	Error df	Sig.	Eta Squared	Noncent. Parameter	Observed Power[b]
Intercept	Pillai's Trace	.960	1879.907[c]	2.000	155.000	.000	.960	3759.814	1.000
	Wilks' Lambda	.040	1879.907[c]	2.000	155.000	.000	.960	3759.814	1.000
	Hotelling's Trace	24.257	1879.907[c]	2.000	155.000	.000	.960	3759.814	1.000
	Roy's Largest Root	24.257	1879.907[c]	2.000	155.000	.000	.960	3759.814	1.000

Effect		Value	F	Hypothesis df	Error df	Sig.	Partial Eta Squared	Noncent. Parameter	Observed Power
POLAFF	Pillai's Trace	.079	3.197	4.000	312.000	.014	.039	12.789	.824
	Wilks' Lambda	.921	3.238[c]	4.000	310.000	.013	.040	12.952	.829
	Hotelling's Trace	.085	3.278	4.000	308.000	.012	.041	13.113	.834
	Roy's Largest Root	.083	6.491	2.000	156.000	.002	.077	12.982	.902
GENDER	Pillai's Trace	.009	.729[c]	2.000	155.000	.484	.009	1.458	.172
	Wilks' Lambda	.991	.729[c]	2.000	155.000	.484	.009	1.458	.172
	Hotelling's Trace	.009	.729[c]	2.000	155.000	.484	.009	1.458	.172
	Roy's Largest Root	.009	.729[c]	2.000	155.000	.484	.009	1.458	.172
POLAFF * GENDER	Pillai's Trace	.042	1.659	4.000	312.000	.159	.021	6.637	.508
	Wilks' Lambda	.958	1.666[c]	4.000	310.000	.158	.021	6.665	.510
	Hotelling's Trace	.043	1.673	4.000	308.000	.156	.021	6.693	.512
	Roy's Largest Root	.043	3.384	2.000	156.000	.036	.042	6.767	.631

a. Design: Intercept+POLAFF+GENDER+POLAFF * GENDER

b. Computed using alpha = .05

c. Exact statistic

EXERCISE FIGURE 8-2. Multivariate analysis of variance. *(continued)*

Tests of Between-Subjects Effects

Source	Dependent Variable	Type III Sum of Squares	df	Mean Square	F	Sig.	Eta Squared	Noncent. Parameter	Observed Power[a]
Corrected Model	Quality of life in past month	16.023[b]	5	3.205	2.449	.036	.073	12.243	.761
	Education in years	68.263[c]	5	13.653	1.056	.387	.033	5.281	.370
Intercept	Quality of life in past month	2474.275	1	2474.275	1890.644	.000	.924	1890.644	1.000
	Education in years	34838.1	1	34838.1	2695.330	.000	.945	2695.330	1.000
POLAFF	Quality of life in past month	7.458	2	3.729	2.849	.061	.035	5.699	.552
	Education in years	62.527	2	31.264	2.419	.092	.030	4.838	.482
GENDER	Quality of life in past month	1.652	1	1.652	1.262	.263	.008	1.262	.201
	Education in years	.510	1	.510	.039	.843	.000	.039	.054

POLAFF * GENDER	Quality of life in past month	8.268	2	4.134	3.159	.045	.039	6.318	.599
	Education in years	.319	2	.160	.012	.988	.000	.025	.052
Error	Quality of life in past month	204.156	156	1.309					
	Education in years	2016.356	156	12.925					
Total	Quality of life in past month	3219.000	162						
	Education in years	44830.3	162						
Corrected Total	Quality of life in past month	220.179	161						
	Education in years	2084.619	161						

a. Computed using alpha = .05

b. R Squared = .073 (Adjusted R Squared = .043)

c. R Squared = .033 (Adjusted R Squared = .002)

Grand Mean

Dependent	Mean	Std. Error
Quality of life in past month	4.29	.099
Education in years	16.08	.310

Political Affiliation

Dependent	Political	Mean	Std. Error
Quality of life in past month	Republican	4.29	.186
	Democrat	4.56	.182
	Independent	4.01	.141
Education in years	Republican	15.71	.584
	Democrat	15.58	.571
	Independent	16.96	.444

EXERCISE FIGURE 8-2. (CONTINUED)

Descriptive Statistics

	Political Affiliation	Gender	Mean	Std. Deviation	N
Quality of life in past month	Republican	Male	4.30	1.30	20
		Female	4.28	1.41	18
		Total	4.29	1.33	38
	Democrat	Male	4.64	1.01	14
		Female	4.47	1.02	34
		Total	4.52	1.01	48
	Independent	Male	3.58	1.10	24
		Female	4.44	1.11	52
		Total	4.17	1.17	76
	Total	Male	4.09	1.22	58
		Female	4.42	1.13	104
		Total	4.30	1.17	162
Education in years	Republican	Male	15.80	3.72	20
		Female	15.61	4.24	18
		Total	15.71	3.92	38
	Democrat	Male	15.57	4.60	14
		Female	15.59	3.77	34
		Total	15.58	3.98	48
	Independent	Male	17.06	2.63	24
		Female	16.87	3.26	52
		Total	16.93	3.06	76
	Total	Male	16.27	3.56	58
		Female	16.23	3.63	104
		Total	16.24	3.60	162

Gender

Dependent Variable	Gender	Mean	Std. Error
Quality of life in past month	Male	4.18	.154
	Female	4.40	.123
Education in years	Male	16.14	.484
	Female	16.02	.387

Education in Years

Scheffe[a,b]

Political affiliation	N	Subset 1
Democrat	48	15.58
Republican	38	15.71
Independent	76	16.93
Sig.		.179

Means for groups in homogeneous subsets are displayed.
Based on Type III Sum of Squares

a. Uses Harmonic Mean Sample Size = 49.745.

b. Alpha = .05.

EXERCISE FIGURE 8-2. (END)

The assumption of equality of covariance matrices has been met (Box's m, $p = .380$). The assumption of homogeneity of variance has also been met for both dependent variables. For quality of life, Levene's $p = .466$, and for education in years, Levene's $p = .125$.

The multivariate tests indicate an overall significant effect (across both dependent variables) for political affiliation. There are no significant effects for gender. One of the three measures is significant for the interaction between political affiliation and gender.

The univariate tests indicate that the only significant result was the interaction between political affiliation and gender in relation to quality of life in the past month. To interpret that result, we constructed the table below from the information in the tables of means for political affiliation and gender and from the table of descriptive statistics. Here we can see that male independents scored the lowest of any group (mean = 3.58). Female independents had a mean score similar to the other groups (mean = 4.44).

EXERCISE TABLE 8-1
Means from Exercise Figure 8-2

Political Affiliation	Gender		
	Male	*Female*	*Row Totals*
Republican	4.30	4.28	4.29
Democrat	4.64	4.47	4.56
Independent	3.58	4.44	4.01
Column Totals	*4.18*	*4.40*	

Analysis of Covariance

BARBARA HAZARD MUNRO

OBJECTIVES FOR CHAPTER 9

After reading this chapter, you should be able to do the following:

1 • Determine when analysis of covariance is appropriate to use.

2 • Explain the relationship between analysis of variance and regression.

3 • Discuss the assumptions, interpretations, and limitations of analysis of covariance.

In the preceding chapters, the statistical methods of analysis of variance (ANOVA)—one-way and complex—are described as techniques to investigate differences among group means. Those tests are used when more than two groups are involved or when we are interested in the effects of several categorical (independent) variables on a "continuous" (dependent) measure.

This chapter presents another ANOVA technique: the analysis of covariance (ANCOVA). This technique combines the ANOVA with regression to measure the differences among group means. The advantages that ANCOVA holds over other techniques are the ability to reduce the error variance in the outcome measure and the ability to measure group differences after allowing for other differences between subjects. The error variance is reduced by controlling for variation in the dependent measure that comes from separate measurable variables that influence all the groups being compared. Such a separate variable is considered to be neither independent nor dependent in the ANOVA. However, it contributes to the variation and reduces the magnitude of the differences among groups. In ANCOVA, the variation from this variable is measured and extracted from the within (or error) variation. The effect is the reduction of error variance and therefore an increase in the power of the analysis. Power is the *likelihood of correctly rejecting the null hypothesis.* With ANCOVA, the control of the extraneous variation will provide a more accurate estimate of the real difference among groups.

THE RESEARCH QUESTION

In general, ANCOVA answers the same research question as ANOVA: Do the experimental groups differ to a greater degree than we would expect by chance alone? However, with ANOVA, two sets of variables are involved in the analysis: the independent variables and the dependent variable. With ANCOVA, a third type of variable is included: the *covariate*.

Vessey, Carlson, and McGill (1994) studied the effectiveness of a distraction technique in reducing a child's perceived pain and behavioral distress during an acute pain experience. They randomly assigned children who were scheduled for a routine venipuncture to an experimental or control group. The experimental group was encouraged to use a kaleidoscope as distraction, and the control group received usual supportive care. Because age was related to behavioral distress from venipuncture, it was entered into the analysis as a covariate. After controlling for age, there was a significant difference between the experimental and control groups in perception of pain and behavioral distress, with the experimental group perceiving less pain and demonstrating less behavioral distress. If they had not included age as a covariate, they would have been unable to explain the variability due to age; it would have been relegated to the "error" term. Thus, their analysis was more powerful in that the error term was reduced, and they were able to validate previous research that indicated that age is an important variable when studying children's responses to painful experiences.

Such an approach is typical of the original purpose for using ANCOVA. Since then, the technique has been used in other ways as well. Frequently, it is used to "equate" groups. In quasiexperimental designs, individuals have not been randomly assigned to groups, and intact groups are often used. A typical example is using already established classes in a school to test different teaching methods. Because the subjects are not randomly assigned, there may be initial differences among groups. In classroom situations, the major concern would be that the groups might differ in scholastic ability. In a hospital situation, one might be concerned that patients in one unit were sicker than those in another unit. If the groups are found to be different, ANCOVA is often used to "equate" them. In the classroom example, scholastic ability would be the covariate, and the effect of scholastic ability would be "removed" before the means of the groups on the dependent variable were compared. In the hospital example, degree of illness might be used as a covariate.

For example, Tappen (1994), in a study of nursing home residents with dementia, compared the effects of skill training, a traditional stimulation approach, and regular care on the ability to perform activities of daily living. On pretest, the individuals in the skill training group on average began treatment at a lower level of functional ability than the other two groups, so she used ANCOVA with the pretest scores as the covariate. With the effect of the pretest scores removed, the effect of treatment on physical self-maintenance was significant. The group receiving skill training showed the largest gain, the stimulation group had a smaller gain, and the control group experienced a decline in their scores. If she had not controlled for initial group differences, her results might have been confounded by the fact that one group was at a lower level at the beginning of the study.

ANCOVA also has been used when random assignment has not "worked." Especially with small samples, an investigator may find that even after random assignment, the groups differ on some important variable. ANCOVA might then be used to equate the groups statistically.

Although ANCOVA has been widely used for such statistical "equalization" of groups, it is not a cure-all and should be used with caution. Some authors condemn its use for anything but the intent to remove another source of variation from the dependent variable. They do not believe that it should be used to equate groups. To use ANCOVA with dissimilar groups, one would have to be able to assert that the groups were essentially equivalent except for the variable(s) being used as covariate(s). This is virtually impossible to know for certain.

TYPE OF DATA REQUIRED

As with ANOVA, one or more categorical variables are independent variables, and the dependent variable is continuous and meets the requirements of normal distribution and equality of variance across groups. In addition, the covariate should be a continuous variable. This is discussed in further detail in the following section.

ASSUMPTIONS

To ensure a valid interpretation of ANCOVA results, several assumptions should be met. These assumptions are based on requirements necessary for the validity of the regression and the ANOVA components of the test. The first three assumptions are those associated with ANOVA:

1. The groups should be mutually exclusive.
2. The variances of the groups should be equivalent (homogeneity of variance).
3. The dependent variable should be normally distributed.

In addition:

4. The covariate should be a continuous variable. If a variable is at the nominal level, it cannot be used as a covariate. (However, a nominal variable may be included as an additional independent variable in ANOVA, rather than as a covariate.)
5. The covariate and the dependent variable must show a linear relationship. When this assumption is violated, the analysis will have little benefit, because there will be little reduction in error variance. The test is most effective when that relation-

ship lies above $r = 0.30$. The stronger the relationship, the more effective the ANCOVA analysis will be; that is, the more the two variables are related, the greater is the reduction in error variance by controlling for the covariate. In cases in which the relationship between the covariate and dependent variable is not linear, one appropriate test would be the complex ANOVA, with the levels of the covariate as another independent variable. Another possibility would be mathematical transformation of the variables to achieve a linear relationship. The transformed variables could then be used in ANCOVA.

Consider an example that demonstrates a violation of this assumption. Suppose we wished to study the effects of two different teaching methods on student performance. Suppose also the investigator wanted to control for the effects of anxiety. Previous research implies there is a U-shaped relationship between anxiety and performance; that is, performance seems to be enhanced by moderate levels of anxiety. However, at high and low levels, performance is hampered. This is depicted in Figure 9-1. Therefore, ANCOVA analysis with level of anxiety as a covariate would violate the assumption of a linear correlation between the covariate and the outcome variable.

One appropriate analysis in this case would be a complex ANOVA with three levels of anxiety as one main effect variable and types of teaching as a second main effect. Another approach would be to use curvilinear regression analysis, in which the anxiety scores could be treated as continuous, rather than categorical, data. For further information on curvilinear regression, see Pedhazur and Schmelkin (1991, Chapter 18).

6. The direction and strength of the relationship between the covariate and dependent variable must be similar in each group. We call this requirement *homogene-*

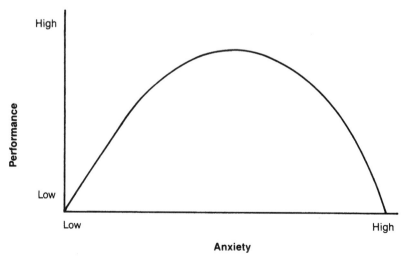

FIGURE 9-1
Possible relationship between performance and anxiety.

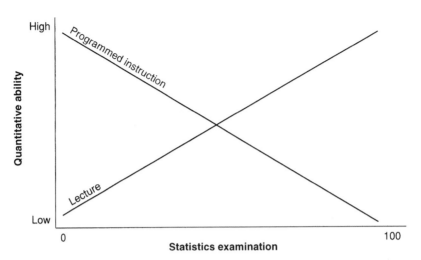

FIGURE 9-2

Lack of homogeneity of regression across two groups.

ity of regression across groups. When there is homogeneity of regression, the regression lines will be parallel. When this assumption is violated, the chance of a type I error is increased. This assumption can be expressed in another way: The independent variable should not have an effect on *the relationship between the covariate and the dependent variable.* Another way to say this is that the covariate has the same effect on the dependent variable in all the groups.

Figure 9-2 demonstrates a violation of the assumption of homogeneity of regression. Note that the lines are not parallel, indicating that the interventions affected the covariate-dependent relationship differentially. Quantitative ability is the covariate (varying from low to high), and the score on the statistics final examination is the outcome measure. There are two groups, one taught by the lecture method and one by programmed instruction. The covariate, quantitative ability does not have the same relationship with the dependent variable in these two groups. In the programmed instruction group, students with higher quantitative ability score lower on the statistics examination (a negative correlation). In the lecture group, the opposite is true; students with higher quantitative ability score higher on the examination.

RELATIONSHIP OF ANOVA AND REGRESSION TO ANCOVA

To understand the rationale behind the mathematical operations involved in ANCOVA, it is necessary to understand the concept of the *residual.* Chapter 11 explains that squaring the correlation coefficient results in a quantity, *r* square, known as a *coefficient of determination.* This coefficient is often used as a measure of the meaningfulness of *r*, because it is a measure of the variance shared by the two variables. To calculate the proportion of variance that is *not shared* by the two variables, we would subtract *r* square from 1. For example, if the correlation between two variables is 0.50, then *r* square = 0.25, and 1 − *r* square = 0.75. We could then state that 25% of the variance was shared by the two variables, and 75% was not shared. This 75% is called the *variance of the residual.* Regression analysis is concerned with the regression sum of squares and the residual sum of squares. With ANOVA, the within sum of squares, or error term, is analogous to the residual sum of squares. Thus, the residual variance is the variation not explained by the variables in the study. With ANCOVA, we use the residuals to determine whether groups differ *after* the effect of some other variable has been removed.

POWER OF THE ANALYSIS

With ANCOVA, one must determine power based on the number of cells in the analysis and on the covariate. Because the covariate reduces the error term, it increases the power of the test. When determining sample size, the investigator must include the expected impact of the covariate on the effect size. Effect and power calculations can be requested with ANCOVA procedures.

EXAMPLE OF A COMPUTER PRINTOUT

The data were collected by doctoral students at Boston College for use in classroom practice. Suppose we wanted to determine if smoking is related to psychological attitudes. We have three mutually exclusive groups in relation to smoking: never smoked, quit smoking, and still smoking. Our outcome measure is the total score on the Inventory of Positive Psychological Attitudes (IPPA; Kass et al., 1991), where the potential range of scores is 30 to 210, with a high score indicating positive psychological attitudes. In preliminary testing, we have determined that the three groups have equivalent variances on the IPPA score (homogeneity of variance assumption). We have also determined that the total IPPA scores for our sample are normally distributed. Additionally, we know that perceived quality of life is related to psychological attitudes. In this questionnaire, quality of life was measured on a six-point scale, where 1 was "very dissatisfied, unhappy most of the time," and 6 was "extremely happy, could not be more satisfied or pleased." The correlation between quality of life and IPPA total score is .56 (p = .000). Thus, the following question could be addressed: After controlling for quality of life, do the three smoking groups differ significantly on positive psychological attitudes? Before running the analysis, there is one remaining assumption to be checked, that of homogeneity of regression.

To adjust for a covariate, the difference between the score of an individual on the covariate and the grand mean of the covariate is weighted by a *common* regression coefficient (*b*). Use of such a common regression coefficient is based on the assumption that there is no interaction between the covariate and the independent variable. If such an interaction exists, ANCOVA should *not* be used.

The question is whether there is an interaction between the independent variable (SMOKE5) and the covariate (QOL14). We need to build a model that will test this interaction before carrying out the ANCOVA. In SPSS for Windows, descriptions of how to conduct the test of the assumption are included in chapters on the General Linear Model (Norusis, 1994).

Because it is important that this assumption be checked, we will walk you through the steps in the process. In this example, in SPSS for Windows, we first selected the Statistics menu, then ANOVA models, and then General Factorial. After identifying IPPATOT as the dependent variable, SMOKE5 as the factor (independent variable), and QOL14 as the covariate, we selected Model and within this menu, selected Custom. Under Build Terms, we highlighted Main Effects. We then clicked on SMOKE5 and QOL14 and moved them to the space for the model on the right side. Next, we changed the Build Terms to Interaction, again highlighted SMOKE5 and QOL14, and moved them over as an interaction term. The resulting model looked like:

SMOKE5
QOL14
SMOKE5 * QOL14

Figure 9-3 contains the results of this analysis. Of interest is the interaction between the main effect, SMOKE5, and the covariate, QOL14. The F associated with the interaction is .21 ($p = .809$). There is *no significant interaction* between the independent variable and the covariate. Thus, the assumption is met, and it is appropriate to conduct the ANCOVA. If the interaction had been *significant,* one could study the effect of quality of life on positive psychological attitudes within each of the three smoking groups.

With the assumptions met, we conduct the ANCOVA. The output is contained in Figure 9-4. The regression effect, which is the effect of the covariate, QOL14, is significant ($F = 71.59$, $p = .000$). After controlling for the covariate, the main effect, SMOKE5, is also significant ($F = 3.76$, $p = .000$). The power for the effect of the covariate is 1.000 and for the smoking group is .681.

Look at the means for the three smoking groups on quality of life. We see that the three groups differ in their scores, with the still smoking group having the lowest quality of life score (3.696) and the never smoked group, the highest (4.477). Now look at the adjusted and estimated means to see what effect controlling for quality of life has on the comparison of the group means on IPPA total. The observed means range from 129.304 for the still smoking group to 156.654 for the nonsmoking group, a 27.35-point difference. After adjusting for the effect of quality of life, the mean score for IPPA total for the nonsmoking group and the quit smoking groups dropped, and the mean for the still smoking group increased. Now, the greatest difference is between the quit smoking group (153.070) and the still smoking group (136.335), a 16.735-point difference. It is the difference between the adjusted means that is being tested for statistical significance in ANCOVA. Post-hoc tests indicate that the
(text continues on page 198)

```
* * * * * * A n a l y s i s   o f   V a r i a n c e -- d e s i g n   1 * * * * * *
Tests of Significance for IPPATOT using UNIQUE sums of squares
Source of Variation        SS        DF        MS       F   Sig of F

WITHIN+RESIDUAL        110608.32      165     670.35
SMOKE5                   1093.33        2     546.67     .82     .444
QOL14                   35922.68        1   35922.68   53.59     .000
QOL14 * SMOKE5            284.50        2     142.25     .21     .809

(Model)                 62474.32        5   12494.86   18.64     .000
(Total)                173082.64      170    1018.13

R-Squared          =    .361
Adjusted R-Squared =    .342
```

The interaction between the independent variable (main effect), SMOKE5 (Smoking status), and the covariate, QOL14 (Quality of life), is not significant ($p = .809$). Thus, the assumption of homogeneity of regression is met.

FIGURE 9-3

Computer output of test of assumption of homogeneity of regression. *(continued)*

```
* * * * * A n a l y s i s   o f   V a r i a n c e  -- design  1 * * * * * * *

Tests of Significance for IPPATOT using UNIQUE sums of squares
Source of Variation        SS        DF        MS        F    Sig of F

WITHIN+RESIDUAL       110892.82      167     664.03
REGRESSION            47539.28        1    47539.28     71.59    .000
SMOKE5                 5000.04        2     2500.02      3.76    .025

(Model)               62189.82        3    20729.94     31.22    .000
(Total)              173082.64      170     1018.13

R-Squared =          .359
Adjusted R-Squared = .348
```

Regression is the effect of the covariate, quality of life, and is significant ($p = .000$). After controlling for the covariate, the smoking groups differ significantly on the total IPPA (inventory of positive psychological attitudes) score ($p = .025$).

FIGURE 9-3 (END)

Effect Size Measures and Observed Power at the .0500 Level

Source of Variation	Partial ETA Sqd	Noncen- trality	Power
Regression	.300	71.592	1.000
SMOKE5	.043	7.530	.681

Variable .. QOL14 -Quality of Life
SMOKE5 -Smoking Status
Never Smoked UNWGT.   4.47664
Quit Smoking UNWGT.   4.36585
Still Smoking UNWGT.   3.69565

Adjusted and Estimated Means
Variable .. IPPATOT   TOTAL IPPA

CELL	Obs. Mean	Adj. Mean	Est. Mean	Raw Resid.	Std. Resid.
1 nonsmokers	156.654	152.334	156.654	.000	.000
2 quit smoking	155.780	153.070	155.780	.000	.000
3 still smoking	129.304	136.335	129.304	.000	.000

Figure 9-4
Computer output of analysis of covariance.

TABLE 9-1
Analysis of Covariance: Post-test Adjusted Means and Standard Deviations (SD)
for Ex-smokers and Smokers

Dependent Variable	Ex-smokers (n = 97)		Smokers (n = 17)		F
	M	(SD)	M	(SD)	
Consumption of sweets*	8.32	(2.82)	6.58	(1.26)	6.12[†]
Number of snack choices**	1.48	(1.40)	.79	(.98)	4.86[†]

*Covariate = habit scores at pretest.   [†]$p < .05$.   **Covariate = number of snacks at pretest.
(From Winkelstein, M. L., & Feldman, R. H. L. [1993]. Psychosocial predictors of consumption of sweets following smoking cessation. Research in Nursing & Health, 16, *102.)*

groups that are not currently smoking score significantly higher on positive psychological attitudes than the smoking group.

EXAMPLE FROM THE LITERATURE

In a study of psychosocial predictors of consumption of sweets following smoking cessation, Winkelstein and Feldman (1993) used ANCOVA to control for the effects of habit and pretest consumption of sweet snacks. Table 9-1 contains a table from the study. The adjusted mean scores for the two groups (ex-smokers and smokers) on each of the dependent variables (consumption of sweets and number of snack choices) are included in the table. We can see that after controlling for the effects of the two covariates, the ex-smokers (those who had stopped smoking 2 weeks earlier) scored significantly higher than the smokers on both outcome measures.

SUMMARY

ANCOVA is an extension of ANOVA that allows us to remove additional sources of variation from the error term, thus enhancing the power of our analysis. This technique is not a cure-all for difficulties with unequal groups and should be used only after careful consideration has been given to meeting the underlying assumptions. It is especially important to check for homogeneity of regression, because if that assumption is violated, ANCOVA can lead to improper interpretation of results.

APPLICATION EXERCISES AND RESULTS

EXERCISES

1. Run the analysis, and describe the results for the following research question.

   After controlling for years of education, does choice about how to spend a $500,000 gift relate to positive psychological attitudes?

Hints:

1. Only three groups have adequate numbers of subjects in the "gift" variable.

2. Be sure to check the assumption of homogeneity of regression.

RESULTS

1. To answer the research question, we ran an analysis of covariance. The covariate was years of education. The independent variable was how one would spend a $500,000 gift with three levels: invest with a broker, buy a vacation home, and pay off mortgage or purchase home. The dependent variable was the total score on the Inventory of Positive Psychological Attitudes in which the potential range of scores is from a low of 30 to a high of 210.

   First, we checked the assumption of homogeneity of regression. The output is contained in Exercise Figure 9-1. We tested to see if there was an interaction between the covariate (EDUC) and the independent variable (GIFT2). Because the interaction was not significant ($p = .328$), the assumption was met.

Tests of Between-Subjects Effects

Dependent Variable: Positive Psychological Attitudes

Source	Type III Sum of Squares	df	Mean Square	F	Sig.	Eta Squared	Noncent. Parameter	Observed Power[a]
Corrected Model	17049.0[b]	5	3409.795	3.629	.004	.108	18.143	.919
Intercept	95142.4	1	95142.4	101.250	.000	.403	101.250	1.000
GIFT2	2105.810	2	1052.905	1.120	.329	.015	2.241	.244
EDUC	8990.073	1	8990.073	9.567	.002	.060	9.567	.867
GIFT2 * EDUC	2113.258	2	1056.629	1.124	.328	.015	2.249	.245
Error	140952	150	939.677					
Total	3741279	156						
Corrected total	158000	155						

a. Computed using alpha = .05

b. R Squared = .108 (Adjusted R Squared = .078)

EXERCISE FIGURE 9-1. Test of the assumption of homogeneity of regression.

Next, we ran the analysis of covariance. The output is contained in Exercise Figure 9-2. In the table of descriptive statistics, we see that the group who would invest the money with a broker had the highest mean score on positive psychological attitudes, and those who would buy a vacation home had the lowest. The assumption of homogeneity of variance was met ($p = .435$).

In the analysis, we see that the covariate education was significantly related to positive psychological attitudes. There was no significant main effect (i.e., the three groups did not differ on their positive psychological attitude scores after controlling for their level of education). Note that the final table of means for the three groups has means that are not the same as those in the descriptive statistics table. These are the adjusted means. After adjusting for years of education, the mean for the invest with a broker group dropped from 158.95 to 157.26; for the vacation home group, the mean rose from 144.83 to 147.33; and for the pay off the mortgage group, the mean rose very slightly, from 147.85 to 147.97. Before adjustment for the covariate, the difference between the highest and lowest score was 14.13. After adjustment, the difference was 9.92.

Between-Subjects Factors

		Value Label
$500,000 gift	1.00	Invest with broker
	2.00	Vacation home
	3.00	Pay off mortgage

Descriptive Statistics

	$500,000 gift	Mean	Std. Deviation	N
Positive Psychological Attitudes	Invest with broker	158.9524	30.8892	63
	Vacation home	144.8250	29.3125	40
	Pay off mortgage	147.8491	33.7829	53
	Total	151.5577	31.9274	156

Levene's Test of Equality of Error Variances[a]

		df1	df2	Sig.
Positive psychological attitudes	.836	2	153	.435

Tests the null hypothesis that the error variance of the dependent variable is equal across groups.

a. Design: Intercept+EDUC+GIFT2

EXERCISE FIGURE 9-2. Analysis of covariance. (*continued*)

Tests of Between-Subjects Effects

Dependent Variable: Positive Psychological Attitudes

Source	Type III Sum of Squares	df	Mean Square	F	Sig.	Eta Squared	Noncent. Parameter	Observed Power[a]
Corrected Model	14935.7[b]	3	4978.572	5.290	.002	.095	15.869	.925
Intercept	96290.8	1	96290.8	102.305	.000	.402	102.305	1.000
EDUC	8948.661	1	8948.661	9.508	.002	.059	9.508	.865
GIFT2	3325.746	2	1662.873	1.767	.174	.023	3.533	.366
Error	143065	152	941.216					
Total	3741279	156						
Corrected total	158000	155						

a. Computed using alpha = .05

b. R Squared = .095 (Adjusted R Squared = .077)

Grand Mean

Dependent Variable: Positive Psychological Attitudes

Mean	Std. Error
150.8538	2.502

$500,000 gift

Dependent Variable: Positive Psychological Attitudes

$500,000	Mean	Std. Error
Invest with broker	157.2591	3.904
Vacation home	147.3346	4.919
Pay off mortgage	147.9678	4.214

EXERCISE FIGURE 9-2. (CONTINUED)

Repeated Measures Analysis of Variance

BARBARA HAZARD MUNRO

OBJECTIVES FOR CHAPTER 10

After reading this chapter, you should be able to do the following:

1 ● Describe the two major ways in which repeated measures ANOVA is used.

2 ● Explain the assumption of compound symmetry.

3 ● Interpret a repeated measures ANOVA computer printout.

4 ● Discuss difficulties that may arise with the use of this technique.

Repeated measures analysis of variance (ANOVA) is an approach that helps us deal with individual differences. These differences usually are part of the error term. Because they increase the error term, they decrease the likelihood of finding a significant result. While individual differences reflect actual differences among individuals, they also reflect the individual's state when the instrument was administered (e.g., tired, bored, angry), environmental factors (e.g., noise, heat, cold), and response styles (e.g., unwillingness to check extreme value). With repeated measures ANOVA, we may be able to measure, and thus control, some of this variation.

THE RESEARCH QUESTION

There are two main types of repeated measures designs (also called within-subjects designs). One type involves taking repeated measures of the same variable(s) over time on a group or groups of subjects. For example, if we were studying hypertension, we would probably want more than one blood pressure reading on our subjects.

The other main type of repeated measures design involves exposing the same subjects to all levels of the treatment. This is often called using subjects as their own controls. Suppose we wanted to test medications to reduce nausea during chemotherapy. We could randomly assign individuals to one of the following three conditions: medication one, medication two, or control.

However, if our subjects varied widely in the amount of nausea they experienced, the within-subject variability would be large. Because the F statistic is based on the ratio of between-group variance to within-group variance, there would have to be a very large between-group difference to attain a significant result; that is, the large variability among the subjects could obscure any real differences between the groups. This would be especially true if the groups were small. One way to remove these individual differences would be to assign each subject to all treatments. Each subject would be exposed to medication one, medication two, and the control condition in random order. Each subject would serve as his or her own control, and the within or error variance would be decreased. This would result in a more powerful test and would decrease the number of subjects needed for the study.

TYPE OF DATA REQUIRED

The between-subjects factors meet the same requirements as other ANOVA models; that is, the categories of each independent variable are mutually exclusive. The within-subjects factors contain repeated measures and are often presented as time 1, time 2, and so forth. This means that we have more than one measure on each subject. The dependent variable must be continuous and meet the assumptions described in the next section.

To test a cognitive remediation intervention on functional outcomes for clients with dementia, Quayhagen, Quayhagen, Corbeil, Roth, and Rodgers (1995) randomly assigned subjects to one of three conditions: active cognitive stimulation training, placebo (passive) activity, or wait-list control condition. Functional outcomes were measured three times: prior to the intervention, after the 12-week treatment phase, and 6 months after completion of treatment. Thus, they had a between-subjects factor, condition, consisting of three levels, and a within subjects factor, time, consisting of three time periods. They could test the effects of treatment, time, and interaction between treatment and time. Because they had more than one dependent variable, they conducted a multivariate repeated measures ANOVA. There were significant condition by time interactions. After the 12-week treatment phase, the experimental group showed improvement, while the other two groups showed declines. By 6 months after treatment, the experimental group had declined to baseline, and the other two groups declined below baseline.

An example of a within-subjects design in which subjects are used as their own control is a study of the measurement of specific gravity in infants' urine (Lybrand, Medoff-Cooper, & Munro, 1990). The urine was collected by two different methods from each baby and measured at three different times. The two methods of collection were from a collecting bag and aspiration from the diaper. The specific gravity was measured after the infant voided, 1 hour after voiding, and 2 hours after voiding. Thus, we have a design with two within-subjects measures. One is the method of collection with two levels, bag and diaper, and the other is time, with three measurements. There were no significant differences for either of the two effects. Thus, whether the urine is measured from the collecting bag or from the diaper, the resulting specific gravity measure is the same, and the measure does not change if it is measured 1 or 2 hours after the infant has voided.

ASSUMPTIONS

The basic assumptions for the *t* test and ANOVA also are necessary here. The dependent variable should be normally distributed, and the homogeneity of variance requirement should be met.

There is one major difference, however. With ANOVA, the observations are independent of each other. This is achieved by randomly assigning subjects to mutually exclusive groups. With repeated measures, however, there is correlation between the measures because they are from the same people. Therefore, the assumption of *compound symmetry* must be met.

There are two parts to this assumption. The first part is the assumption that the correlations across the measurements are the same. Suppose you measured a variable three times. You could then calculate the correlation between the first measure and the second, between the first and the third, and between the second and the third. All three of these correlations should be about the same, or $r_{12} = r_{13} = r_{23}$.

The second part of the assumption is that the variances should be equal across measurements. With three measurements, the variance of 1 = variance of 2 = variance of 3. The assumption of compound symmetry is critical. The general robustness of the ANOVA model does not withstand much violation of this assumption.

POWER AND SAMPLE SIZE CONSIDERATION

Because repeated measures generally reduce the error term, they enhance the power of the analysis, resulting in the need for fewer subjects.

REPEATED MEASURES OVER TIME

The simplest example of such an analysis is presented in Chapter 6, in which we discussed the use of the correlated *t* test to compare satisfaction with current weight to satisfaction with weight at age 18. Because the two measures of satisfaction were taken from the same subjects, the two scores were correlated. The correlated *t* test was appropriate, because it removes from the comparison of the two group means the correlation between the two measures. This increases the power of the comparison of the two means. We can extend this concept to situations with more than one group and to situations in which subjects are measured several times on the same variable.

Suppose that instead of one group measured twice, we had a true experimental design with subjects assigned randomly to an experimental group and to a control group. If we measured these subjects pre-experiment and postexperiment, we could no longer use the correlated *t* test. We would now have two groups that were measured twice. This is called a *mixed design* because we have between- and within-subjects measures. First, we have two different groups: the experimental and the control group. These two groups constitute the between-group measure. Comparing these groups answers the question of whether the experimental condition had an effect on the outcome. The second part of the design, the within-group component, concerns the fact that each group is measured twice on the same variable. The question answered here is whether there is a difference between the pretest and posttest measures. Because there are two independent variables, we also would have an interaction effect (i.e., is there an interaction between study group and time?).

Another example is presented in Figure 10-1. We want to study the effectiveness of various treatment modalities on hypertension, and we want to examine the effects over time. We randomly assign individuals with hypertension to one of three groups: drug therapy, relaxation therapy, or control. Each subject is in only one group. All subjects' blood pressure is measured at the following intervals: 1 week, 1 month, 3 months, and 6 months.

If we were to use regular one-way ANOVA to analyze these data, we would have to calculate four ANOVAs, one for each time the blood pressure was measured. The individual differences would be part of the error term.

If we use repeated measures ANOVA, we have two independent variables (rather than one independent variable measured against four different measures of the same variable). One independent variable is treatment group, with three levels. The oth-

	Treatment group			
	Drug therapy (DT) $n = 10$	Relaxation therapy (RT) $n = 10$	Control (C) $n = 10$	Row $\bar{X}_s$
1 week	$\bar{X}_{DT}$, 1 week	$\bar{X}_{RT}$, 1 week	$\bar{X}_C$, 1 week	$\bar{X}$ 1 week
1 month	$\bar{X}_{DT}$, 1 month	$\bar{X}_{RT}$, 1 month	$\bar{X}_C$, 1 month	$\bar{X}$ 1 month
3 months	$\bar{X}_{DT}$, 3 months	$\bar{X}_{RT}$, 3 months	$\bar{X}_C$, 3 months	$\bar{X}$ 3 months
6 months	$\bar{X}_{DT}$, 6 months	$\bar{X}_{RT}$, 6 months	$\bar{X}_C$, 6 months	$\bar{X}$ 6 months
Column $\bar{X}_s$	$\bar{X}_{DT}$	$\bar{X}_{RT}$	$\bar{X}_C$	

(The leftmost label for the rows 1 week–6 months is "Time".)

FIGURE 10-1
A mixed design.

er independent variable is time, with four levels. With the repeated measures approach, we can answer three main questions:

1. Do the three groups have significantly different blood pressures after treatment? All blood pressure recordings would be included here; that is, the time component is ignored, and the question is answered by comparing the three column means, $\bar{X}DT$, $\bar{X}RT$, and $\bar{X}C$ (see Fig. 10-1). If the overall F is significant, post-hoc tests would be used to find differences between pairs of scores.
2. Are there significant differences in blood pressure across the four time periods? Treatment group is ignored here, and the mean blood pressure is calculated for each of the time periods. In our example, the row means would be compared.
3. Is there an interaction between treatment type and time? Twelve means would be compared to answer this question (three levels of first independent variable times and four levels of second). In Figure 10-1, those means are shown in the cells. This would tell us whether different approaches worked better at one point than another.

Example of Computer Analysis

Figure 10-2 contains the output produced by SPSS for Windows. It is an extension of the example given in Chapter 6 for the correlated *t* test, in which we compared two measures of satisfaction with weight. The within-subjects factor (FACTOR1) has two levels, satisfaction with weight at age 18 (SATIS12) and current satisfaction with weight (SATIS11). We have added a between-subjects factor, gender, with two levels, male and female. The outcome measures are satisfaction with weight on a 10-point scale in which 1 is very dissatisfied, and 10 is very satisfied.

In the table of descriptive statistics, comparing the totals for the two time periods, we see that overall, subjects were more satisfied with their weight at age 18 (mean = 7.19) than with their current weight (mean = 6.06). We also see that within each time period, men were more satisfied with their weight than women. For example, on satisfaction with weight at age 18, the group mean for men was 7.82 and for women, 6.88.

Levene's Tests of Equality of Error Variances are listed for each of the repeated measures. These test whether subjects' mean scores have equal variances at each of the time periods. Because the *p* values are greater than .05, we know that the groups do not differ significantly in terms of variance.

Next, Box's Test of Equality of Covariance Matrices is given as the test to determine if the variance–covariance matrices are equal across all levels of the between-subjects factor. The *p* values of 0.800 indicate that the assumption has been met.

Look at the Test of Between-Subjects Effects. For GENDER1, $F = 4.873$, and $p = .029$. There is an overall difference between males and females. The power for this comparison is .593. Men reported significantly higher satisfaction with their weight across both time periods.

Before deciding which results to report for the within-subjects effects, we need to determine whether or not the assumption of compound symmetry has been met. According to Finn and Mattsson (1978), "In practice, behavioral data rarely meet the assumption of compound symmetry" (p. 83). They also state, "It is a critical assumption in the univariate analysis of repeated measures data, and is one that is not required by the corresponding 'multivariate' analysis" (p. 82). By "multivariate," Finn and Mattsson (1978) are referring to the use of more than one dependent variable in the analysis. In our example, the univariate approach is one between-subjects factor, gender, and one within-subjects factor, time, with two satisfaction with weight measures. The multivariate approach, which is less powerful than the univariate approach, would be to have one between-subjects factor, gender, no within-subjects factor, and two dependent variables, the two satisfaction measures. The multivariate approach is more robust.

Thus, if the compound symmetry requirement is *not* met, the multivariate results may be reported, rather than the univariate results. According to Finn and Mattsson (1978), "The multivariate approach to the analysis of repeated measures is not only less restrictive, but usually more realistic. Especially in longitudinal data, we expect the correlations will not be uniform. If, however, the assumptions of the univariate model are met, the univariate analysis should be used, because it is more powerful and requires fewer subjects" (p. 80).

One approach, if the assumption of compound symmetry is not met, is to use the multivariate approach. There are other approaches, however. Adjustments can be made in the degrees of freedom in the univariate approach to decrease the likelihood of type I error. This is done through the use of an "epsilon" correction. Epsilon is multiplied by the degrees of freedom in the numerator and denominator, and the new degrees of freedom are used to test the *F* value for significance.

SPSS for Windows (1996) provides three possible values of epsilon. They report, "The Greenhouse-Geisser epsilon is conservative, especially for a small sample size. The Huynh-Feldt epsilon is an alternative that is not as conservative as the Greenhouse-Geisser epsilon; however it may be a value greater than 1. . . . The lower-bound epsilon . . . represents the most conservative approach possible, since it indicates the most extreme possible departure from sphericity (p. 102)."

Mauchly's test of sphericity tests the assumption of compound symmetry. If the *p* value is greater than .05, the assumption is met. If it is less than .05, the assumption has been violated, and you should report either the multivariate results or those based on corrected degrees of freedom.

In our example, Mauchly's test of sphericity is not significant, indicating that the assumption has been met. The univariate approach is appropriate in this case. Note that all of the epsilon values equal 1.000. This is further indication that the univariate approach is appropriate, because multiplying the degrees of freedom by one will not change any of the values. When corrections are made using epsilon, the resulting degrees of freedom are smaller, thus requiring a larger value of *F* for significance.

The multivariate tests are given first. Because the assumptions were met for the univariate model, the multivariate results would not be appropriate to report. Pow-

(text continues on page 212)

Descriptive Statistics

	gender	Mean	Std. Deviation	N
satisfaction with weight at age 18	Male	7.82	2.59	57
	Female	6.88	2.58	113
	Total	7.19	2.62	170
satisfaction with current weight	Male	6.49	2.72	57
	Female	5.85	2.79	113
	Total	6.06	2.77	170

Within-Subjects Factors

Measure: MEASURE 1

FACTOR1	Dependent Variable
1	SATIS12
2	SATIS11

Between-Subjects Factors

		Value Label
gender	1	Male
	2	Female

Box's Test of Equality of Covariance Matrices[a]

Box's M	1.021
F	.335
df1	3
df2	318072
Sig.	.800

Tests the null hypothesis that the observed covariance matrices of the dependent variables are equal across groups.

a. Design:
Intercept+GENDER1
Within Subjects
Design:
FACTOR1

Levene's Test of Equality of Error Variances[a]

	F	df1	df2	Sig.
satisfaction with weight at age 18	.820	1	168	.367
satisfaction with current weight	.224	1	168	.637

Tests the null hypothesis that the error variance of the dependent variable is equal across groups.

a. Design: Intercept+GENDER1
Within Subjects Design: FACTOR1

Tests of Between-Subjects Effects

Measure: MEASURE_1
Transformed Variable: Average

Source	Type III Sum of Squares	df	Mean Square	F	Sig.	Eta Squared	Noncent. Parameter	Observed Power[a]
Intercept	13852.7	1	13852.7	1409.256	.000	.893	1409.256	1.000
GENDER1	47.900	1	47.900	4.873	.029	.028	4.873	.593
Error	1651.406	168	9.830					

a. Computed using alpha = .05

gender

Measure: MEASURE_1

gender	Mean	Std. Error
Male	7.16	.294
Female	6.36	.209

Mauchly's Test of Sphericity[a]

Measure: MEASURE_1

Within Subjects Effect	Mauchly's W	Approx. Chi-Square	df	Sig.	Epsilon[b] Greenhouse-Geisser	Huynh-Feldt	Lower-bound
FACTOR1	1.000	.000	0		1.000	1.000	1.000

Tests the null hypothesis that the error covariance matrix of the orthonormalized transformed dependent variables is proportional to an identity matrix.

a. Design: Intercept+GENDER1
   Within Subjects Design: FACTOR1

b. May be used to adjust the degrees of freedom for the averaged tests of significance. Corrected tests are displayed in the layers (by default) of the Tests of Within Subjects Effects table.

Because Mauchly's Test is not significant, univariate results are appropriate (i.e., assumption of compound symmetry has been met).

FIGURE 10-2
Computer printout of repeated measures over time. (*continued*)

Multivariate Tests[a]

Effect		Value	F	Hypothesis df	Error df	Sig.	Eta Squared	Noncent. Parameter	Observed Power[b]
FACTOR1	Pillai's Trace	.122	23.451[c]	1.000	168.000	.000	.122	23.451	.998
	Wilks' Lambda	.878	23.451[c]	1.000	168.000	.000	.122	23.451	.998
	Hotelling's Trace	.140	23.451[c]	1.000	168.000	.000	.122	23.451	.998
	Roy's Largest Root	.140	23.451[c]	1.000	168.000	.000	.122	23.451	.998
FACTOR1 * GENDER1	Pillai's Trace	.002	.396[c]	1.000	168.000	.530	.002	.396	.096
	Wilks' Lambda	.998	.396[c]	1.000	168.000	.530	.002	.396	.096
	Hotelling's Trace	.002	.396[c]	1.000	168.000	.530	.002	.396	.096
	Roy's Largest Root	.002	.396[c]	1.000	168.000	.530	.002	.396	.096

a. Design: Intercept+GENDER1
Within Subjects Design: FACTOR1

b. Computed using alpha = .05

c. Exact statistic

Tests of Within-Subjects Effects

Measure: MEASURE_1

Sphericity Assumed

Source	Type III Sum of Squares	df	Mean Square	F	Sig.	Eta Squared	Noncent. Parameter	Observed Power[a]
FACTOR1	105.501	1	105.501	23.451	.000	.122	23.451	.998
FACTOR1 * GENDER1	1.783	1	1.783	.396	.530	.002	.396	.096
Error(FACTOR1)	755.794	168	4.499					

a. Computed using alpha = .05

FACTOR1

Measure: MEASURE_1

FACTOR1	Mean	Std. Error
1	7.35	.210
2	6.17	.225

Level 1 = satisfaction with weight at age 18
Level 2 = satisfaction with current weight

FIGURE 10-2 (END)

er is very high for the within-subjects analysis and very low for the test of the interaction between gender and satisfaction with weight.

The univariate Tests of Within-Subjects Effects are given next. FACTOR1, or the within-subjects factor, is significant at the .000 level. Overall, subjects differ on their satisfaction with their weight at the two time periods. Looking at the means below, we see that subjects reported significantly higher satisfaction with their weight at age 18 (mean = 7.35) than currently (mean = 6.17).

There is no interaction between gender and time in relation to satisfaction with weight. In the table of means for time period by gender, we see that both groups reported higher satisfaction with their weight at age 18.

SUBJECTS EXPOSED TO ALL TREATMENT LEVELS

An example is given in Figure 10-3. Ten subjects are exposed to four different methods of pain control. The dependent variable is a rating by the patient of his or her perceived level of pain. This rating is taken four times, once after each treatment. Note that each cell contains only one score. Subject 1's rating of perceived pain after exposure to drug therapy (6) is the only score in the upper left cell. Because

	Treatments			
Subjects	Drug therapy	Laughter therapy	Therapeutic touch	Distraction
1	6	5	8	9
2	7	8	10	9
3	4	4	6	7
4	1	2	4	5
5	3	2	3	3
6	5	6	8	7
7	2	3	7	6
8	4	3	8	7
9	0	1	4	6
10	5	4	7	5
Col $\bar{X}_s$	3.7	3.8	6.5	6.4

FIGURE 10-3
Within-subjects design.

there is only one score in each cell, there is no variability within the cells of this design.

The total variation consists of between-subjects variation and within-subjects variation. Between-subjects variation consists of the differences among the 10 subjects in this design. Testing the significance of that amount of variation would tell us whether the row means differed significantly from each other. We are not interested in this because it tells us only whether the subjects differed from each other. We want to know whether there were differences among the treatments. By calculating the between-people variation, however, we are able to remove that source of variation from the error term. If the variability among subjects is large, the error term would be substantially reduced.

The second main source of variation is the within-subject variation. This measures how much each subject's scores varied across the treatment levels. We are interested in this. Do the subjects have lower ratings of pain with some treatments than with others? There are two components to this within-people variation. One is due to the effect of treatment, and the other is due to uncontrolled factors that influence how a subject rates his or her pain at any time.

Example of Computer Analysis of Within-Subjects Design

Figure 10-4 contains the computer output produced by analysis of the data in Figure 10-3.

There are four measures, one for each treatment: DRUG, LAUGHTER, TT (therapeutic touch), and DISTRACT (distraction); there is one within-subjects factor with four levels.

The means, standard deviations, and number in each cell are the same as in Figure 10-3. Because the Mauchly sphericity test is not significant ($p = 0.469$), the assumption of compound symmetry has been met, and the univariate test is appropriate (and more powerful).

In the table of the multivariate tests, note the measures of power. The univariate tests indicate that there is a significant overall difference among the four treatment groups ($p = 0.000$). Follow-up tests are necessary to determine where the differences lie.

Paired t tests can compare each pair of means. As would be expected from looking at the means, paired t tests demonstrate that the drug and laughter therapy group means were significantly lower than the means for therapeutic touch and distraction. Thus, we would report that drug therapy and laughter therapy are related to significantly lower reports of pain than therapeutic touch and distraction.

PROBLEMS WITH USE OF REPEATED MEASURES

When subjects are exposed to more than one treatment, we need to consider that previous treatments may still be having an effect. In drug trials, for example, time is allowed for one drug to "wash out" before a second drug is tested. Adequate time

(text continues on page 216)

Descriptive Statistics

Within-Subjects Factors

Measure: MEASURE 1

FACTOR1	Dependent Variable
1	DRUG
2	LAUGHTER
3	TT
4	DISTRACT

Measure: MEASURE 1

	Mean	Std. Deviation	N
DRUG THERAPY	3.7000	2.2136	10
LAUGHTER THERAPY	3.8000	2.0976	10
THERAPEUTIC TOUCH	6.5000	2.2236	10
DISTRACTION	6.4000	1.8379	10

Mauchly's Test of Sphericity[a]

Measure: MEASURE 1

Within Subjects Effect	Mauchly's W	Approx. Chi-Square	df	Sig.	Epsilon[b]		
					Greenhouse-Geisser	Huynh-Feldt	Lower-bound
FACTOR1	.551	4.602	5	.469	.709	.935	.333

Tests the null hypothesis that the error covariance matrix of the orthonormalized transformed dependent variables is proportional to an identity matrix.

a. Design: Intercept
   Within Subjects Design: FACTOR1

b. May be used to adjust the degrees of freedom for the averaged tests of significance. Corrected tests are displayed in the layers (by default) of the Tests of Within Subjects Effects table.

Multivariate Tests[a]

Effect		Value	F	Hypothesis df	Error df	Sig.	Eta Squared	Noncent. Parameter	Observed Power[b]
FACTOR1	Pillai's Trace	.867	15.185[c]	3.000	7.000	.002	.867	45.554	.992
	Wilks' Lambda	.133	15.185[c]	3.000	7.000	.002	.867	45.554	.992
	Hotelling's Trace	6.508	15.185[c]	3.000	7.000	.002	.867	45.554	.992
	Roy's Largest Root	6.508	15.185[c]	3.000	7.000	.002	.867	45.554	.992

a. Design: Intercept
   Within Subjects Design: FACTOR1

b. Computed using alpha = .05

c. Exact statistic

Tests of Within-Subjects Effects

Measure: MEASURE_1
Sphericity Assumed

Source	Type III Sum of Squares	df	Mean Square	F	Sig.	Eta Squared	Noncent. Parameter	Observed Power[a]
FACTOR1	73.000	3	24.333	25.269	.000	.737	75.808	1.000
Error(FACTOR1)	26.000	27	.963					

a. Computed using alpha = .05

FIGURE 10-4
Computer output of within-subjects design.

215

should be allowed to prevent carry-over effects. Pilot testing can be used to determine whether carry-over is a problem.

The latency effect is more subtle and involves an interaction with a previous treatment. Would exposure to one treatment have an enhancing or depressing effect on a subsequent treatment?

Repeated exposure to measures may result in an increase in the outcome measure that is related to the subject learning about the measure, rather than a real change. Because subjects are measured repeatedly, such things as sensitization to the instruments may cause difficulties. Scores on an anxiety scale may vary due to repeated exposure to the scale, rather than to real changes in anxiety. Even physiological measures may reflect this. For example, vital signs may increase with a new situation, then decrease with repeated measures. Practice with previous tests may increase scores on later tests. Subjects may be bored by repeated measures and be careless with later tests.

If such sequence effects are relatively small, repeated measures designs can be used. Randomizing the order in which the subjects are exposed to the treatments tends to spread the sequence effects over all the treatment levels and prevents them from being a confounding influence on only certain levels (Winer, 1971).

EXAMPLE FROM THE LITERATURE

Figure 10-5 is from the Quayhagen et al. (1995) study mentioned previously in this chapter. The purpose of the study was to test a cognitive remediation intervention on functional outcomes for clients with dementia. The experimental condition was active cognitive stimulation training. The placebo was passive activity, and the control was a wait-list condition. Functional outcomes were measured three times: prior to the intervention, after the 12-week treatment phase, and 6 months after com-

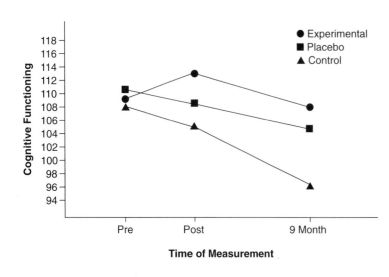

FIGURE 10-5
Mean condition differences in cognitive functioning for care receivers. (From Quayhagen, M. P., Quayhagen, M., Corbeil, R. R., Roth, P. A., & Rodgers, J. A. [1995]. A dyadic remediation program for care recipients with dementia. *Nursing Research*, 44(3), 157.)

pletion of treatment. Thus, they had a between-subjects factor, condition, consisting of three levels, and a within-subjects factor, time, consisting of three time periods. They could test the effects of treatment, time, and interaction between treatment and time. There were significant condition-by-time interactions. After the 12-week treatment phase, the experimental group showed improvement, while the other two groups showed declines. By 6 months after treatment, the experimental group had declined to baseline, and the other two groups declined below baseline.

SUMMARY

Repeated measures ANOVA is a particularly interesting technique because health care providers tend to take repeated measures on clients, and it often makes sense to do so with research subjects as well. There are stringent requirements for this analysis, however. If the requirements cannot be met and we have enough subjects, it is possible to use a multivariate approach or the epsilon correction.

APPLICATION EXERCISES AND RESULTS

EXERCISES

1. Run the appropriate analysis to answer the following questions, and write up the results:

   a. Do never married people rate their quality of life differently than married people?

   b. Do people rate their quality of life differently currently than at age 18?

   c. Is there an interaction between marital status and rating of quality of life?

   HINT: Recode MARITAL into a new variable where Never Married = 0, Married = 1, and everyone else is assigned to the missing values category.

2. Are there significant differences in the ratings of the subjects in this study on the following items within the IPPA scale: reaction to pressure (IPA2), making mistakes (IPA10), defined goals in life (IPA13), and feeling loved (IPA28)?

RESULTS

1. A repeated measures analysis of variance was run to answer these questions. The output is contained in Exercise Figure 10-1. There was one between-subjects factor, marital status, with two levels, never married and married, and one within-subjects factor, quality of life (QOL), with two levels, QOL at age 18 and currently.

   The assumption of equality of covariance matrices was met. Because Mauchly's test of sphericity was not significant, the univariate results are reported. For the within-subjects effects, there was no significant difference between ratings of QOL at the two time periods. Looking at the means, we see that the mean at age 18 was 4.42 and currently was 4.48. There was no significant interaction between QOL and marital status ($p = .632$).

(text continues on page 221)

Within-Subjects Factors

Measure: MEASURE_1

QOL	Dependent Variable
1	QOL18
2	QOLCUR

Between-Subjects Factors

		Value Label
Recoded Marital status	.00	Never married
	1.00	Married

Box's Test of Equality of Covariance Matrices[a]

Box's M	2.261
F	.739
df1	3
df2	135538
Sig.	.529

Tests the null hypothesis that the observed covariance matrices of the dependent variables are equal across groups.

a. Design: Intercept+MS
Within Subjects Design: QOL

Multivariate Tests[a]

Effect		Value	F	Hypothesis df	Error df	Sig.	Eta Squared	Noncent. Parameter	Observed Power[b]
QOL	Pillai's Trace	.002	.230[c]	1.000	134.000	.632	.002	.230	.076
	Wilks' Lambda	.998	.230[c]	1.000	134.000	.632	.002	.230	.076
	Hotelling's Trace	.002	.230[c]	1.000	134.000	.632	.002	.230	.076
	Roy's Largest Root	.002	.230[c]	1.000	134.000	.632	.002	.230	.076
QOL * MS	Pillai's Trace	.002	.230[c]	1.000	134.000	.632	.002	.230	.076
	Wilks' Lambda	.998	.230[c]	1.000	134.000	.632	.002	.230	.076
	Hotelling's Trace	.002	.230[c]	1.000	134.000	.632	.002	.230	.076
	Roy's Largest Root	.002	.230[c]	1.000	134.000	.632	.002	.230	.076

a. Design: Intercept+MS
Within Subjects Design: QOL

b. Computed using alpha = .05

c. Exact statistic

Mauchly's Test of Sphericity[a]

Measure: MEASURE_1

Within Subjects Effect	Mauchly's W	Approx. Chi-Square	df	Sig.	Epsilon[b] Greenhouse-Geisser	Huynh-Feldt	Lower-bound
QOL	1.000	.000	0	.	1.000	1.000	1.000

Tests the null hypothesis that the error covariance matrix of the orthonormalized transformed dependent variables is proportional to an identity matrix.

a. Design: Intercept+MS
   Within Subjects Design: QOL

b. May be used to adjust the degrees of freedom for the averaged tests of significance. Corrected tests are displayed in the layers (by default) of the Tests of Within Subjects Effects table.

Tests of Within-Subjects Effects

Measure: MEASURE_1
Sphericity Assumed

Source	Type III Sum of Squares	df	Mean Square	F	Sig.	Eta Squared	Noncent. Parameter	Observed Power[a]
QOL	.199	1	.199	.230	.632	.002	.230	.076
QOL * MS	.199	1	.199	.230	.632	.002	.230	.076
Error(QOL)	115.856	134	.865					

a. Computed using alpha = .05

EXERCISE FIGURE 10-1. Repeated measures analysis of variance, between- and within-subjects factors, Exercise 1. *(continued)*

219

Levene's Test of Equality of Error Variances[a]

	F	df1	df2	Sig.
quality of life at age 18	.751	1	134	.388
quality of life in past month	1.123	1	134	.291

Tests the null hypothesis that the error variance of the dependent variable is equal across groups.

a. Design: Intercept+MS
Within Subjects Design: QOL

Tests of Between-Subjects Effects

Measure: MEASURE_1
Transformed Variable: Average

Source	Type III Sum of Squares	df	Mean Square	F	Sig.	Eta Squared	Noncent. Parameter	Observed Power[a]
Intercept	4600.881	1	4600.881	2841.903	.000	.955	2841.903	1.000
MS	.117	1	.117	.072	.789	.001	.072	.058
Error	216.938	134	1.619					

a. Computed using alpha = .05

Grand Mean

Measure: MEASURE_1

Mean	Std. Error
4.45	.083

Recoded Marital Status

Measure: MEASURE_1

Recoded	Mean	Std. Error
never married	4.43	.139
married	4.47	.093

QOL

Measure: MEASURE_1

QOL	Mean	Std. Error
1	4.42	.107
2	4.48	.100

EXERCISE FIGURE 10-1. (END)

The assumption of homogeneity of variance for the between-subjects factors was met. There was no significant difference between married and never married people in their reported quality of life ($p = .789$). Looking at the means, we see that the never married group had a mean score of 4.43 and the married group, 4.47.

2. A repeated measures analysis of variance was run to answer the research question. The outcome is contained in Exercise Figure 10-2 (see pp. 222–223). There were no between-subjects factors. There were four within-subjects factors. All items were rated on a seven-point scale.

We see in the table of descriptive statistics that subjects scored themselves lowest on reaction to pressure and highest on feeling loved. Because Mauchly's test of sphericity was significant ($p = .006$), either the multivariate tests or the univariate tests with the epsilon correction is appropriate. Note that in this printout, the corrected tests are provided by default in the within-subjects effects table. "Attitude" was the name given by the researcher to designate the within-subjects factor. There is a significant effect for attitude ($p = .000$; i.e., there were significant differences across these four measures). To determine which pairs of means differ significantly, we would have to run paired t tests.

Descriptive Statistics

Within-Subjects Factors

Measure: MEASURE_1

ATTITUDE	Dependent Variable
1	IPA2
2	IPA10
3	IPA13
4	IPA28

	Mean	Std. Deviation	N
Reaction to pressure	4.12	1.76	177
Making mistakes	4.89	1.68	177
Defined goals for life	5.11	1.72	177
Feeling loved	5.82	1.47	177

Multivariate Tests[a]

Effect		Value	F	Hypothesis df	Error df	Sig.	Eta Squared	Noncent. Parameter	Observed Power[b]
ATTITUDE	Pillai's Trace	.478	53.082[c]	3.000	174.000	.000	.478	159.247	1.000
	Wilks' Lambda	.522	53.082[c]	3.000	174.000	.000	.478	159.247	1.000
	Hotelling's Trace	.915	53.082[c]	3.000	174.000	.000	.478	159.247	1.000
	Roy's Largest Root	.915	53.082[c]	3.000	174.000	.000	.478	159.247	1.000

a. Design: Intercept
Within Subjects Design: ATTITUDE

b. Computed using alpha = .05

c. Exact statistic

EXERCISE FIGURE 10-2. Repeated measures analysis of variance, within-subjects design. *(continued)*

Mauchly's Test of Sphericity[a]

Measure: MEASURE_1

| Within Subjects Effect | Mauchly's W | Approx. Chi-Square | df | Sig. | Epsilon[b] | | |
					Greenhouse-Geisser	Huynh-Feldt	Lower-bound
ATTITUDE	.910	16.430	5	.006	.947	.964	.333

Tests the null hypothesis that the error covariance matrix of the orthonormalized transformed dependent variables is proportional to an identity matrix.

a. Design: Intercept
   Within Subjects Design: ATTITUDE

b. May be used to adjust the degrees of freedom for the averaged tests of significance. Corrected tests are displayed in the layers (by default) of the Tests of Within Subjects Effects table.

Tests of Within-Subjects Effects

Measure: MEASURE_1
Sphericity Assumed

Source	Type III Sum of Squares	df	Mean Square	F	Sig.	Eta Squared	Noncent. Parameter	Observed Power[a]
ATTITUDE	260.373	3	86.791	49.268	.000	.219	147.804	1.000
Error(ATTITUDE)	930.127	528	1.762					

a. Computed using alpha = .05

Tests of Between-Subjects Effects

Measure: MEASURE_1
Transformed Variable: Average

Source	Type III Sum of Squares	df	Mean Square	F	Sig.	Eta Squared	Noncent. Parameter	Observed Power[a]
Intercept	17620.1	1	17620.1	3072.227	.000	.946	3072.227	1.000
Error	1009.410	176	5.735					

a. Computed using alpha = .05

EXERCISE FIGURE 10-2. (END)

Grand Mean

Measure:
MEASURE_1

Mean	Std. Error
4.99	.090

Correlation

Barbara Hazard Munro

OBJECTIVES FOR CHAPTER 11

After reading this chapter, you should be able to do the following:

1 • Explain when to use correlational techniques to answer research questions or test hypotheses.

2 • Be able to read a computer printout reporting correlations.

3 • Report a correlation coefficient in terms of its statistical significance and meaningfulness.

4 • Understand measures of relationship other than the Pearson Product Moment Correlation Coefficient.

5 • Know when it is appropriate to use multiple correlation, partial correlation, and semipartial correlation.

THE RESEARCH QUESTION

Correlational techniques are used to study relationships. They may be used in exploratory studies, in which one intent is to determine whether relationships exist, and in hypothesis-testing studies, in which we test a hypothesis about a particular relationship.

Lee (1991) conducted a descriptive study to explore the relationship of hardiness and current life events to perceived health in rural adults. One question she addressed was, "What relationship exists between the personality characteristic of hardiness and self-perception of health?" The correlation between hardiness and perceived health was -0.37, with a p value <0.001. What does that tell you about the relationship between these two variables? What does the negative sign indicate?

What does a value of 0.37 mean? What does the p value indicate? One aim of this chapter is to help you answer such questions.

To interpret correlation coefficients, you must know how the variables are measured. A negative sign indicates that individuals who score high on one of these variables tend to score low on the other. Does this mean that those with high hardiness scores have lower perceived health? Not in this case, because the variable "hardiness" was scored in such a way that a high score indicated low hardiness. Thus, subjects in this study who rated themselves higher on hardiness also tended to rate themselves higher on health status. To judge the strength of the relationship, one must consider the actual number of the correlation coefficient (0.37) and the associated p value (<0.001). We discuss a measure of the "meaningfulness" of the coefficient and the effect of the number of subjects on the p value in subsequent sections of this chapter.

The term *correlation* is used in everyday language. In this chapter, it concerns a relation that can be measured mathematically; we can calculate a number representing how strong a relation is. However, a correlation that shows that two variables are related does *not* mean that one variable *caused* the other. It is a mistake to infer causation from correlation alone. For example, there is a relation between the number of police cars at an accident and the amount of damage done to the vehicles and people involved. However, the police cars did not cause the damage. Therefore, although a relationship may exist, other factors also may affect the variables under study.

TYPE OF DATA REQUIRED

The Pearson Product Moment Correlation Coefficient (r) is the most usual method by which the relation between two variables is quantified and is the focus of this chapter. A brief description of other formulas, most of which have been derived from the Pearson r, is given. To calculate r, there must be at least two measures on each subject. It is often assumed that both of these measures must be at the interval level. In most cases, however, valid results also may be obtained with ordinal data. Moreover, we can code categorical variables for use with r and with regression equations. Mathematically, it is possible to use any level of data when calculating r, but factors other than the level of the data must be considered when deciding whether a correlation coefficient is appropriate.

For example, Cole and Slocumb (1995) examined the relationships between safe sexual behavior and predisposing factors in a sample of heterosexual males. See Table 11-1 for a table from their study. A "zero-order" correlation simply means a correlation between two variables. Later we talk about partial and semipartial correlations that are "higher order" correlations in that more than two variables are involved.

All of the variables were continuous. Safe sexual behavior was measured by a 4-point, 24-item scale. We see that safe sex behavior (number 6) is significantly correlated with internal health locus of control (number 2) and attitudes toward con-

TABLE 11-1
Zero-Order Correlations Among Predisposing Factors and Safe Sex Behavior

	1	2	3	4	5	6
1. Self-esteem	1.00					
2. Internal health LOC	.21*	1.00				
3. Chance health LOC	−.14*	.21*	1.00			
4. Perceived susceptibility	−.17†	−.08	.04	1.00		
5. Attitudes toward condoms	.08	.02	−.15†	.05	1.00	
6. Safe sex behavior	−.08	.16†	.01	−.05	.38*	1.00

Note: LOC = locus of control.

*$p \leq .01$. †$p \leq .05$

(From Cole, F. L., & Slocumb, E. M. [1995]. Factors in influencing safer sexual behaviors in heterosexual late adolescent and young adult collegiate males. Image, 27(3), 217–224.)

doms (number 5). Males with an internal orientation to the control of health and a positive attitude toward condoms were more likely to practice safe sexual behaviors. The other correlations between safe sexual behavior and predisposing factors were not significant.

Note two additional features of this table. First, only the bottom triangle is filled out. If the top portion would be filled out, it would duplicate the information contained in the bottom triangle. If you are not familiar with correlation matrices, take a moment to figure out why this is true. Next, note that there are 1's in the diagonal of the table. This is because, assuming no measurement error, each variable correlates perfectly with itself. The diagonals become important when we discuss factor analysis and provide information about replacing the diagonals with other numbers.

ASSUMPTIONS

Although we can calculate correlations with data at all levels, certain assumptions must be made if we are to generalize beyond the sample statistic, that is, if we are to make inferences about the population itself:

1. The sample must be representative of the population to which the inference will be made.
2. The variables that are being correlated, say X and Y, must each have a normal distribution; that is, the distribution of their scores must approximate the normal curve.
3. For every value of X, the distribution of Y scores must have approximately equal variability. This is called the *assumption of homoscedasticity*.
4. The relationship between X and Y must be linear; that is, when the two scores for each individual are graphed, they should tend to form a straight line. The points will not all fall on this line, but they should be scattered closely around it. The

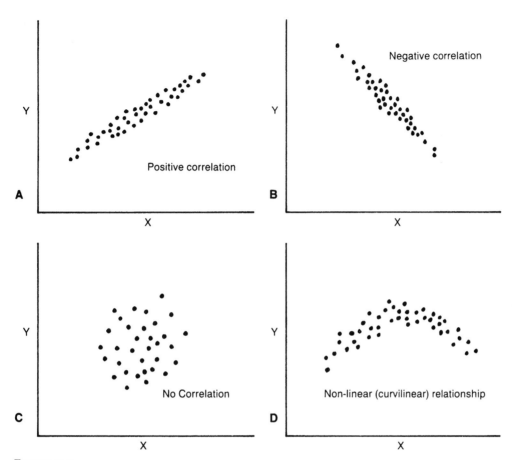

FIGURE 11-1
Linear and nonlinear relationships.

technique for graphing the relationship between two variables is demonstrated in the next section of this chapter. In Figure 11-1, *A* and *B* demonstrate linear relationships, and *D* shows a curvilinear relationship. A technique for measuring curvilinear relationships is presented later in this chapter.

POWER ANALYSIS

Cohen (1987) defines a small effect as a correlation coefficient, *r*, equal to .10; a moderate effect as *r* = .30, and a large effect as *r* = .50. For a two-tailed test with an alpha of .05, and an effect size of .30, we would need 84 subjects for a power of .80. A one-tailed test would change the requirement to 68 subjects for the same power (Cohen, 1987). What happens when we have a small sample (e.g., 20 subjects)? For a two-tailed test, with an effect size of .30 and an alpha of .05, our power would only be .25. Again, this demonstrates the importance of using adequate numbers of subjects to detect significant results.

CORRELATION COEFFICIENT

The correlation coefficient r allows us to state mathematically the relationship that exists between two variables. The correlation coefficient may range from $+1.00$ through 0.00 to -1.00. A $+1.00$ indicates a perfect positive relationship, 0.00 indicates no relationship, and -1.00 indicates a perfect negative relationship.

The correlation coefficient also tells us the *type* of relationship that exists, that is, whether the relationship is *positive* or *negative*. The relationship between job satisfaction and job turnover has been shown to be negative (we say that an *inverse* relationship exists between them). These terms mean that as one variable increases, the other decreases. People with higher job satisfaction have lower rates of job turnover and vice versa. Similarly, those with higher college grades have lower dropout rates. There is a positive relationship between graduate requirement examination (GRE) scores and graduate grades; that is, those with higher GRE scores usually have higher grades.

If you were to look at scores on two variables, as in Table 11-2, you might observe that those who scored high on one measure tended to score high on the other, and those who did poorly on one measure did poorly on the other. (It is common to use X to designate the independent variable and Y for the dependent variable.) In this example, however, it is not necessary to think of one as independent and the other as dependent. The two sets of scores might represent a quiz and an examination given to students in some class, with no notion of one causing the other.

In addition to "eyeballing" these figures, you might graph the data to see what they look like. Such a graph is called a *scatter diagram* (Fig. 11-2). To draw such a

TABLE 11-2
Subjects' Scores on Two Measures

Subjects	X	Y
1	2	1
2	5	6
3	7	9
4	3	2
5	10	8
6	1	3
7	9	10
8	4	3
9	8	9
10	6	7

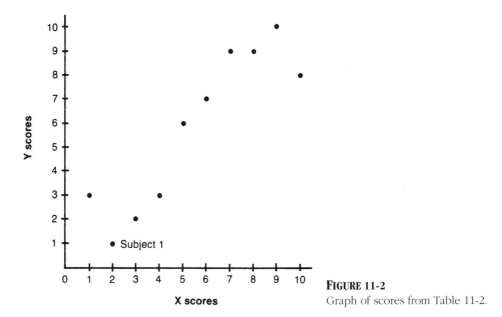

FIGURE 11-2
Graph of scores from Table 11-2.

graph, you plot the pair of scores for each subject. For subject 1, the X score was 2, so you move to 2 on the horizontal scale where the X scores are plotted. The Y score was 1, so you move straight up from the 2 on the horizontal axis to the spot opposite the 1 on the vertical axis where the Y scores are plotted. The dot that represents subject 1's scores is labeled in the graph. All other scores are plotted in the same way. In this example, the scores extend diagonally from the lower left to the upper right corner of the graph. Such a configuration indicates a positive relationship between the two scores: Low scores on X tend to go with low scores on Y and vice versa. If there were a negative relationship, high scores on one variable with low scores on the other, the dots on the graph would go from the upper left to the lower right. When no relationship exists, the dots are scattered into a central cluster, like a target (see Fig. 11-1*C*). Although the graph indicates a positive relationship between the two variables, it does not tell us how strong the relationship is. To make such a determination, we need to calculate a correlation coefficient, r.

Computer Analysis

Figure 11-3 contains output created by SPSS for Windows, 7.0 through the correlation program. We have five variables: smoking history is ordinal, scored from 0 to 2, where 0 is never smoked, 1 is quit smoking, and 2 is still smoking; depressed state of mind is also ordinal, ranging from 1, rarely, to 4, routinely; overall state of health is a 10-point rating scale where 1 is very ill and 10 is very healthy; quality of life in the past month is a 6-point scale from 1, very dissatisfied, unhappy most of the time, to 6, extremely happy, could not be more satisfied or pleased. The total score on the Inventory of Positive Psychological Attitudes (Kass et al., 1991) ranges from 30 to 210.

Correlations

		Smoking history	Depressed state of mind	Overall state of health	Quality of life in past month	Total IPPA
Pearson Correlation	Smoking history	1.000	.283**	-.231**	-.150*	-.226**
	Depressed state of mind	.283**	1.000	-.460**	-.498**	-.698**
	Overall state of health	-.231**	-.460**	1.000	.501**	.552**
	Quality of life in past month	-.150*	-.498**	.501**	1.000	.564**
	Total IPPA	-.226**	-.698**	.552**	.564**	1.000
Sig. (2-tailed)	Smoking history	.	.000	.002	.046	.003
	Depressed state of mind	.000	.	.000	.000	.000
	Overall state of health	.002	.000	.	.000	.000
	Quality of life in past month	.046	:000	.000	.	.000
	Total IPPA	.003	.000	.000	.000	.
N	Smoking history	177	177	176	176	174
	Depressed state of mind	177	177	176	176	174
	Overall state of health	176	176	176	176	173
	Quality of life in past month	176	176	176	176	173
	Total IPPA	174	174	173	173	174

**. Correlation is significant at the 0.01 level (2-tailed).

*. Correlation is significant at the 0.05 level (2-tailed).

FIGURE 11-3

Correlation coefficient produced by SPSS Windows 7.0.

This printout provides three pieces of information in three different sections of the table. In the first section, correlation coefficients are reported. The second section contains p values based on a two-tailed level of significance (you can request one-tailed values). The third section contains the number of subjects included in each analysis. Note that these numbers are somewhat different, because a pairwise deletion was used. That means that subjects were included whenever values were recorded for them on the two variables being correlated. In listwise deletion, subjects would have been excluded if data were missing on any of the five variables in the table.

If our question was which of these variables were significantly related to total IPPA score, what would the answer be? Take a minute to look at the table. We would say that all four variables were significantly related to total IPPA at the .01 level. Specifically, smoking history and depression were negatively related to positive attitude score, indicating that people who smoked more and who were more depressed reported lower levels of positive attitudes. Overall state of health and quality of life in the past month were positively related, indicating that higher levels of health and quality of life are related to more positive attitudes. You might want to look through the table for other significant relationships.

Relationships Measured With Correlation Coefficients

When using the formula with z-scores, r is the average of the cross-products of the z-scores ($r = [\Sigma zXzY]/n$). (Hopefully, this will be clear when we have taken you through this process.)

A perfect positive relationship, $+1.00$, is demonstrated in Table 11-3. The five subjects took a quiz, X, on which the scores ranged from 6 to 10 and an examination, Y, on which the scores ranged from 82 to 98. You can see that the subjects have the same *rank* on both measures. Subject 1 had the lowest score on both tests, and subject 2 had the next lowest scores on both, and so forth.

TABLE 11-3
A Perfect Positive Relationship Between Two Variables

Subjects	X	Y	zX	zY	zXzY
1	6	82	−1.42	−1.42	2.0
2	7	86	−0.71	−0.71	0.5
3	8	90	0.00	0.00	0.0
4	9	94	0.71	0.71	0.5
5	10	98	1.42	1.42	2.0

$\bar{X} = 8, s = 1.41$ $\quad$ $\bar{Y} = 90, s = 5.66$ $\quad\quad$ $\Sigma zXzY = 5.00$

$$r = \frac{\Sigma zXzY}{n} = \frac{5.00}{5} = 1$$

Because the means and standard deviations (*sd*) of the two tests are different, we cannot directly compare the scores from the two tests. We can, however, transform the scores to *z*-scores with a mean of zero and a standard deviation of 1. In Chapter 3, the formula for converting a score to a *z*-score was given as:

$$z = \frac{X - \bar{X}}{sd}$$

in which

X = individual's score

$\bar{X}$ = mean

sd = standard deviation.

In Table 11-3, the *z*-scores for the *X* variable are listed under *zX*, and the *z*-scores for the *Y* variable are under *zY*. We can now compare the *z*-scores for *X* and *Y* and see that each subject received matching *z*-scores for the two tests. This is a perfect positive correlation.

The correlation is the mean of the cross-product of the *z*-scores for each subject. This is a measure of how much each pair of scores varies together. The cross-products are labeled as *zXzY* in the table. For subject 2, the cross-product is calculated as -0.071×-0.071 and is 0.50. To take the average of the cross-products, add them and divide by the number of cross-products. Thus, the formula for *r* is $(\Sigma zXzY)/n$. The sum of the cross-products $(\Sigma zXzY)$ is 5; dividing that by 5 (the number of cross-products) results in an *r* equal to 1. The scores are plotted in Figure 11-4. When the dots are joined they form a straight line, which indicates a perfect relationship.

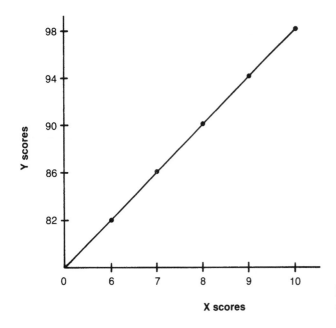

FIGURE 11-4
Graph of scores from Table 11-4.

TABLE 11-4
A Perfect Negative Correlation Between Two Variables

Subjects	X	Y	zX	zY	zXzY
1	6	98	−1.42	1.42	−2.0
2	7	94	−0.71	0.71	−0.5
3	8	90	0.00	0.00	0.0
4	9	86	0.71	−0.71	−0.5
5	10	82	1.42	−1.42	−2.0

$\bar{X} = 8, s = 1.41$ $\bar{Y} = 90, s = 5.66$ $\Sigma zXzY = -5.00$

$$r = \frac{\Sigma zXzY}{n} = \frac{-5.00}{5} = -1.00$$

To demonstrate a perfect negative correlation, reverse the scores on the Y variable (Table 11-4). Subject 1 still gets the lowest score on X but now also gets the highest score on Y. Carrying out the same procedure, the sum of the cross-products is −5; thus, $r = -5/5$, or −1, a perfect negative correlation. Figure 11-5 shows the graph of these scores.

In Table 11-5, the Y scores are scrambled in such a way that there is no relationship between the X and Y scores. These scores are plotted in Figure 11-6.

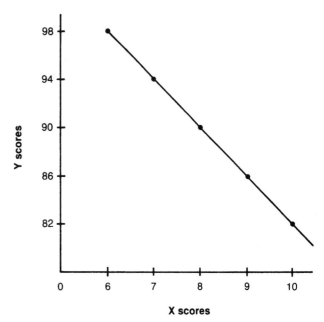

FIGURE 11-5
Graph of scores in Table 11-5.

TABLE 11-5
A Demonstration of No Relationship Between Two Variables

Subjects	X	Y	zX	zY	zXzY
1	6	94	−1.42	0.71	−1.0
2	7	82	−0.71	−1.42	1.0
3	8	90	0.00	0.00	0.0
4	9	98	0.71	1.42	1.0
5	10	86	1.42	−0.71	−1.0

$\bar{X} = 8, s = 1.41$ $\bar{Y} = 90, s = 5.66$ $\Sigma zXzY = 0.00$

$$r = \frac{\Sigma zXzY}{n} = \frac{0.00}{5} = 0.00$$

Strength of the Correlation Coefficient

How large should r be for it to be useful? As is often the case, it depends. Alternate forms of a test should be measuring the same thing, so the correlation between them should be high. With tests (such as GREs), the results of which are used in important decision making, the correlations between two forms of the same test must be very high, approximately 0.95. However, when studying the relationships among various aspects of human behavior, we may be happy with a correlation of 0.50. Some "descriptors" that can be attached to rs of varying strengths are listed below. The *di-*

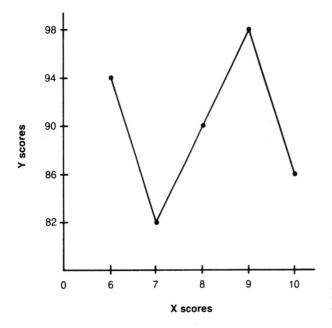

FIGURE 11-6
Graph of scores in Table 11-6.

rection of the relationship does not affect the *strength* of the relationship. A correlation of −0.90 is just as high, or just as "strong," as an *r* of +0.90. The following categories include + and − *r*s:

0.00–0.25	little if any
0.26–0.49	low
0.50–0.69	moderate
0.70–0.89	high
0.90–1.00	very high

Significance of the Correlation

If you want to generalize the *r* that you calculate from the sample to the correlation of these two variables in the population, you must determine the level of probability of *r*, that is, the probability that *r* occurred by chance alone. You may use either a one- or two-tailed test for significance, depending on whether you hypothesized about the relationship. When you use statistical programs for the computer, the exact probability of *r* may be retrieved. When you calculate *r* by hand, you can consult a table, such as that in Appendix E. The level of statistical significance is greatly affected by the size of the sample, *n*. It makes sense that if *r* is based on a sample of 1,000, there is a much greater likelihood that it represents the *r* of the population than if *r* was based on a sample of 10. With a two-tailed test and a sample of 100, an *r* of 0.20 is statistically significant at the 0.05 level, but with a sample of 10, the correlation must be 0.632 or larger to be significant. With large samples, *r*s that are described as demonstrating "little if any" relationship are statistically significant. To reiterate, the statistical significance implies that the *r* did not occur by chance; the relationship actually is greater than zero. However, a "highly significant" correlation may be quite small. For this reason, many people also speak about the *meaningfulness* of *r*.

Meaningfulness of the Correlation Coefficient

The coefficient of determination, $r2$, often is used as a measure of the "meaningfulness" of *r*. This is a measure of the amount of variance the two variables share. The circle containing X represents all the variability or variance of X, and the other circle represents the total variance for Y. The overlapping area indicates their shared variance. This area can be determined by squaring the correlation coefficient *r*. To determine the meaningfulness of an *r* of 0.20, square the coefficient: $r^2 = (0.20)^2 =$

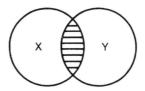

0.04, or 4%. You can then say that the variance shared between these two variables equals 4%. When reporting this, researchers usually say that the independent variable, X, accounts for 4% of the variance of the dependent variable. Obviously, this is not very much, because another 96% of variance is not accounted for. To account for approximately half of the variance, you would need an r of 0.70 (because 0.70^2 = 0.49, or 49%).

Confidence Intervals

We constructed confidence intervals around mean scores and stated that 95% (or 99%) of the confidence intervals would include the population mean. We also may construct confidence intervals around r. This is another way of determining the meaning of the r you calculate.

Transforming r Values

Methods for testing differences between means and developing confidence intervals are based on the characteristics of the normal curve. When a distribution is asymmetric, these methods are not appropriate. When the value of r in the population exceeds approximately 0.25, the sampling distribution becomes skewed and becomes more skewed as the value of r increases (Thorndike, 1988). Thus, before rs in different samples can be compared and before confidence intervals can be constructed, the r values must be transformed to values for which distribution will be symmetric. This transformation is known as Fisher's z. Appendix F contains a table that can be used to transform r values into z_r values.

When comparing r values from two different groups, you would transform the r values to z_r values, and then apply the t test (or analysis of variance) to the z_r values to determine whether they were statistically different. You would also transform r values to z_rs before attempting to average them. We demonstrate the use of Fisher's z_r values in constructing confidence intervals.

Calculation of Confidence Intervals

To set up the confidence interval around a given r, r must first be transformed into a *Fisher's* z_r using the table in Appendix F. For example, assume that we had 103 subjects and an r of 0.9.

The first step is to convert r to z_r. In Appendix F, note that an r of 0.9 equals a z_r of 1.472.

The second step is to determine the standard error. The formula for the standard error is $1/\sqrt{n-3}$. In this example, that is $1/\sqrt{103-3} = 0.1$.

The third step is to determine the confidence interval to choose. The 95% and 99% levels are commonly used. The formulas follow:

$$95\% = Z_r \pm (1.96) \text{ (standard error)}$$
$$99\% = Z_r \pm (2.58) \text{ (standard error)}$$

For our example, they become the following:

$$95\% = 1.472 \pm (1.96)\ (0.1) = 1.276 \text{ and } 1.668$$
$$99\% = 1.472 \pm (2.58)\ (0.1) = 1.214 \text{ and } 1.730$$

The fourth step is to transform the z_rs back to rs using Appendix F. When using the table, you will see that not every possible z_r is listed. Select the one closest to the number you calculated.

a. 95%: z_rs = 1.276 and 1.668; after transformation back to rs, they become 0.855 and 0.930, respectively.

b. 99%: z_rs = 1.214 and 1.730; after transformation back to rs, they become 0.840 and 0.940, respectively.

The fifth step is to set up the confidence intervals.

Note that the confidence intervals are not symmetric around the r value.

Level	Confidence Interval for r
a. 95%	0.855–0.930
b. 99%	0.840–0.940

BRIEF DESCRIPTION OF OTHER MEASURES OF RELATIONSHIP

There are measures other than the Pearson r for measuring relationships. An overview is given here, but computational formulas are not presented. Three "short-cut" versions of r are *phi, point-biserial,* and *Spearman rho.*

Short-Cut Versions of r

Many researchers assume that short-cut versions of r are different from Pearson's r and that applying r and one of these formulas to a set of data would result in different results. Actually, these measures usually give the same result as r. The only advantage of using them is when doing hand calculations. They are really short-cut versions of r that can be used with specific types of data.

Phi

When both variables being correlated are *dichotomous,* that is, each has only two levels, a short-cut version of r can be used. Examples of dichotomous variables include gender (male and female), a yes or no response choice, and pass or fail. When using the computer to analyze your data, you can use r and will get exactly the same result as if you had used phi. See Chapter 5 for a more complete description of phi.

Point-Biserial and Spearman Rho

When you want to correlate one dichotomous variable with one continuous variable, you can use the point-biserial formula. When you have two sets of ranks, you can use the Spearman rho formula. You might ask two groups to rank a list of stressors from most stressful to least stressful. You could compare the rankings of the two groups by using the Spearman rho formula. Spearman rho is often called a *non-parametric* test, as though it were distribution free, which is not true. It is better thought of as a short-cut version of *r*.

Nonparametric Measures

Kendall's Tau

This measure is a nonparametric measure and is not a short-cut formula for *r*. It was developed as an alternate procedure for Spearman rho. It is sometimes used when measuring the relation between two ranked (ordinal) variables. Kendall's tau might be an alternative if your data seriously violated the assumptions underlying *r*. It can be calculated using most of the major computer packages, such as SAS or SPSS.

Contingency Coefficient

One nonparametric technique can be used to measure the relationship between two nominal level variables. The variables need not be dichotomous but may have multiple levels. For example, this technique could be used to determine the relationship between race and political affiliation.

To calculate this coefficient, you must use the chi-square statistic, which is discussed in Chapter 5.

Estimating r

Two formulas are not short-cut versions of *r* but estimate results that might be obtained using *r*. Nunnally and Bernstein (1994) recommend that these techniques should *not* be used. Because they are sometimes reported in the literature and often mentioned in statistics texts, they are outlined here.

Biserial

This technique can be used when one variable is dichotomized and the other is continuous. *Dichotomized* means that the variable has been made dichotomous, cut into two levels from a variable that would have been naturally continuous. For example, scores could be divided into high and low, creating a dichotomized variable. A biserial correlation estimates what the correlation would be if you changed the dichotomized variable into a continuous variable (perhaps by including the entire range of scores). Nunnally and Bernstein (1994) argue against such a use, stating that the resulting coefficient is usually artificially high.

Tetrachoric

This coefficient estimates r from the relationship between two dichotomized variables. If there are serious problems with estimating r from one dichotomized variable (biserial), there are obviously even more difficulties with estimating r from two dichotomized variables.

"Universal" Measure

We have been discussing the relationship between two variables that have a linear relationship. When we graph these relationships, they suggest a straight line across the graph. Although the relationship may be positive or negative, it is the same across all the scores. An example of a nonlinear relationship can be seen in Figure 11-1D. In this case, low scores on the X variable are related to low scores on the Y variable, but high scores on X also are related to low scores on Y. Such a relationship is called *curvilinear*. An example might be the possible relationship between anxiety and test scores. In this graph, those with moderate anxiety could perform the best on tests. Those with very low or very high anxiety perform poorly. There is a real advantage to having data plotted to determine whether a nonlinear relationship exists, because r cannot be used to test such a relationship.

Eta

Eta, sometimes called the *correlation ratio,* can be used to measure a nonlinear relationship. The range of values for eta is from 0 to +1. It can be used with all variables, whether nominal or continuous. Eta is closely related to r and has been called a "universal" relationship because it can be used regardless of the form of the relationship (Nunnally & Bernstein, 1994). When it is used with two continuous variables that have a linear relationship, it reduces to r.

PARTIAL CORRELATION

When discussing research design, we confront the notion of "control." How do we "control" variance that will distract or mislead us? There are several ways. If we are concerned about the impact of a variable, such as age, we might use random assignment of subjects to groups as a method of control, we might select only one age group, or we might match subjects by age before assigning them to groups. There also are statistical measures of control: We can record the age of the subjects and use that as a variable in the study. One method of statistical control is *partial correlation.*

This technique also allows us to describe the relationship between two variables (or more, if you go to multiple partial correlation) after statistically controlling for the influence of some third variable. When studying research design, you learned that the relationship between two variables may be unclear because of the confounding influence of another variable. For example, if you calculate the correlation between mental age and height in children 1 to 10 years of age, you will find a high correlation. Does that mean that height causes intelligence? The key factor is age, not height. Once you control for age, the relationship between height and mental age becomes trivial.

One study was conducted to determine whether the number of hours studied was related to grades; the researchers found a negative correlation. This does not mean that studying less results in higher grades. Once they controlled for intelligence, the researchers found a significant positive relation between grades and hours of study. (Although that study indicates that "smarter" people study fewer hours, more recent evidence suggests that in most cases, brighter students study more.)

Partial correlations may be written as $r_{12.3}$. This indicates that you are measuring the correlation between variables 1 and 2 with the effect of variable 3 removed from *both* the variables being correlated. Consider the example of college grades (variable 1) with hours of study (variable 2) and intelligence (variable 3). If we used partial correlation to study this relationship, the correlation between intelligence and grades (r_{13}) is removed, and the correlation between intelligence and hours of study (r_{23}) also is removed. The confounding influence of intelligence is thus removed statistically, and the relationship between grades and hours of study can be measured accurately. Partial correlation also may be written as $r_{y1.2}$, which would indicate the correlation of an independent variable, 1, with a dependent variable, y, with the effect of variable 2 removed from the independent and dependent variables.

SEMIPARTIAL CORRELATION

This is the correlation of two variables with the effect of a third variable removed from only *one* of the variables being correlated. It is closely tied to multiple correlation, as is discussed in the next section. Semipartial correlation may be written as $r_{1(2.3)}$ or $r_{y(1.2)}$. The first way indicates the correlation between variables 1 and 2 with the effect of variable 3 removed from 2 alone; the second way indicates the correlation between the dependent variable, y, and an independent variable, 1, with the effect of variable 2 removed from 1 alone. The following diagram explains further.

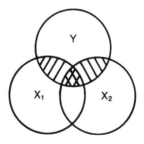

The circles represent the amount of variance of each of the variables. Remember that the variance shared by two variables is measured by r^2. If we take variable X_1 into account first, the variance accounted for in Y equals the variance contributed by X_1 (r^2_{y1}), plus the unique variance accounted for by X_2. That unique variance is the variance shared between Y and X_2 after the effect of X_1 on X_2 has been removed (or after the cross-hatched area has been subtracted). The squared semipartial correlation between X_2 and Y is the unique variance contributed by X_2 ($r^2_{y(2.1)}$). Therefore, in this case, R^2 (the squared multiple correlation, which is explained more fully in the following section) = the r^2 between X_1 and Y + the semipartial correlation squared between X_2 and Y, or $R^2 = r^2_{y1} + r^2_{y(2.1)}$.

MULTIPLE CORRELATION

We have been discussing correlation as measuring the relationship between two variables. This concept can be extended to one in which the relationship is measured between one variable and a combination of other variables. When discussing r, we were talking about one independent variable (X) and one dependent variable (Y). In multiple correlation (R), we are talking about more than one independent variable (X_1, X_2, X_3, and so on) and one dependent variable (Y). It is also possible to have more than one dependent variable (Y_1, Y_2, Y_3, and so on); this is called *canonical correlation* and is discussed in Chapter 12.

The multiple correlation, R, can go from 0 to 1. There are no negative Rs because the method of least squares is used to calculate R, and squaring numbers eliminates negatives. R^2 is the amount of variance accounted for in the dependent variable by the combination of independent variables. When reporting multiple correlations, R^2, rather than R, is often presented.

As we demonstrated in the discussion of semipartial correlation, the calculation of the squared multiple correlation, R^2, may require more than simply adding the squared correlation of each independent variable with the dependent variable. This is because if there were no correlation between the independent variables, the correlations might be as follows:

	X_1	X_2	Y
X_1	1.00	0.00	0.40
X_2	0.00	1.00	0.30

This could be depicted as:

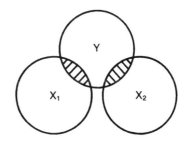

In this case, there is no overlap between variables X_1 and X_2. They are not correlated; thus, each accounts for a different portion of the variance in Y. We could add up their squared correlation (r^2s) with Y ($[0.40]^2$s + $[0.30]^2$) and determine that $R_2 = 0.25$.

Usually in behavioral research, however, the independent variables are correlated among themselves as depicted in the following:

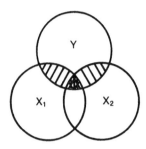

In this case, there is correlation between X_1 and X_2, and if you add up the squared correlation of X_1 with Y and the squared correlation of X_2 with Y, you would add in the cross-hatched area twice. The variance accounted for in Y is actually all that is explained by one of the variables plus the *additional* variance explained by the second variable. The additional variance is measured by the squared semipartial correlation of the second variable with the dependent variable. If X_1 is counted first, it accounts for all of its shared variance with Y, and X_2 adds the variance that it alone contributes (its shared variance with Y minus the cross-hatched area). The first variable gets "credit" for the first piece of variance accounted for, even though it shares some of that with X_2. The order of entry of variables into a multiple correlation may be important when understanding the relationships being studied. This is discussed in more detail in Chapter 12. Multiple correlation is a technique for measuring the relationship between a dependent variable and a weighted combination of independent variables.

EXAMPLE FROM THE LITERATURE

Table 11-6 contains a correlation matrix from an article by Friedman and King (1994). Three variables, symptom severity, emotional support, and negative affect, are significantly related to satisfaction with life. However, we cannot add up the squared correlations for each of these variables to determine the multiple correlation of these variables with satisfaction with life. Note that the relationship between two of these predictor variables, symptom severity and negative affect is .47, which is significant at the .001 level. Thus, there is considerable overlap between these two variables. Multiple regression, discussed in the next chapter, is used to clarify these relationships.

TABLE 11-6
Correlation Matrix of Study Variables (N = 80)

	1	2	3	4	5	6
1. Symptom severity		.05	.02	.47**	.00	−.47**
2. Tangible support			.37†	−.23*	.20	.06
3. Emotional support				−.14	.37**	.31†
4. Negative affect					.06	−.45**
5. Positive affect						.05
6. Satisfaction with life						

*$p < .05$.   †$p < .01$.   **$p < .001$.

(From Friedman M. M., & King K. B. [1994]. The relationship of emotional and tangible support to psychological well-being among older women with heart failure. Research in Nursing & Health, 17, 437).

SUMMARY

Correlation is a procedure for quantifying the relationship between two or more variables. It measures the strength and indicates the direction of the relationship. Multiple correlation measures the relationship between one variable and a weighted composite of the other variables. Partial correlation is a statistical method for describing the relationship between two variables, with the effect of another confounding variable removed. In semipartial correlation, the influence of a third variable is removed from only one of the variables being correlated.

APPLICATION EXERCISES AND RESULTS

EXERCISES

1. What are the correlations between the following variables: age, years of education, smoking history, satisfaction with current weight, overall state of health, confidence during stressful situations, and life purpose and satisfaction?

RESULTS

1. The correlations are contained in Exercise Figure 11-1. Many questions could be answered. For example, we might look at what variables are related to overall state of health. We would see that age and smoking history are inversely related (i.e., those who are older and smoke more report lower levels of health). Higher levels of education, satisfaction with current weight, confidence, and life satisfaction are all positively related to overall health.

Correlations

		Subject's age	Education in years	Smoking History	Satisfaction With Current Weight	Overall State of Health	Confidence During Stressful Situations	Life Purpose and Satisfaction
Pearson Correlation	Subject's age	1.000	-.063	.114	-.200**	-.228**	-.053	-.081
	Education in years	-.063	1.000	-.137	.065	.269**	.246**	.281**
	Smoking history	.114	-.137	1.000	.037	-.244**	-.140	-.290**
	Satisfaction with current weight	-.200**	.065	.037	1.000	.467**	.261**	.249**
	Overall state of health	-.228**	.269**	-.244**	.467**	1.000	.455**	.579**
	Confidence during stressful situations	-.053	.246**	-.140	.261**	.455**	1.000	.800**
	Life purpose and satisfaction	-.081	.281**	-.290**	.249**	.579**	.800**	1.000
Sig. (two-tailed)	Subject's age		.420	.140	.009	.003	.489	.300
	Education in years	.420		.079	.408	.000	.001	.000
	Smoking history	.140	.079		.633	.001	.064	.000
	Satisfaction with current weight	.009	.408	.633		.000	.000	.001

Sig. (2-tailed)							
Overall state of health	.003	.000	.001	.000	.	.000	.000
Confidence during stressful situations	.489	.001	.064	.000	.000	.	.000
Life purpose and satisfaction	.300	.000	.000	.001	.000	.000	.
N							
Subject's age	170	165	169	168	169	170	167
Education in years	165	168	166	166	167	168	165
Smoking history	169	166	175	173	174	175	172
Satisfaction with current weight	168	166	173	175	175	175	172
Overall state of health	169	167	174	175	176	176	173
Confidence during stressful situations	170	168	175	175	176	177	174
Life purpose and satisfaction	167	165	172	172	173	174	174

**. Correlation is significant at the 0.01 level (2-tailed).

EXERCISE FIGURE 11-1. Correlation coefficients.

Regression

Barbara Hazard Munro

Objectives for Chapter 12

After reading this chapter, you should be able to do the following:

1 • Know when it is appropriate to use regression techniques.

2 • Understand the statistics generated by the regression procedure.

3 • Set up and solve a prediction equation.

4 • Explain the difference between testing the significance of R^2 and the significance of a *b*-weight.

5 • Code categorical variables.

6 • Discuss methods for selecting variables for entry into a regression equation.

7 • Understand the statistics generated by a canonical correlation.

8 • Interpret the results section of research studies that report these techniques.

The Research Question

We are constantly interested in predicting one thing based on another. We want to predict the weather to plan our weekend. We want to predict how well a student will do in nursing practice. We want to predict how long a patient may remain ill. Countless predictions are necessary for us to move through life.

A brilliant statistical invention is regression, which permits us to make predictions from some known evidence about some unknown future events. Only about a century old, regression is the basis of many statistical methods, and in this book, there is nothing more important to understand.

Regression makes use of the correlation between variables and the notion of a straight line to develop a prediction equation. Once a relationship has been established between two variables, it is possible to develop an equation that will allow you to predict the score of one of the variables, given the score of the other. In the case of a multiple correlation, regression is used to establish a prediction equation in which the independent variables are each assigned a weight based on their relationship to the dependent variable. For example, in the study of factors influencing safer sexual behaviors in heterosexual late adolescent and young adult collegiate males (Cole & Slocumb, 1995) discussed in Chapter 11, the authors used multiple regression to assess the importance of the predictor variables. With the correlations described in Chapter 11, Cole and Slocumb found two variables related to safe sex behavior, internal health locus of control and attitudes toward condoms. However, the multiple regression results found that in addition to these two variables, self-esteem was significantly negatively related to safe sex behaviors.

Regression is a useful technique that allows us to *predict* outcomes and *explain* the interrelationships among variables. The type of data required and the underlying assumptions are the same for regression as for correlation. We repeat them here for your convenience. Information about testing assumptions is provided later in this chapter in the discussion of the testing of residuals.

TYPE OF DATA REQUIRED

To calculate r, there must be at least two measures on each subject. It is often assumed that both of these measures must be at the interval level. In most cases, however, valid results also may be obtained with ordinal data. Moreover, we can code categorical variables for use with r and with regression equations. Mathematically, it is possible to use any level of data when calculating r, but factors other than the level of the data must be considered when deciding whether a correlation coefficient is appropriate.

ASSUMPTIONS

Although we can calculate correlations with data at all levels, certain assumptions must be made if we are to generalize beyond the sample statistic, that is, if we are to make inferences about the population itself:

1. The sample must be representative of the population to which the inference will be made.
2. The variables that are being correlated, say X and Y, must each have a normal distribution; that is, the distribution of their scores must approximate the normal curve.
3. For every value of X, the distribution of Y scores must have approximately equal variability. This is called the *assumption of homoscedasticity.*

4. The relationship between X and Y must be linear; that is, when the two scores for each individual are graphed, they should tend to form a straight line. The points will not all fall on this line, but they should be scattered closely around it.

POWER ANALYSIS

Multiple regression is a useful technique, but there are numerous examples of its misuse. A major problem is including too many variables for the number of subjects. Computer programs provide an adjusted R and the actual R^2. It is a more conservative estimate given the number of subjects and variables. It also has been called a *shrinkage formula,* because it predicts how much the R^2 is likely to shrink. There are several formulas for this adjustment; one is given here:

$$\text{Adjusted} \quad R^2 = 1 - (1 - R^2)\ \frac{n - 1}{n - k - 1}$$

The formula is based on the number in the sample (n) and the number of independent variables (k). The more variables compared to subjects, the greater the shrinkage will be. If you put in the same number of subjects as independent variables, you will get a perfect R (1) no matter which variables you use. (However, the *adjusted R* will be zero.) Thus, you must always consider the number of subjects and independent variables. Very high and seemingly impressive R^2s may be an artifact of too few subjects. Nunnally and Bernstein (1994) state that one should have at least 10 subjects per predictor "in order to even hope for a stable prediction equation" (p. 201).

Cohen (1987) provides a formula for determining sample size, given an effect size index, which he calls L. He defines a small effect as an R^2 of 0.02, a moderate effect as an R^2 of 0.13, and a large effect as an R^2 of 0.30. The formula is:

$$N = \frac{L(1 - R^2)}{R^2} + u + 1,$$

where N = total sample size

   L = effect size index

   u = number of independent variables

L can be obtained from a table and is defined by Cohen as a function of power and number of independent variables at a given level of alpha. For our example, we select a power of 0.80, an alpha of 0.05, a moderate effect size, and two different numbers of independent variables to determine appropriate sample sizes.

For three independent variables, the value of L is 10.90, and the formula is:

$$N = \frac{10.90(1 - 0.13)}{0.13} + 3 + 1$$

$$N = 77.$$

For six independent variables, the value of L is 13.62, and the formula is:

$$N = \frac{13.62(1 - 0.13)}{0.13} + 6 + 1$$

$$N = 98$$

Software programs also can calculate sample size. Sample size must be determined prior to data collection to ensure an adequate sample to conduct the proposed analyses.

It is possible to increase the accuracy of the prediction by adding predictor variables to the equation. The best additional variables to add are highly correlated with the dependent variable but not highly correlated with the other independent variables. Usually four or five predictors are enough. Adding more than that adds little to the R^2 because of intercorrelations among the predictors.

Because the analysis uses error variance and true variance, the multiple correlation is usually inflated by such error variance. In addition to the shrinkage formula, another way to evaluate the R^2 is to calculate it with a second sample. This is called *cross-validation*. A weakness of multiple regression is a tendency to throw variables into the equation. There should be some rationale for each variable included.

SIMPLE LINEAR REGRESSION

We begin by explaining *simple* regression. A correlation between two variables is used to develop a prediction equation. The techniques described in this chapter are for predictions based on a *linear* relationship between variables. If the relationship is curvilinear, other techniques, such as trend analysis, must be used.

If the correlation between two variables were perfect ($+1$ or -1), we would be able to make a perfect prediction about the score on one variable, given the score on the other variable. We never get perfect correlations, so we are never able to make perfect predictions. The higher the correlation, the more accurate the prediction. If there were no correlation between two variables, knowing the score of one would not help in estimating the score on the other. When you have no information to aid you in predicting a score, your best guess for any subject would be the mean, because that is the center of the data.

To be able to make predictions, the relationship between two variables, the independent (X) and the dependent (Y), must be measured. If there is a correlation, a regression equation can be developed that will allow prediction of Y given X. For example, in the study previously mentioned, Cole and Slocumb (1995) regressed safe sex behavior on predisposing factors, which included attitude toward condoms, internal health locus of control, self-esteem, chance health locus of control, and perceived susceptibility. They reported a multiple R of .46. R squared was .21, indicating that 21% of the variance in safe sex behavior was explained by the predictors ($p = 0.01$). Seventy-nine percent of the variation was not explained by this model.

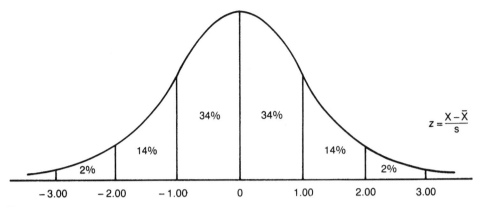

FIGURE 12-1
Normal curve with standardized scores.

Understanding Regression Through the Use of Standard Scores

In previous chapters, standard scores (z-scores) are used to explain the concepts of standard deviation and correlation. Remember that once scores have been converted to z-scores, they have a mean of 0 and a standard deviation of 1 (Fig. 12-1). Direct comparisons between sets of z-scores can be made, because they are measured on the same scale. Given z-scores, the formula for a prediction (regression) equation is simple. It is $Y' = rX$, where Y' is the predicted score, and X is the "known" or predictor variable. Given a perfect positive correlation, $Y' = X$. For example, someone with a z-score of +2 on X would also score +2 on Y.

$$Y' = (1)(2)$$

Chapter 11 shows that with a perfect positive correlation ($r = +1$), everyone receives exactly the same z-score on Y as on X. With a perfect negative correlation ($r = -1$), each subject receives exactly the opposite z-score on Y as on X. For example, someone with a -3 on X would get a +3 on Y'.

$$Y' = (-1)(-3) = +3$$

As previously mentioned, if there is *no* correlation between the variables, *no* prediction can be made, and our "best guess" for Y' is the mean. Using the formula for Y', with $r = 0$ and $X = +3$, we calculate Y' as $(0)(3) = 0$. Zero is, of course, the mean of a z-score distribution. These extreme cases, perfect correlations and zero correlations, however, are uncommon in the world of research. Therefore, consider what happens with more reasonable correlations. Suppose an individual, Jill, scored +2 on X. Given the following rs, what Y score would you predict for Jill? Work these equations before continuing.

$$r = -0.20$$
$$r = 0.60$$
$$r = 0.20$$
$$r = -0.60$$

For $r = -0.20$, our equation would be $Y' = (-0.20)(2)$ or -0.40. The other answers are, respectively, 1.20, 0.40, and -1.20. If you predicted each Y score correctly, you have mastered this simplest type of prediction, for which you have only the standard scores and the correlation coefficient.

Regression literally means a falling back toward the mean. With perfect correlations, there is no falling back; the predicted score is the same as the predictor. With less than perfect correlations, there is some error in the measurement, and we would expect that in the case of an individual who received an extremely high score, chance may have been working in her favor; therefore, on a second measure, her score would be somewhat less—it would have fallen back toward the mean. In the same way, an individual with an extremely low score perhaps had all the fates against her and on a second measure would do better, thus moving her score closer to the mean.

Each prediction regresses toward the mean, depending on the strength of the correlation. If there is no correlation ($r = 0$), $Y' = 0$ (the mean). As the correlation

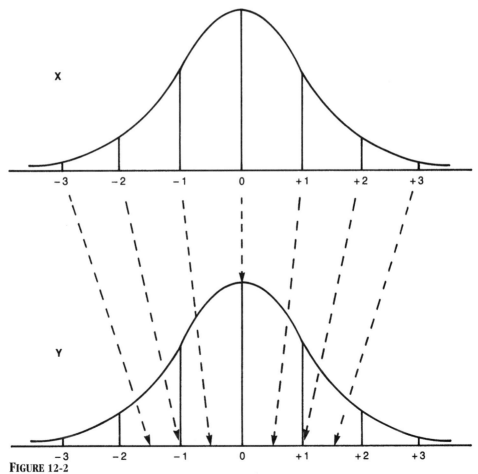

FIGURE 12-2
Predicting from X to Y, with $r = 0.50$.

rises toward 1, Y' moves proportionately outward from the mean, toward the position of the X predictor. The correlation coefficient tells us exactly what percentage of this distance Y' moves. Figure 12-2 shows predictions based on an r of 0.50. Note on the figure that all the predicted scores (Y's) are halfway between the mean and the X-score. This is because the correlation is 0.5. (If the correlation had been 0.7, the Y'-scores would have moved 0.7 times the distance between the mean and X.) If the X-score is above the mean, the predicted score will be lower than the X-score and closer to the mean. With an r of 0.5 and an X-score of $+2$, $Y' = (0.5)(2) = 1$. With a correlation of 0.5, an individual who was 2 standard deviations above the mean would be predicted to be 1 standard deviation above the mean on Y.

If the X-score is below the mean, the predicted score is higher and closer to the mean. An X-score of -3 would result in a predicted score of $(0.5)(-3) = -1.5$. Remember that these are predictions based on a correlation of 0.5, so you would not be able to predict perfectly an individual's score. The person's actual score will differ from the predicted score. This discrepancy between predicted and actual scores reflects the error in the prediction and is discussed more fully in the next section of this chapter. Because most measures will not be in z-scores, we now present the more general regression equation.

Regression Equation

The regression equation is the equation for a straight line and is written as:

$$Y' = a + bX$$

Y' is the predicted score.

Given data on X and Y from a sample of subjects called the *regression sample,* a and b can be calculated. With these two measures Y can be predicted, given X. The letter a is called the *intercept constant* and is the value of Y when $X = 0$. It is the point at which the regression line intercepts the Y axis. The letter b is called the *regression coefficient* and is the rate of change in Y with a unit change in X. It is a measure of the slope of the regression line.

An example is given in Figure 12-3. The intercept constant, a, is equal to 3; you can see that is the value of Y when $X = 0$. It is the point at which the regression line connects with the Y axis. The regression coefficient, b, $= 0.5$. This means that the value of Y goes up 0.5 of a point for every 1-point change in X. When $X = 0$, $Y = 3$, and when X goes up to 1, Y goes up to 3.5. As you will see when we are calculating a and b, a is based on the means of the two variables, and b is based on the correlation between them.

The regression line is the "line of best fit" and is formed by a technique called the *method of least squares.* The concept of least squares is presented in Chapter 2 with a discussion of characteristics of the mean. Because the mean is (in one sense) the center of the data, the sum of the deviations of the scores around the mean, $\Sigma(X - \bar{X})$, is 0. Also, if you square these deviations and add them, that number will be smaller than the sum of the squared deviations around any other measure of central tendency. In the same way, the regression line passes through the exact center

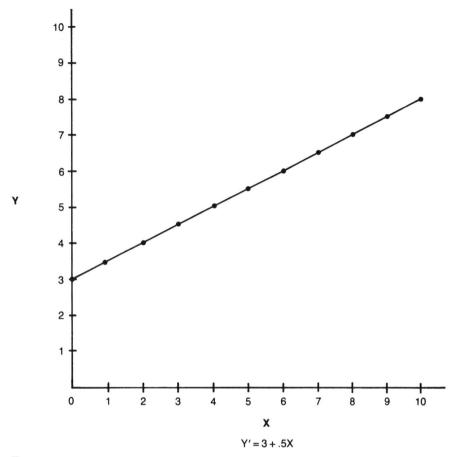

$$Y' = 3 + .5X$$

FIGURE 12-3
The regression line.

of the data in the scatter diagram. Therefore, it is the "line of best fit." There are deviations around the regression line, just as there are deviations around the mean. The regression line represents the predicted scores (Y's), but because a prediction is not perfect, the actual scores (Ys) would deviate somewhat from the predicted scores. Because the regression line passes through the center of the pairs of scores, if you add up the deviations from the regression line ($Y - Y'$), they will equal 0. Also, if you square those deviations and add them, the sum of the squared deviations around the regression line is smaller than the sum of the squared deviations around any other line drawn through the scatter diagram.

If Cole and Slocumb (1995) applied their prediction equation to the patients in their sample, they would find that the clients' *actual* score on safe sex behavior (Y) would vary from their *predicted* (Y') score. Because the correlations between the predictors and the outcome measure were not perfect, there is error in the prediction. Even using the sample on which the prediction equation was calculated, there will be differences between Y and (Y'). $Y - Y'$ equals the deviations from the predicted scores just as $X - \bar{X}$ equals the deviations around the mean. The regression equation minimizes the squared differences of the predicted score from the actual score.

Given a regression equation of $Y' = 4 + 0.2X$ and three individuals with scores on X of 5, 10, and 20, respectively, the predicted scores for the three would be calculated as follows:

$$a + \quad bX \quad = Y'$$

1. $4 + (0.2)\ (5) = 5$
2. $4 + (0.2)(10) = 6$
3. $4 + (0.2)(20) = 8$

Confidence Intervals

Because there is error in predictions, we need to know how accurate a prediction is. The standard error of estimate can be used to construct confidence intervals around predicted scores. The standard error of estimate is the standard deviation of the errors of prediction. We use that in the same way that we use the standard errors of the mean and the correlation coefficient to construct confidence intervals. Given a predicted score, we can then say that 95% or 99% of the confidence intervals will capture the actual score. (See Chapters 3 and 4 for a more complete description of confidence intervals.)

MULTIPLE REGRESSION

Multiple regression is possible when there is a measurable multiple correlation between a group of predictor variables and one dependent variable. The prediction equation is:

$$Y' = a + b_1 X_1 + b_2 X_2 + b_3 X_3 + \ldots b_k X_k$$

There is still one intercept constant, a, but each independent variable (e.g., X_1, X_2, X_3) has a separate b-weight. Given a prediction equation of:

$$Y' = 2 + 0.5 X_1 + 0.2 X_2 + 0.4 X_3$$

and three individuals with the following scores:

X_1	X_2	X_3
1. 8	4	7
2. 12	3	5
3. 10	6	9

their predicted scores would be calculated as:

---

1. $2 + (0.5) (8) + (0.2)(4) + (0.4)(7) = 9.6$
2. $2 + (0.5)(12) + (0.2)(3) + (0.4)(5) = 10.6$
3. $2 + (0.5)(10) + (0.2)(6) + (0.4)(9) = 11.8$

If adding extra variables increases the amount of variance accounted for in the dependent variable, that will also increase the accuracy of our prediction. Multiple regression simply extends the multiple correlation into the computation of the regression equation.

SIGNIFICANCE TESTING

When doing a simple linear regression, the correlation between the two variables is tested for significance, and r^2 represents meaningfulness. With multiple correlation, we are interested not only in the significance of the overall R and the amount of variance accounted for (R^2), but also in the significance of each of the independent variables. Just because R^2 is significant does not mean that all the independent variables are contributing significantly to the explained variance. In multiple regression, the multiple correlation is tested for significance, and each of the b-weights also is tested for significance. Testing the b-weight tells us whether the independent variable associated with it is contributing significantly to the variance accounted for in the dependent variable.

The F-distribution is used for testing the significance of the R^2s, and either the F- or t-distribution is used to test the significance of the bs. See Appendix D for the F-distribution. When using the computer-packaged programs, the Fs or ts and associated probabilities are printed out. The F-distribution is used for demonstration here.

When testing for the significance of R^2s, the degrees of freedom (df) are calculated as $k/(n - k - 1)$. In other words, there are two dfs; a numerator, k, and a denominator, $n - k - 1$. The k stands for the number of independent variables, and n stands for the number of subjects. When testing the significance of a b-weight, the df is $1/(n - k - 1)$.

We start with examples of testing the Fs associated with R^2s for significance. If we had two independent variables and a sample size of 63, the df would be $2/(63 - 2 - 1)$, or $2/60$. In Appendix D, the dfs for the numerator are listed across the top of the page. The numerator also is known as the greater mean square. The dfs for the denominator are listed down the left side of the page. The denominator also is called the *lesser mean square*. In our example, there are 2 dfs in the numerator and 60 dfs in the denominator. The tabled values for $2/60$ df, which must be equaled or exceeded, are 3.15 at the 0.05 level and 4.98 at the 0.01 level. Note that the 0.05 level is in light print, and the 0.01 level is in dark print. An F of 4.50

would be significant at the 0.05 level but not at the 0.01 level. Two additional examples follow:

F	k	n	df	p
4.05	3	129	3/125	<0.01
2.00	6	207	6/200	ns

To test the *b*-weights, the procedure is the same except that the numerator of the *df* is always 1. Some examples for testing *b*-weights follow:

F	k	n	df	p
5.25	2	68	1/65	<0.05
8.00	3	154	1/150	<0.01

COMPUTER ANALYSIS

The question to be addressed is whether smoking history, depressed state of mind, overall state of health, and quality of life in the past month predict a score on the Inventory of Positive Psychological Attitudes (IPPA). Figure 12-4 contains the correlations presented in the previous chapter (see Fig. 11-3). Note again the correlations of the four variables: smoking history, depressed state of mind, overall state of health, and quality of life in the past month with total IPPA. The correlations range from a high of −.698 to a low of −.226. All are significant at the .01 level. Because we can see that all of the variables are significantly related to each other, we will use multiple regression to determine how well the combination of independent variables explains the variance in the total IPPA score. The research question is, "What is the multiple correlation between a set of four predictors, which includes smoking history, depressed state of mind, overall state of health, and quality of life in the past month, and the outcome, positive psychological attitude?" To answer this question, the total IPPA score is regressed on the four predictor variables.

The output from this analysis is contained in Figure 12-5. There are three tables produced by SPSS 7.0 for Windows. The first contains the Model Summary, where we see that R = .764, R square is .583, and the adjusted R square is .573; thus, this analysis accounted for 57% of the variance. All of the variables were entered together (Method=Enter).

The ANOVA table is next, and there we see that the overall analysis is significant at the .000 level. Note that rather than sum of squares for between and within, we see sum of squares for regression and residual.

The coefficients are presented in the third table. The unstandardized coefficients (*b*-weights) are presented first, then the standardized or beta coefficients. Because

Correlations

		Smoking history	Depressed state of mind	Overall state of health	Quality of life in past month	Total IPPA
Pearson Correlation	Smoking history	1.000	.283**	-.231**	-.150*	-.226**
	Depressed state of mind	.283**	1.000	-.460**	-.498**	-.698**
	Overall state of health	-.231**	-.460**	1.000	.501**	.552**
	Quality of life in past month	-.150*	-.498**	.501**	1.000	.564**
	Total IPPA	-.226**	-.698**	.552**	.564**	1.000

FIGURE 12-4
Correlations from Figure 11-3.

Model Summary[a,b]

	Variables					Std. Error
Model	Entered	Removed	R	R Square	Adjusted R Square	of the Estimate
1	quality of life in past month, smoking history, overall state of health, depressed state of mind [c,d]		.764	.583	.573	20.7913

a. Dependent Variable: TOTAL IPPA

b. Method: Enter

c. Independent Variables: (Constant), quality of life in past month, smoking history, overall state of health, depressed state of mind

d. All requested variables entered.

FIGURE 12-5
Computer output of multiple regression. (*continued*)

ANOVA[a]

Model		Sum of Squares	df	Mean Square	F	Sig.
1	Regression	101626	4	25406.6	58.774	.000[b]
	Residual	72622.8	168	432.279		
	Total	174249	172			

a. Dependent Variable: TOTAL IPPA

b. Independent Variables: (Constant), quality of life in past month, smoking history, overall state of health, depressed state of mind

Coefficients[a]

Model		Unstandardized Coefficients		Standardized Coefficients	t	Sig.	95% Confidence Interval for B	
		B	Std. Error	Beta			Lower Bound	Upper Bound
1	(Constant)	137.078	11.046		12.410	.000	115.272	158.884
	Smoking history	−.179	2.187	−.004	−.082	.935	−4.497	4.139
	Depressed state of mind	−21.750	2.700	−.492	−8.057	.000	−27.080	−16.420
	Overall state of health	3.303	.907	.220	3.642	.000	1.513	5.093
	Quality of life in past month	5.579	1.651	.208	3.379	.001	2.320	8.839

a. Dependent Variable: TOTAL IPPA

FIGURE 12-5 (CONTINUED)

the *b*-weight reflects the actual measure with its associated mean and standard deviation, it is not directly interpretable. Beta reflects the weight associated with standardized scores (z-scores) on the variables. It is a partial correlation coefficient, a measure of the relationship between an independent and a dependent variable with the influence of the other independent variables held constant. Of the four predictors, three contribute significantly to the variance in total IPPA. They are depressed state of mind ($p = .000$), overall state of health ($p = .001$), and quality of life in the past month ($p = .000$).

Smoking history had a correlation of $-.226$ with total IPPA score, which is significant at the .01 level (see Fig. 12-4), but when the other predictor variables are accounted for, the partial correlation (beta) between smoking history and total IPPA is only $-.002$ ($p = .964$). Why is this so? Smoking history is significantly correlated with each of the other predictor variables; thus, beyond what it shares with those variables, it does not account for any of the variance in IPPA total. The standard error is a measure of the difference between predicted and actual scores and can be used to construct confidence intervals around the *b*-weights.

For this analysis, we would report that the regression of IPPA total (positive psychological attitudes) on four predictor variables, which included smoking history, depressed state of mind, overall state of health, and quality of life in the past month, accounted for 57% of the variance and was significant at the .000 level. Smoking history was not significantly related to positive psychological attitudes. There was a negative relationship between depressed state of mind and total IPPA ($p = .000$), indicating that people who were more depressed reported lower levels of positive psychological attitudes. Overall state of health ($p = .001$) and quality of life in the past month ($p = .000$) were positively related to positive psychological attitudes. Confidence intervals are provided for each *b* value.

The prediction equation based on this table is:

$$\text{Predicted score for TOTAL IPPA} = 137.038 - .179(\text{smoking history})$$
$$- 21.750(\text{depressed state of mind})$$
$$+ 3.303(\text{overall state of health})$$
$$+ 5.579(\text{quality of life}).$$

CODING

Nominal level variables can be included in a regression analysis, but they must be coded to allow for proper interpretation. You might collect information on the marital status of your subjects, and when entering the information into the computer, you decide on some arbitrary code numbers, such as single $= 1$, married $= 2$, and divorced $= 3$. If you entered that variable into a regression equation, it would be treated as though the numbers really meant something, that 2 was twice as big as 1, and so on. Such coding is *not recommended*. Instead, coding methods have been developed to allow us to enter such variables; three of these techniques, *dummy, effect,* and *orthogonal,* are presented here.

In all the coding methods, variables are coded into *vectors,* and the rule is that $n - 1$ vectors are used to describe the categories. If the variable has two categories, such as gender, one vector ($2 - 1 = 1$) is enough. If there were four categories, three vectors would be required, and so on.

Dummy Coding

This system uses 1s and 0s. If gender is a variable, you could code all males as 1 and all females as 0 (or vice versa). Correlational techniques applied to such a variable would tell you whether or not the gender of the individual was related to some measure. The 1 and 0 indicate that you belong to the chosen group or you do not. There is no distinction among members of a group; that is, all the 1s are considered equally male and all the 0s equally female. Suppose you had three groups, experimental group 1, experimental group 2, and a control group. You would need $n - 1$ ($3 - 1$) vectors to describe those categories (Table 12-1). To code those groups, start with the first vector, which we label $X1$. All the subjects in the first experimental group get a 1 on that vector, and all others get a 0. On the second vector, $X2$, all subjects in the second experimental group get a 1, and all the other subjects get a 0. The control group has received 0s on both vectors. On these two vectors, each group has a different pattern; that is, the first experimental group has 1,0; the second experimental group has 0,1; and the control group has 0,0.

This form could be extended for any number of categories. When the regression is run, the vectors $X1$ and $X2$ are entered to represent group membership. When such dummy coding is used, the intercept constant, a, in the prediction equation equals the mean of the dependent variable for the group that is assigned 0s throughout. In our example, that would be the control group. Therefore, in this form of analysis, we are testing the means of the other groups against the mean of a control group. In addition to a, the prediction equation would contain a b-weight for each of the vectors; that is, the prediction equation would look like:

The regression weight, b_1, represents the difference between the group assigned 1s on $X1$ and the group assigned 0s throughout. In our example, testing b_1 for significance would be testing to see whether there is a significant difference between the first experimental group and the control group on some dependent variable, Y.

$$Y' = a + b_1X_1 + b_2X_2$$

Testing b_2 for significance tells us if there is a significant difference between the second experimental group and the control group. Although it is most clear when used with a control group, dummy coding may be used to code categorical variables, whether or not a control group exists. You can use dummy coding for ethnicity, marital status, and so on, but you must understand what testing the b-weights means. In addition to comparing a group with the control group, you may want to compare it

TABLE 12-1
Dummy Coding

	Vectors	
Groups	*X1*	*X2*
Experimental 1	1	0
Experimental 2	0	1
Control	0	0

with some other group. In our example, you may want to compare experimental group 1 with experimental group 2. To do that, you would need to use a method that allows you to make multiple comparisons between means.

Effect Coding

Effect coding looks like dummy coding except that the last group gets −1s throughout, instead of 0s (Table 12-2). Five categories of marital status are coded into four vectors. We proceed in the same way as with dummy coding, but we give the last group −1 on each vector. Vectors $X1$ through $X4$ would then be entered into the regression equation to represent marital status.

When using effect coding, the a in the prediction equation represents the mean of the dependent variable. It is not the mean of one particular group on the dependent variable, but the overall mean for all the subjects in the analysis. This is called the *grand mean*. What you are testing with this type of coding is how each group's mean differs from the grand mean.

In our example, the regression equation would be:

If you tested b_1 for significance, you would be testing to see whether the mean score on the dependent variable for single people differed from the overall or grand mean. We could compare the means for single, married, divorced, and widowed against the grand mean, but what about the separated group? There is no b-weight

$$Y' = a + b_1X_1 + b_2X_2 + b_3X_3 + b_4X_4$$

to represent the fifth group. That b-weight can be calculated easily when you know that all the b-weights add up to zero; in the example, this is $b_1 + b_2 + b_3 + b_4 + b_5 = 0$. Given the b-weights for the first four categories from the regression, the fifth b-weight can be obtained by subtracting the sum of the first four from zero. For example, if the b-weights were $b_1 = 1$, $b_2 = 3$, $b_3 = -2$, $b_4 = 2$, then $1 + 3 + (-2)$

TABLE 12-2
Effect Coding

Marital Status	Vectors			
	X1	*X2*	*X3*	*X4*
Single	1	0	0	0
Married	0	1	0	0
Divorced	0	0	1	0
Widowed	0	0	0	1
Separated	−1	−1	−1	−1

+ 2 = 4, and 0 − 4 = −4. So the *b*-weight for the "separated" category would be −4. To compare specific pairs of means, a test for multiple comparisons between means must be applied.

Orthogonal Coding

When you hypothesize ahead of time, you are able to use more powerful statistical tests. Orthogonal coding allows you to code your hypotheses so they can be tested. To use this technique, you must have hypothesized a priori (i.e., before the data were collected). Here, orthogonal means that the comparisons that you want to test are independent of each other; that is, knowing the answer to one does not give you the answer to the other.

To have comparisons that are independent, only $n - 1$ comparisons can be made; that is, if there were three groups (experimental 1, experimental 2, and control), there could only be two orthogonal contrasts. Suppose that you were trying to decrease the number of postoperative complications, and you had three groups. Subjects in experimental group 1 were given special preoperative instruction by a nurse and a booklet to which they could refer later. Experimental group 2 received instruction only, and the control group just received the usual care. You would want to know whether the special instructions reduced postoperative complications and whether providing a booklet and instruction was better than instruction alone. We could compare the mean for experimental groups 1 and 2 with the mean of the control group to see whether there was a difference between experimental and control groups. We also could compare the means of the two experimental groups to see whether the booklet made a difference. Table 12-3 contains the vectors necessary to code such a contrast. On vector $X1$, subjects in both experimental groups receive a −1, and the control group subjects receive a 2. That contrast tests the difference between the mean number of postoperative complications for all the experimental subjects and the mean for the control group subjects. Testing b_1 for significance would tell you whether that difference was statistically significant. The second contrast is given in vector $X2$. The first experimental group is compared with the second. Test-

TABLE 12-3
Orthogonal Coding

Groups	Vectors	
	X1	X2
Experimental 1	−1	1
Experimental 2	−1	−1
Control	2	0

ing b_2 for significance would tell you whether there was a significant difference in the mean number of postoperative complications between those within the experimental group who received the booklet and those who did not. To ensure that hypothesized contrasts are orthogonal, three tests must be applied:

1. There must be only $n - 1$ contrasts.
2. The sum of each vector must equal zero. In the example, the sum of $X1$ is (-1) $+ (-1) + 2 = 0$, and the sum of $X2$ is $1 + (-1) + 0 = 0$.
3. The sum of the cross-products must equal zero. In the example, $(-1 \times 1) + (-1 \times -1) + (2 \times 0) = 0$.

Table 12-4 shows some other examples of possible contrasts, given three groups. Are they all orthogonal? The vectors $X1$ and $X2$ reflect an orthogonal contrast, as do the vectors $Y1$ and $Y2$. Vectors $Z1$ and $Z2$ do not reflect an orthogonal contrast; group 1 is compared to group 2 and to group 3. The sum of the cross-products does not equal zero $([-1 \times 1] + [0 \times -1] + [1 \times 0] = -1)$.

In the regression equation with orthogonal coding, a is the grand mean of the dependent variable, and each b represents a hypothesized contrast.

Summary of Coding

Regardless of the method of coding used, the overall $R2$ will remain the same, and so will its significance. Predictions based on the resulting prediction equations will be identical. The differences lie in the meaning attached to testing the b-weights for significance. With dummy coding, the b-weight represents the difference between the mean of the group represented by that b and the group assigned 0s throughout.

In effect coding, the bs represent the difference between the mean of the group associated with that b-weight and the grand mean. With orthogonal coding, the b-weight measures the difference between two means specified in a hypothesized contrast.

TABLE 12-4
Contrasts

| | *Pairs of Vectors* | | | | | |
Group	*X1*	*X2*	*Y1*	*Y2*	*Z1*	*Z2*
1	2	0	−1	1	−1	1
2	−1	1	2	0	0	−1
3	−1	−1	−1	−1	1	0

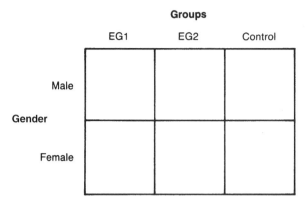

FIGURE 12-6
Design of study.

Coding Interactions

As pointed out in Chapter 8, you can study the interaction among variables. Interactions among variables may be coded and entered into the regression equation. Suppose you had two categorical variables to code: group membership and gender. Dummy coding will be used in this example, but any of the coding methods could be used. Figure 12-6 shows the basic design of the study. There are six mutually exclusive groups. We can now look at the effects of group membership, the effects of gender, and whether there is any interaction between group and gender. For example, does the booklet reduce postoperative complications for women but not for men? Coding of an interaction is demonstrated in Table 12-5. (M and F are used for male and female.) The six groups formed by the design are listed. First, we code group membership. To do that, ignore the gender variable. We need two group vectors and will call them $G1$ and $G2$. All EG1 subjects will be assigned 1 on $G1$; all

TABLE 12-5
Coding Interactions

Groups	Vectors				
	G1	*G2*	*S1*	*I1*	*I2*
EG1, M	1	0	1	1	0
EG1, F	1	0	0	0	0
EG2, M	0	1	1	0	1
EG2, F	0	1	0	0	0
Control, M	0	0	1	0	0
Control, F	0	0	0	0	0

other subjects will be assigned 0. All EG2 subjects will receive a 1 on $G2$; all other subjects will receive a 0. Only one vector ($S1$) is needed to code gender. Males are assigned 1s; females are assigned 0s.

In this example, there are two vectors for group and one for gender, so there must be two (2 × 1) vectors to code the interaction between these two variables. These vectors are labeled $I1$ and $I2$. For $I1$, multiply $G1$ by $S1$, and for $I2$, multiply $G2$ by $S1$.

As shown in these examples, coding is the way categorical variables and interactions are entered into the regression equation.

MULTIPLE COMPARISONS AMONG MEANS

None of the coding methods allows us to make all the comparisons among mean scores that we might like. If we have three groups, A, B, and C, and use dummy coding, we can compare the means of A and B with the mean of the control group C to see whether they are statistically different; however, we cannot compare the means of A and B by testing the b-weights. With effect coding, we could compare the means of each of the three groups with the grand mean, but we could not compare A with B, A with C, and so on. With orthogonal coding, we are restricted to $n - 1$ orthogonal hypothesized contrasts.

As is discussed in Chapter 7, some contrasts can be measured "after the fact," that is, after the overall F is found to be significant. Using these *post hoc* tests, we can then compare each group with every other group or compare two groups with one group and so on. Given our two experimental groups (preoperative teaching plus booklet and preoperative teaching alone) and a control group, we could compare each experimental group with the control group, the two experimental groups, the two experimental groups together with the control group, and so forth. Measures for multiple comparisons among means allow us to explore all interesting differences in our data once we have an overall F that is significant. To test for these post hoc comparisons, you could use the analysis of variance program in your statistical software.

SELECTING VARIABLES FOR REGRESSION

Because there is so much intercorrelation among variables used in behavioral research, we may want to select a subset of variables that does the best job of predicting a particular outcome. Usually, we want to find the smallest group of variables that will account for the greatest proportion of variance in the dependent variable. Using such information, we can make practical decisions. If two predictors are equally good, we will probably decide to use the one that is easiest to administer, most economical, and so forth. Outlined here are some of the commonly used methods for selecting variables, including *standard, hierarchical,* and *stepwise*.

Standard

All the independent variables are entered at once. This is the method used in the computer analyses presented in this chapter, and in SPSS, is called ENTER. All variables are evaluated in relation to the dependent variable and the other independent variables through the use of partial correlation coefficients.

Hierarchical

The researcher may want to force the order of entry of variables into the equation. Suppose you want to know whether a particular intervention would improve pregnancy outcomes. You already have some givens, such as age, socioeconomic status, and nutritional status, and you would like to know whether your intervention makes a difference over and above factors that you cannot change. You might then enter the givens first and add your intervention last. As is shown in Chapter 15, this technique is used in developing *path* models. The variables may be entered one at a time or in subsets, but there should always be a theoretical rationale for the order of entry.

For example, Picot (1995) used hierarchical multiple regression to study the coping of African-American caregivers. The caregiving demands variables were entered first, then the perceived rewards and costs, and finally the household income and quality of social support. The variables accounted for 43% of the variance in emotive coping.

Stepwise

Forward Solution

The independent variable that has the highest correlation with the dependent variable is entered first. The second variable entered is the one that will increase the R^2 the most over and above what the first variable contributed. We have four independent variables, and we calculated the correlations between each independent variable and the dependent variable and found the highest correlation to be 0.50. That independent variable enters the equation and accounts for 0.50^2, or 25%, of the variance. Now we want to know which of the three remaining variables will add the most to the 25% that is already explained. We cannot simply select the one with the next highest correlation with the dependent variable, because there is intercorrelation among the independent variables. Therefore, we, or more likely the computer, calculate partial correlations between each of the three remaining independent variables and the dependent variable. Thus, the effect of the first variable is removed from the correlation. The variable that has the highest partial correlation with the dependent variable enters next. Then the partials between the two remaining independent variables and the dependent variable, taking out the effects of the first two variables in the equation, are to be calculated. The one with the highest partial correlation is entered next. Various criteria may be set for entry into the regression equation. The 0.05 level of significance is often used. In that case, a variable has to contribute a significant ($p = 0.05$) amount of variance to be included in the analysis. Once none of the remaining independent variables can contribute significantly to the R^2, the analysis is ended.

Backward Solution

In this method, we start with the overall R^2 generated by putting all of our independent variables in the equation. Then each variable is deleted one at a time to see whether the R^2 drops significantly. Each variable is tested to see what would happen if it were the last one entered into the equation. With four independent variables, the following differences would be tested:

$$R^2 y.1234 - R^2 y.234 \quad \text{tests for variable 1}$$
$$R^2 y.1234 - R^2 y.134 \quad \text{tests for variable 2}$$
$$R^2 y.1234 - R^2 y.124 \quad \text{tests for variable 3}$$
$$R^2 y.1234 - R^2 y.123 \quad \text{tests for variable 4}$$

If for any of these variables there is a significant drop in R^2, that variable is contributing significantly and will not be removed. If all the variables contribute significantly, the analysis would end with all four variables remaining in the equation. If one is not significant, there would be three variables left in the equation. Then, each of those three variables would be tested to see whether it would contribute significantly if entered last. The analysis continues until all variables in the equation contribute significantly if entered last.

Stepwise Solution

The stepwise solution combines the forward solution with the backward solution and therefore overcomes difficulties associated with each. With the forward solution, once a variable is in the equation, it is not removed. No attempt is made to reassess the contribution of a variable once other variables have been added. The backward solution remedies that problem, but the order of entry is not clear (i.e., Which variable enters first and contributes most to the explained variance?).

With the stepwise solution, variables are entered in the method outlined under the heading Forward Solution and are assessed at each step using the backward method to determine whether their contribution is still significant, given the effect of other variables in the equation.

Summary of Methods of Entry

Selecting a method for entering variables into the equation is an important decision, because the results will differ depending on the method selected. Stepwise methods were in vogue in the 1970s, but they are less popular today. Because the order of entry is based on statistical, rather than theoretical, rationale, the technique is criticized for capitalizing on chance. This is because the entry is based on the correlations among the variables, and these correlations are not stable with time because error is involved in their measurement. This becomes more of a problem when dealing with variables with low reliability.

Nunnally and Bernstein (1994) state that stepwise solutions are particularly problematic when testing hypotheses. The possibility of making a type 1 error expands dramatically with increased numbers of predictors. They believe it is preferable to combine stepwise and hierarchical approaches. Variables are not to be "dumped" into an analysis and "large samples are an absolute necessity" (p. 195). They urge a ratio of 50 subjects to one variable if you want to use as many as 10 variables. They stress the need to examine the beta weights and R and to cross-validate results.

ISSUES RELATED TO REGRESSION

Multicollinearity

A problem for behavioral researchers is the interrelatedness of the independent variables. These variables provide very similar information, and evaluation of results is problematic. Schroeder (1990) provides detail on diagnosing and dealing with multicollinearity. Indications of the problem include high correlations between variables (>0.85); substantial R^2 but statistically insignificant coefficients; unstable regression coefficients (i.e., weights that change dramatically when variables are added or dropped from equation); unexpected size of coefficients (much larger or smaller than expected); and signs (+ or −) that are unexpected (Lewis-Beck, 1980).

The *tolerance* of a variable is used as a measure of collinearity. It is the proportion of the variance in a variable that is not accounted for by the other independent variables (Norusis, 1996a). To obtain measures of tolerance, each independent variable is treated as a dependent variable and is regressed on the other independent variables. A high multiple correlation indicates that the variable is closely related to the other independent variables. If the R^2 were 1, then the independent variable would be completely related to the others. Tolerance is simply $1 - R^2$; therefore, a tolerance of 0 ($1 - 1 = 0$) indicates perfect collinearity. The variable is a perfect linear combination of the other variables. Tolerances may be requested as part of the output in the regression procedure. By default, tolerances are set as criteria for entry into regression equations. These values may be changed by the investigator.

The *variance inflation factor* is the reciprocal of tolerance (Norusis, 1996a). Therefore, variables with high tolerances have small variance inflation factors and vice versa.

Figure 12-7 adds the collinearity statistics to the coefficients that were presented in Figure 12-5. The tolerance values go from a low of .657 to a high of .906. Because the tolerance equals $1 - R$ squared, a tolerance of .657 for quality of life in the past month means that 34.3% ($1 - .657 = .343$) of the variance in this variable is shared with the other predictors. Because the other values for tolerance are even higher, multicollinearity is not a problem in this analysis.

Coefficients[a]

Model		Unstandardized Coefficients		Standardized Coefficients	t	Sig.	95% Confidence Interval for B		Collinearity Statistics	
		B	Std. Error	Beta			Lower Bound	Upper Bound	Tolerance	VIF
1	(Constant)	137.078	11.046		12.410	.000	115.272	158.884		
	Smoking history	-.179	2.187	-.004	-.082	.935	-4.497	4.139	.906	1.104
	Depressed state of mind	-21.750	2.700	-.492	-8.057	.000	-27.080	-16.420	.664	1.505
	Overall state of health	3.303	.907	.220	3.642	.000	1.513	5.093	.679	1.472
	Quality of life in past month	5.579	1.651	.208	3.379	.001	2.320	8.839	.657	1.522

a. Dependent Variable: TOTAL IPPA

FIGURE 12-7
Collinearity statistics.

Testing Assumptions by Analyzing Residuals

You should check the data before they are submitted to a regression procedure. Frequency distributions are assessed for outliers and for violation of normality of distributions. Scattergrams between variables are helpful to assess the shape of the relationship. Additionally, an important tool for checking the assumptions is residual analysis. Verran and Ferketich (1987) present an overview of the use of residual analysis to test linear model assumptions.

The residual is the difference between the actual and the predicted score. If the analysis were perfect, there would be no residuals; they would be zero.

Normal Distribution

If the relationships are linear and the dependent variable is normally distributed for each value of the independent variable, then the distribution of the residuals should be approximately normal (Norusis, 1996a). This can be assessed by using a histogram of the standardized residuals. See Figure 12-8 for an example. The normal curve is interposed on the standardized residuals. On the total IPPA score, the residuals are fairly normally distributed, with one peak .25 of a standard deviation above the mean.

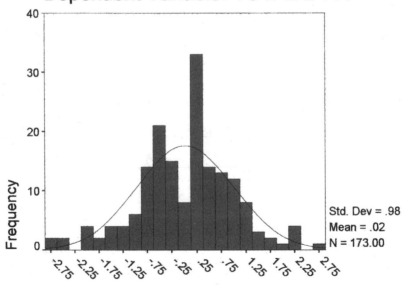

FIGURE 12-8
Histogram of residuals.

It is possible to transform the data mathematically, if residual analysis indicates violation of the assumption of normality.

Homoscedasticity

To check this assumption, the residuals can be plotted against the predicted values and against the independent variables. When standardized predicted values are plotted against observed values, the data would form a straight line from lower left corner to upper right corner, if the model fit the data exactly. Although the regression line is not drawn, if you took a ruler and drew a line from lower left to upper right hand corner, you would have it. In Figure 12-9, we demonstrate plotting residuals against one of our independent variables, overall state of health. Note that the actual scores vary around the prediction line, but in general, they cluster fairly close to the line.

When the residuals are from a normal distribution, the plotted values fall close to the line in the normal probability plot (Norusis, 1996a). Figure 12-10 contains an example from our analysis. Note that just below .25 and .50 there are fewer negative residuals than would be expected in a normal distribution.

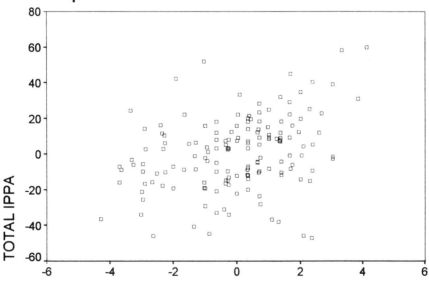

FIGURE 12-9

Plot of residuals against independent variable.

Normal P-P Plot

Dependent Variable: TOTAL IPPA

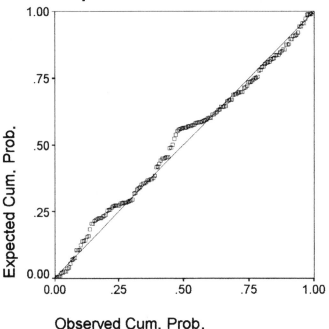

FIGURE 12-10

Normal probability plot.

Example From the Literature

Table 12-6 contains results of a study on personality, appraisal, and adaptational outcomes in human immunodeficiency virus–seropositive men and women (Anderson, 1995). Here we present the results from the men and for the outcome measure, activity disruption. First, look at the correlations of the variables with activity disruption. You can see that the predictor variables, socioeconomic status (SES), self-esteem, optimism, and threat appraisal, are all significantly correlated with activity disruption. Because SES was significantly correlated with three of the four outcome variables (all but mood disturbance), it was entered first in the equation. The person variables were entered on step 2, threat appraisal on step 3, and the interactions of the person variables and SES on step 4. The output from the hierarchical regression shows that SES accounted for 15% of the variance, the person variables in step 2 added an additional 24% to the explained variance, threat appraisal only added 1%, and the interactions added an additional 7%. The betas for step 4 show that the SES by self-esteem interaction was significant. To explain that interaction, Anderson compared high SES men with low SES men and found that among men with low SES,

TABLE 12-6
Correlation Matrix for Variables in Men (n = 77)

	2	3	4	5	6	7	8
1. Socioeconomic status	.26*	.25*	−.07	−.39**	−.16	.41**	.30†
2. Self-esteem		.63**	−.59**	−.58**	−.71**	.60**	.71**
3. Optimism			−.53**	−.40**	−.55**	.52**	.64**
4. Threat appraisal				.40**	.57**	−.47**	−.56**
5. Activity disruption					.71**	−.54**	−.65**
6. Mood disturbance						−.53**	−.65**
7. Life satisfaction							.75**
8. Purpose in life							

*$p < .05$.   †$p < .01$.   **$p < .001$, two-tailed.

*Moderating Effect of Socioeconomic Status (SES) on Person Variables
in Activity Disruption Among Men (n = 77)*

	R	R^2	F of Equation	R^2 Change	Betas			
					Step 1	Step 2	Step 3	Step 4
Step 1								
SES	.39	.15	13.20	.15	−.39†	−.25*	−.27*	−.23*
Step 2								
Self-esteem						−.50†	−.44†	−.42*
Optimism	.63	.39	15.71†	.24†		−.02	.01	−.12
Step 3								
Threat appraisal	.63	.40	12.11†	.01			.13	.12
Step 4								
SES by self-esteem								.43*
SES by optimism	.69	.47	10.58†	.07*				−.19

*$p < .01$.   †$p < .001$.
(From Anderson, S. E. H., [1995]. Personality, appraisal, and adaptational outcomes in HIV seropositive men and women. Research in Nursing & Health, 18, *303–312.)*

those with low self-esteem had greater disruption in usual activities than did those with high self-esteem. This study is a good example of moderating and mediating effects through the use of hierarchical regression. We suggest that you look at the article.

Summary

Multiple regression may be used for explanation and prediction. It is a flexible technique that allows the use of categorical and continuous variables. Overall, this is one of the most powerful techniques in our field, and if used wisely, it can be of great assistance in studying many problems related to human behavior and the health professions.

CANONICAL CORRELATION

When calculating a multiple correlation, you have more than one independent variable but only one dependent variable. Often, however, we are interested in more than one dependent variable. We could run separate regressions for each dependent variable, but that would not allow us to explore all the variation in the data. A method that takes all the information into account, thus giving a better understanding of all the relationships, is *canonical correlation*. This technique measures the relationship between a *set* of independent variables and a *set* of dependent variables. The method of least squares is used to give two composites, one for the independent variables, sometimes called the variables "on the left," and one for the dependent variables, or variables "on the right." (Many authors reserve the term *multivariate analysis* for situations in which there is more than one dependent variable.) Due to the complexity of the analysis, this technique was rarely used until sophisticated computer software became available. Use of the technique is increasing, and overviews of the method have been presented in the literature. For example, Wikoff and Miller (1991) discussed the use of canonical analysis in a "Methodology Corner" in *Nursing Research*. Although the variables are weighted through the procedure of canonical correlation, the main emphasis of this technique is on assessing relationships, rather than on prediction. More than one canonical correlation coefficient can be generated from a single analysis, because each coefficient represents the relationship between one factor in one of the groups of variables and a related factor in the other group. In this way, canonical correlation is like factor analysis. As is demonstrated in Chapter 14, there may be several factors in a group of variables. If there are three factors in one set of variables and three related factors in the second group of variables, three canonical correlation coefficients might emerge, one for each pair of factors. There cannot be more canonical correlation coefficients (Rcs) than there are variables in the smaller set. For example, if you had four independent variables ($X1$, $X2$, $X3$, $X4$) and three dependent variables ($Y1$, $Y2$, $Y3$), the most Rcs that could be calculated is three. The variance accounted for by each Rc is unique. The first canonical correlation accounts for the largest amount of variance, the second accounts for the second largest amount, and so on. The procedure ends when no significant Rcs are left.

A *canonical variate* is a weighted composite of the variables in a set. It is a "new" variable or construct derived from the original variables. *Canonical weights,* which are in standard score form, are generated for each variable. Like standardized regression coefficients (betas), they are used more for explanation than for prediction. Because they are in standard score form, they indicate the relative importance of the variable with which they are associated. They must be interpreted with caution, however. Canonical weights, like the betas in regression equations, may be unstable because they may vary a great deal from one analysis to another. Because of this, many researchers prefer to interpret loadings called *structure coefficients.* These loadings represent the correlation between the canonical variates and the real (or original) variables. If there is a high correlation between the new variable (canonical variate) and the original variables, the canonical variate represents what the original variables were measuring. Loadings or structure coefficients of 0.30 or higher are treated as meaningful (Pedhazur, 1982). They are interpreted like the loadings in factor analysis. The higher loadings give meaning to the canonical correlation and are used to name it. The square of a loading is the proportion of variance accounted for, so you can say how much of the variance is accounted for by an *Rc.*

To test the significance of a canonical correlation, Wilks' lambda (λ) is used. Lambda varies from 0 to 1 and stands for the error variance, the variance *not* accounted for by the independent variables. Thus, it is interpreted in an opposite way to the squared multiple correlation, R^2. A 1 means that the independent variables are *not* accounting for any of the variance in the dependent variable, and a 0 means that the independent variables are accounting for *all* of the variance. The *smaller* the lambda, the *greater* the variance accounted for. A $1 - \lambda$ would be equivalent to R^2. A chi-square statistic (called *Bartlett's test*) is used to test the significance of lambda.

The redundancy of the variables is often mentioned when canonical correlation results are presented. The higher the redundancy, or correlation, among a group of variables, the better the ability to predict from one group to another.

Computer Analysis

We extend the example used earlier in this chapter for the regression analysis (see Fig. 12-5). There we use total IPPA as the dependent variable. In this analysis, we use the two subscales within the IPPA, life satisfaction and confidence, as the outcome measures. The independent variables will remain the same. Figure 12-11 contains the printout.

All of the multivariate tests of significance indicate that the analysis was significant. If there were only one dependent variable, all four of these measures would be equivalent to the overall *F* statistic in ANOVA or multiple regression. With more than one dependent variable, however, they are not always equivalent. Which one should you use? Norusis (1994) states that two factors should be taken into account, power and robustness. In terms of power, from most to least powerful, the tests are Pillai's, Wilks', Hotelling's, and Roy's. (See the section on Multivariate Analysis of Variance in Chapter 8 for more detail on these measures.) In addition to being the most powerful, Pillai's trace also is the most robust; that is, it best withstands violations of the assumptions. The power and effect sizes were requested in this analysis.

Two canonical correlations are produced, equal to the number of variables in the smaller set (two dependent variables). Eigenvalues are measures of the explained variance. In general, an eigenvalue must equal at least 1 to represent a significant portion of the variance. See Chapter 14 for more information on this measure. The first canonical correlation squared (Rc^2) equals 0.579, which indicates that it explains 57.9% of the variance. The second canonical correlation explains about 8% (0.077) of the variance. Both canonical correlations are significant ($p = .000$ and .004).

```
EFFECT .. WITHIN+RESIDUAL Regression
Multivariate Tests of Significance (S = 2, M = 1/2, N = 81 )

Test Name          Value   Approx. F Hypoth. DF   Error DF  Sig. of F

Pillais           .65539   20.10601      8.00     330.00      .000
Hotellings       1.45629   29.67191      8.00     326.00      .000
Wilks             .38903   24.73407      8.00     328.00      .000
Roys              .57862
Note.. F statistic for WILKS' Lambda is exact.


- - - - - - - - - - - - - - - - - - - - - - - - - - - - - - - - - -
Multivariate Effect Size and Observed Power at .0500 Level

TEST NAME    Effect Size    Noncent.      Power

Pillais           .328      160.848       1.00
Hotellings        .421      237.375       1.00
Wilks             .376      197.873       1.00


- - - - - - - - - - - - - - - - - - - - - - - - - - - - - - - - - -
Eigenvalues and Canonical Correlations

Root No.     Eigenvalue      Pct.    Cum. Pct.  Canon Cor.   Sq. Cor

     1          1.373       94.290     94.290       .761       .579
     2           .083        5.710    100.000       .277       .077


- - - - - - - - - - - - - - - - - - - - - - - - - - - - - - - - - -
Dimension Reduction Analysis

Roots        Wilks L.        F Hypoth. DF   Error DF  Sig. of F

1 TO 2         .38903   24.73407      8.00     328.00      .000
2 TO 2         .92323    4.57360      3.00     165.00      .004

Both canonical correlations are significant.


- - - - - - - - - - - - - - - - - - - - - - - - - - - - - - - - - -
EFFECT .. WITHIN+RESIDUAL Regression (Cont.)
Univariate F-tests with (4,165) D. F.

Variable    Sq. Mul. R  Adj. R-sq.  Hypoth. MS     Error MS            F

CONFID        .46140      .44834   4215.08815    119.28275     35.33695
LIFE          .56343      .55285   8603.92581    161.61449     53.23734

Variable     Sig. of F

CONFID         .000
LIFE           .000
```

FIGURE 12-11

Computer output of canonical correlation.

```
EFFECT .. WITHIN+RESIDUAL Regression (Cont.)
Raw canonical coefficients for DEPENDENT variables
          Function No.

Variable                 1           2

CONFID                .019       -.107
LIFE                  .040        .073
```

Raw coefficients are like b-weights in regression.

```
Standardized canonical coefficients for DEPENDENT variables
          Function No.

Variable                 1           2

CONFID                .277      -1.568
LIFE                  .769       1.394
```

Standardized coefficients are like betas in regression.

```
Correlations between DEPENDENT and canonical variables
          Function No.

Variable                 1           2

CONFID                .875        .483
LIFE                  .985        .174
```

The correlations (structure coefficients) are usually interpreted.

```
Variance in dependent variables explained by canonical variables

CAN. VAR.   Pct Var DE Cum Pct DE Pct Var CO Cum Pct CO

       1       86.808     86.808     50.229     50.229
       2       13.192    100.000      1.013     51.242
```

FIGURE 12-11 (CONTINUES)

The univariate F-tests are the regressions of each dependent variable taken separately on the independent variables. Both of those regressions are significant.

Next the coefficients associated with the dependent variables are presented. The raw canonical coefficients are equivalent to the b-weights in regression and can be used to calculate predicted scores based on subjects' actual scores.

The standardized canonical coefficients are like the beta weights in regression. They are based on the standard scores of the variables and indicate the relative importance of each variable.

The correlations between the dependent and canonical variables are sometimes called structure coefficients and are what are usually interpreted when assessing the

```
Raw canonical coefficients for COVARIATES
        Function No.

COVARIATE               1          2

SMOKE5               -.046     -1.147
DEPRESS8             -.801      1.215
HEALTH13              .129       .058
QOL14                 .298       .420
```

Independent variables are labeled covariates.

```
Standardized canonical coefficients for COVARIATES
        CAN. VAR.

COVARIATE               1          2

SMOKE5               -.033      -.821
DEPRESS8             -.564       .856
HEALTH13              .276       .124
QOL14                 .347       .490


- - - - - - - - - - - - - - - - - - - - - - - - - - - - -

Correlations between COVARIATES and canonical variables
        CAN. VAR.

Covariate               1          2

SMOKE5               -.338      -.730
DEPRESS8             -.897       .294
HEALTH13              .719       .191
QOL14                 .819       .257


- - - - - - - - - - - - - - - - - - - - - - - - - - - - -

Variance in covariates explained by canonical variables

CAN. VAR.   Pct Var DE Cum Pct DE Pct Var CO Cum Pct CO

    1         30.482     30.482     52.681     52.681
    2          1.385     31.867     18.039     70.720
```

FIGURE 12-11 (END)

relationships between the two sets of variables. Values greater than 0.30 are treated as meaningful.

Next, the coefficients for the independent variables (called COVARIATES on the printout) are presented. Again, there are three types of coefficients: raw, standardized, and correlation.

What would be examined to interpret these results in relation to the variables

```
Correlations between COVARIATES and canonical variables
          CAN. VAR.

Covariate            1           2

SMOKE5            -.338       -.730

DEPRESS8          -.897        .294
HEALTH13           .719        .191
QOL14              .819        .257


Correlations between DEPENDENT and canonical variables
          Function No.

Variable             1           2

CONFID             .875        .483
LIFE               .985        .174
```

FIGURE 12-12
Coefficients for interpretation of canonical correlation.

are the correlations between the variables and the canonical variables. They are reproduced in Figure 12-12.

Using the rule that coefficients greater than 0.30 are meaningful, we can say that the first canonical variate indicates that smoking less, being less depressed, and having better health and higher quality of life are associated with being more confident and having higher life satisfaction. On the second canonical variate, smoking status and confidence are the only variables with loadings greater than .30. People who smoke more report lower levels of confidence.

Example From the Literature

In a study designed to determine the degree to which components of Pender's Health Promotion Model explained health promotion practices in a sample of older people, Duffy (1993) used canonical correlation for hypothesis testing. Table 12-7 contains the results. The six dimensions of health-promoting lifestyle comprised the outcome set, and 11 variables were contained in the predictor set. The predictors were divided into modifying factors—age, gender, education, marital status, annual income and race—and individual perceptions—self-esteem, internal health locus of control, chance health locus of control, powerful others health locus of control, and current health scale. Given six variables in the dependent set and 11 in the independent set, the most canonical variates that could be extracted was six. Of those, three accounted for significant portions of the variance and are included in the table. "The first canonical variate, explaining 61.5 percent of variance, indicated that subjects who reported their current health as good, had high self-esteem, and believed their health was under their own personal control rather than under the control of powerful others were more likely to report frequent or routine practice of self-actualization, nutrition,

TABLE 12-7
Canonical Correlational Analysis Summary Table Between HPM
Modifying Factors and Individual Perceptions (SET 1) and
*Health Promotion Mean Subscale Scores (Set 2) (n = 383)**

Variable Sets	Canonical Variate		
	1	*2*	*3*
SET 1			†
HPM modifying factors			
Age	.13	.07	.61*
Gender (1 = male, 2 = female)	.28	.49*	.31*
Education	.11	.01	.17
Marital status (1 = married,	−.13	.18	.31*
0 = all others)			
Annual income	−.11	.32*	.33*
Race (1 = white, 2 = black)	−.05	.27	−.04
HPM Individual Perceptions			
Self-esteem	.69*	.43*	−.05
Internal health LOC	.34*	−.13	.23
Chance health LOC	−.28	.27	−.38*
Powerful others health LOC	−.38*	−.04	.26
HPQ current health scale	.80*	−.41*	.05
Redudancy	.15	.08	.08
Total	.31		
SET 2			
Mean HPLP Sub Scales			
Self-actualization	.88*	.29	.08
Health responsibility	.19	−.21	.47*
Nutrition	.59*	−.49*	.11
Exercise	.38*	−.62*	.51*
Stress management	.44*	.18	.43*
Interpersonal support	.50*	.01	−.32*
Redundancy	.09	.02	.01
Total	.12		
Canonical correlation	.57	.36	.24
variance explained	61.5%	19.6%	7.8%
Total variance explained		88.7%	
Total redundancy		43.0%	

95 cases rejected due to missing data.

†*Cutoff = .30*

(From Duffy, M. E. [1993]. Determinants of health-promoting lifestyles in older persons. Image, 75(1), 27.)

interpersonal support, stress management, and exercise health promotion activities. The second variate, explaining 19.6 percent of variance, suggested that males with higher annual incomes as well as higher self-esteem but poorer current health were less likely to report engaging in the frequent or routine practice of exercise and good nutrition. The third variate, which accounted for 7.8 percent of variance, reported that older old subjects who had higher annual incomes, were married, and not likely to leave control of their health to chance or fate were more likely to engage in the regular health promotion practices of exercise, health responsibility, and stress management but not in interpersonal support activities" (Duffy, 1993, p.27).

SUMMARY

Canonical correlation is an extension of multiple regression that enables the researcher to include more than one dependent variable in the analysis. It is a powerful technique that helps us study the complex relationships that exist in health care research.

APPLICATION EXERCISES AND RESULTS

EXERCISES

1. What is the multiple correlation of three sets of predictors and overall state of health? The first set of predictors includes age and years of education. The second set contains confidence and life satisfaction. The third set contains smoking history and satisfaction with current weight.

2. What is the canonical correlation between the following two sets of variables: the predictor set, age, education, smoking history, depressed state of mind, exercise, and current quality of life; and the outcome set, positive psychological attitudes and overall state of health.

RESULTS

1. A hierarchical multiple regression was run to answer the question. The results are contained in Exercise Figure 12-1. The variables were entered in three steps. Education and age were entered in the first set and accounted for 12% of the variance ($p = .000$). Confidence and life purpose were entered in the second set and accounted for an additional 26% of the variance (R square = .379, $p = .000$). Satisfaction with current weight and smoking history were entered in the third set and accounted for an additional 10% of the variance ($p = .000$). The three sets accounted for 48% of the variance in overall state of health. In the final model, only life purpose ($p = .000$) and satisfaction with current weight ($p = .000$) accounted for significant portions of the variance.

   An examination of the tolerances in Model 3 indicates that two of the variables, confidence and life satisfaction, have low tolerances, indicating multicollinearity. Because tolerance is equal to $1 - R$ square, the tolerance for life satisfaction indicates that 68% of the variance is shared with other variables. For confidence, 65% of the variance is shared. Because these are two subscales from one instrument, it is not surprising that they are high-

Model Summary[a,b]

Model	Variables Entered	Variables Removed	R	R Square	Adjusted R Square	Std. Error of the Estimate
1	Education in years, Subject's age [c,d]	.	.342	.117	.106	2.01
2	Confidence during stressful situations, Life purpose and satisfaction [e,d]	.	.616	.379	.364	1.69
3	Satisfaction with current weight, Smoking history [f,d]	.	.696	.484	.465	1.55

a. Dependent Variable: overall state of health

b. Method: Enter

c. Independent Variables: (Constant), education in years, subject's age

d. All requested variables entered.

e. Independent Variables: (Constant), education in years, subject's age, Confidence during stressful situations, Life purpose and satisfaction

f. Independent Variables: (Constant), education in years, subject's age, Confidence during stressful situations, Life purpose and satisfaction, satisfaction with current weight, Smoking History

EXERCISE FIGURE 12-1. Hierarchical multiple regression, Exercise 1. (*continued*)

ANOVA[a]

Model		Sum of Squares	df	Mean Square	F	Sig.
1	Regression	86.388	2	43.194	10.743	.000[b]
	Residual	651.351	162	4.021		
	Total	737.739	164			
2	Regression	279.909	4	69.977	24.455	.000[c]
	Residual	457.830	160	2.861		
	Total	737.739	164			
3	Regression	357.335	6	59.556	24.736	.000[d]
	Residual	380.404	158	2.408		
	Total	737.739	164			

a. Dependent Variable: overall state of health

b. Independent Variables: (Constant), education in years, subject's age

c. Independent Variables: (Constant), education in years, subject's age, Confidence during stressful situations, Life purpose and satisfaction

d. Independent Variables: (Constant), education in years, subject's age, Confidence during stressful situations, Life purpose and satisfaction, satisfaction with current weight, Smoking History

EXERCISE FIGURE 12-1. (CONTINUES)

ly correlated. In Exercise Figure 11-1, we can see that the correlation between these two variables is .80. Thus, it would be better to use one or the other of these variables or to use the total IPPA score, rather than the two subscale scores.

2. The results of the canonical correlation are contained in Exercise Figure 12-2. The multivariate results all indicate that the overall analysis is significant. We have included just the correlations between the variables and the canonical variables, because they are what is usually interpreted. We would interpret the first canonical variate as indicating that people who are better educated, nonsmokers, not depressed, regular exercisers, and report high quality of life are healthier and have more positive psychological attitudes. The second canonical variate indicates that people who are older, more depressed, and exercise less are less healthy.

Coefficients[a]

Model		Unstandardized Coefficients		Standardized Coefficients	t	Sig.	Collinearity Statistics	
		B	Std. Error	Beta			Tolerance	VIF
1	(Constant)	6.595	.873		7.554	.000		
	Subject's age	-3.5E-02	.012	-.212	-2.862	.005	.996	1.004
	Education in years	.149	.043	.256	3.458	.001	.996	1.004
2	(Constant)	2.350	.903		2.602	.010		
	Subject's age	-2.9E-02	.010	-.178	-2.840	.005	.991	1.009
	Education in years	6.3E-02	.038	.108	1.668	.097	.918	1.089
	Confidence during stressful situations	-3.5E-03	.015	-.024	-.235	.815	.359	2.785
	Life purpose and satisfaction	6.3E-02	.012	.554	5.269	.000	.351	2.849

3							
(Constant)	1.584	.882		1.796	.074		
Subject's age	-1.8E-02	.010	-.106	-1.807	.073	.943	1.060
Education in years	6.3E-02	.035	.108	1.813	.072	.914	1.094
Confidence during stressful situations	-8.6E-03	.014	-.060	-.614	.540	.347	2.885
Life purpose and satisfaction	5.4E-02	.011	.474	4.691	.000	.320	3.127
Smoking history	-.298	.181	-.101	-1.646	.102	.868	1.152
Satisfaction with current weight	.263	.047	.340	5.587	.000	.880	1.136

a. Dependent Variable: overall state of health

EXERCISE FIGURE 12-1. (END)

```
EFFECT .. WITHIN+RESIDUAL Regression
Multivariate Tests of Significance (S = 2, M = 1 1/2, N = 74 1/2)

Test Name          Value  Approx. F Hypoth. DF    Error DF  Sig. of F

Pillais           .75114  15.23689    12.00        304.00      .000
Hotellings       1.72906  21.61326    12.00        300.00      .000
Wilks             .33490  18.32119    12.00        302.00      .000
Roys              .61012
Note.. F statistic for WILKS' Lambda is exact.

- - - - - - - - - - - - - - - - - - - - - - - - - - - - - - - - - -
Multivariate Effect Size and Observed Power at .0500 Level

TEST NAME    Effect Size    Noncent.      Power

Pillais            .376     182.843       1.00
Hotellings         .464     259.359       1.00
Wilks              .421     219.854       1.00

- - - - - - - - - - - - - - - - - - - - - - - - - - - - - - - - - -
Eigenvalues and Canonical Correlations

Root No.    Eigenvalue      Pct.   Cum. Pct.  Canon Cor.    Sq. Cor

    1          1.565       90.505    90.505      .781         .610
    2           .164        9.495   100.000      .376         .141

- - - - - - - - - - - - - - - - - - - - - - - - - - - - - - - - - -


Correlations between DEPENDENT and canonical variables
        Function No.

Variable             1           2

HEALTH             .765        -.644
IPPATOT            .956         .294

- - - - - - - - - - - - - - - - - - - - - - - - - - - - - - - - - -


Correlations between COVARIATES and canonical variables
        CAN. VAR.

Covariate            1           2

AGE               -.168         .620
EDUC               .404        -.162
SMOKE             -.326         .184
DEPRESS           -.876        -.333
EXER               .631        -.535
QOLCUR             .821        -.040
```

EXERCISE FIGURE 12-2. Canonical correlation, Exercise 2.

Logistic Regression

Barbara Hazard Munro

OBJECTIVES FOR CHAPTER 13

After reading this chapter, you should be able to do the following:

1 • Determine when it is appropriate to use logistic regression.

2 • Interpret a computer printout of a logistic regression analysis.

3 • Evaluate research reports using this technique.

As described in the previous chapter, multiple regression is used extensively by researchers. It allows us to find the best fitting and most parsimonious model to describe the relationship between the dependent variable and a set of independent or predictor variables.

Although the independent variables can be of differing levels of measurement (nominal to ratio), the dependent variable is supposed to be continuous and meet the assumptions underlying the technique. Suppose, however, the outcome measure is categorical. For example, in medical and epidemiologic studies, outcomes may be occurrence or nonoccurrence, mortality (dead or alive), and so forth. It is possible to code a dichotomous outcome variable as 1 or 0 and run a regression. In that case, the statistics generated will be the same as if you ran a *discriminant function analysis*. With more than two outcome categories, multiple regression cannot be used, and discriminant function or some other technique must be used. Until recently, discriminant function analysis often was used to develop a model when the outcome measure was categorical. Today, more people are reporting logistic regression, especially when the outcome measure is dichotomous. People who have studied the methods report that logistic regression is better suited to the data, and the results include odds ratios that lend interpretability to the data.

The odds of an outcome being present as a measure of association has found wide use, especially in epidemiology, because it approximates how much more likely (or unlikely) it is for the outcome to be present given certain conditions. For example, when looking at lung cancer in smokers and nonsmokers, an odds ratio of 2 indicates that smokers had twice the incidence of lung cancer in the study population. The odds ratio approximates another indicator called relative risk. Before describing logistic regression, we present an overview of discriminant function analysis as reported in the literature.

DISCRIMINANT FUNCTION ANALYSIS

The Research Question

Discriminant function analysis allows us to distinguish among groups based on some predictor variables. The mathematical function that combines information from predictor variables to obtain the maximum discrimination among groups is called the *discriminant function*. With two groups, the results are the same as using multiple regression with a dummy-coded dependent variable.

Type of Data Required

This technique tells us which set of predictors will most clearly distinguish among these groups. For example, in a study of adaptation to chronic illness, Pollock, Christian, and Sands (1990) used discriminant function analysis to determine what factors differentiated among the following groups: rheumatoid arthritis, hypertension, and multiple sclerosis. They found that health promotion activities, psychological distress, physiological adaptation, and dependence on medications correctly classified 73% of the sample.

When we use this technique, we are interested in explanation and prediction. We want to know which factors are most related to these groups and how well they can predict group membership. The aim of the procedure is to find a way to maximize the discrimination among groups. As with canonical correlation, more than one statistic may be derived. The most discriminant functions that can be derived are one less than the number of categories in the dependent variable or the number of independent variables, whichever is smaller. The first discriminant function derived from the data explains most of the between-group variance. The second discriminant function explains the next largest piece of variance, and so on. These functions are not correlated with each other. All the variables may be entered at once, or a stepwise procedure may be used to select the most discriminating variables. Eigenvalues and their associated canonical correlations are used to judge the most discriminating variables. Eigenvalues represent the amount of variance explained by a discriminant function.

As with multiple regression, each variable is weighted, and these weights may be used to calculate a discriminant score for each subject. The mean of the discriminant scores for a given group, for example, the rheumatoid arthritis group (Pollock et al., 1990), is called the *centroid*.

The discriminant functions are calculated by a method similar to factor analysis. Principal components analysis is used on a matrix of indices of discrimination between and within groups. This type of analysis discriminates among subjects, rather than among variables. Rotation may be used to increase the interpretability of the functions.

Wilks' lambda (Λ) is used to measure the association between the independent and dependent variables. Using the discriminant function scores, the members of the known groups are classified to see how well the system works. We want to know what percent is classified correctly and what percent is classified incorrectly.

The analysis produces *raw coefficients* (like *b*s in multiple regression), *standardized coefficients* (like betas), and *structure coefficients* (like those in canonical correlation). The raw coefficients are commonly used for calculating scores for each individual. The standardized coefficients represent the relative importance of the independent variables with which they are associated. Like betas, they should be interpreted with caution, however, because they tend to be unstable.

The correlations between the discriminant score for each individual and the scores on the original variables are called *structure coefficients,* or *loadings.* The square of that coefficient is the proportion of variance in a particular variable explained by the discriminant functions. Structure coefficients of 0.30 or greater are considered meaningful (Pedhazur, 1982). These coefficients are used to interpret the discriminant functions.

Figure 13-1 contains results from the Pollock et al. (1990) study. Two discriminant functions were produced. The Figure (*A*) indicates that the first function discriminates between the rheumatoid arthritis group (RA) and the hypertension group (HPT). (Their centroids are the farthest apart on that dimension.) Using the criterion of 0.30 or greater for the correlation of the predictor variables with the discriminant functions, dependence on medications (0.98) is the variable contributing to the discriminating power of the first function (*B*). The RA group was much more dependent on medications than the HPT group. Maximal separation on the second function occurs between the RA group and the multiple sclerosis group (MS). Psychological distress (0.41) and physiological adaptation (0.72) are contributing to this discrimination. The RA group had lower scores on physiological adaptation, and the MS group had higher psychological distress. The classification results are shown in *C.* Overall, 73% of the cases were correctly classified.

Assumptions

When studying this method of analysis, the general conclusion is that discriminant function estimators are sensitive to the assumption of normality. In particular, the estimators of the coefficients for non-normally distributed variables are biased away from zero. The practical implication for dichotomous independent variables is that the discriminant function estimators will overestimate the magnitude of the association (Hosmer & Lemeshow, 1989).

According to Norusis (1994), when the dependent variable has only two values—either the event occurs or it does not—the assumptions underlying regression analy-

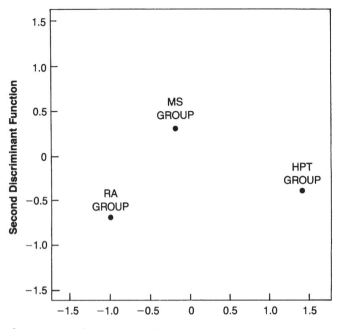

Plot of Three Group Centroids on Two Discriminant Functions Derived From Four Predictor Variables

A   First Discriminant Function

Results of Discriminant Function Analysis of Predictor Variables for Three Diagnostic Groups (N = 208)

Predictor Variables	Correlations of Predictor Variables with Discriminant Functions	
	1	2
HLPRACT–Health Promotion	.24	.24
PSYDIS–Psych. Distress	.02	.41
PAXTOT–Physiological Adapt.	.17	.72
MEDS–Dependence on Meds.	.98	−.11

B

Discriminant Function Classification Results (N = 208)

Actual Group	No. of Cases	Predicted Group Membership		
		2	3	4
Group 2	43	34	3	6
Hypertension		79.1%	7.0%	14.0%
Group 3	42	3	32	7
Rheumatoid arthritis		7.1%	76.2%	16.7%
Group 4	123	6	31	86
Multiple sclerosis		4.9%	25.2%	69.9%
Percent of "grouped" cases correctly classified: 73.08				

C Note: Three cases had at least one missing discriminating variable.

FIGURE 13-1

From Pollock, Christian, and Sands (1990, pp 302–303).

sis are violated because the distribution of errors is not normal but binomial (because the outcome is either 1 or 0). Discriminant analysis does allow direct prediction of group membership, but the assumption of multivariate normality of the independent variables and equal variance–covariance matrices in the two groups are required for the prediction rule to be optimal. "Logistic regression requires far fewer assumptions than discriminant analysis; and even when the assumptions required for discriminant analysis are satisfied, logistic regression still performs well" (Norusis, 1994, p. 1). In logistic regression, estimates of the probability of an event are given. This provides information not obtainable from regression weights. The method of least squares is used in regression. The coefficients minimize the squared distances between the observed and predicted scores. In logistic regression, the *maximum-likelihood method* is used. This means that the coefficients make our observed results most likely. The logistic model is nonlinear; when graphed, the data assume an S-shaped curve. Therefore, an iterative algorithm is necessary for parameter estimation. This technique is used more often now that the computer software is available.

ODDS RATIOS VERSUS RELATIVE RISK

Before giving an example of logistic regression, we need to explain some of the terms used with this analysis. An *odds ratio* is defined as the probability of occurrence over the probability of nonoccurrence. Table 13-1 contains fictional data to demonstrate calculations of an odds ratio. We see that of 450 women, 95 had a low birth weight infant (LBW), and 355 did not. Also, 200 of the women had prenatal care, and 250 did not.

Table 13-2 contains probabilities based on the data in Table 13-1. The probability of having an LBW infant if no prenatal care was received is calculated as the number of LBW infants in the no prenatal care group over the total number who received no prenatal care (75/250). The resulting probability is 0.3. In the same way, the probability of a normal weight baby with no prenatal care is the number of normal weight babies over the total number in the no prenatal care group. Therefore, for women who have not received prenatal care, the probability of having a normal weight baby is 0.7 and of having an LBW infant is 0.3. For those receiving prenatal care, the prob-

TABLE 13-1
Low Birth Weight

	Yes	*No*	*Row Totals*
Prenatal Care			
No	75	175	250
Yes	20	180	200
	—	—	—
	95	*355*	*450*

TABLE 13-2
Probabilities

Probability of Low Birth Weight (LBW) With No Prenatal Care

LBW
No prenatal care $\dfrac{75}{250} = 0.3$

Probability of Normal Birth Weight With No Prenatal Care

Normal weight
No prenatal care $\dfrac{175}{250} = 0.7$

Probability of LBW With Prenatal Care

LBW
Prenatal care $\dfrac{20}{200} = 0.1$

Probability of Normal Birth Weight With Prenatal Care

Normal weight
Prenatal care $\dfrac{180}{200} = 0.9$

abilities are 0.1 for LBW and 0.9 for normal weight. (Remember these numbers were contrived for this example.)

The odds of an event are the probability of occurrence over the probability of nonoccurrence. The odds of these events are presented in Table 13-3. The odds of having an LBW infant with no prenatal care is 0.43 and with prenatal care is 0.11. The odds ratio, which is the ratio of one probability to the other, is calculated as 3.91 in Table 13-4. We can say that the odds of having an LBW infant are almost four times greater when the woman has no prenatal care.

TABLE 13-3
Odds

Odds of low birth weight (LBW) infant, when no prenatal care:

$$\frac{\text{Probability of occurrence}}{\text{Probability of nonoccurrence}} = \frac{0.3}{0.7} = 0.43$$

Odds of LBW infant, with prenatal care:

$$\frac{\text{Probability of occurrence}}{\text{Probability of nonoccurrence}} = \frac{0.1}{0.9} = 0.11$$

TABLE 13-4
Odds Ratio

Ratio of one probability to the other

$$\frac{0.43}{0.11} = 3.91$$

Odds ratios are used to estimate what epidemiologists call relative risk. A risk is the number of occurrences out of the total. Relative risk is the risk given one condition versus the risk given another condition. Table 13-5 contains the calculation of the risks of LBW, with and without prenatal care. Table 13-6 contains a calculation of the relative risk. The relative risk is three times higher for women with no prenatal care. The odds ratio is at least equal to relative risk but often overestimates it, especially if the occurrence of the event is not rare. Here the odds ratio was 3.91, and the relative risk was 3. Because odds ratios are generated by the logistic regression procedure, it is important to understand what they are and not confuse them with actual measures of relative risk.

LOGISTIC REGRESSION

The Research Question

Logistic regression is used to determine which variables affect the probability of a particular outcome. For example, Hoshowsky and Schramm (1994) used logistic regression to determine the variables that most predicted the development of intraoperative pressure sores. They found that time on the operative table was most predictive. The odds of developing a pressure sore were five times higher for people who were on the table more than 4 hours.

TABLE 13-5
Risks of Low Birth Weight

Without prenatal care:

$$\frac{75}{250} = 0.3$$

With prenatal care:

$$\frac{20}{200} = 0.1$$

TABLE 13-6
Relative Risk

$$\frac{0.3}{0.1} = 3.0$$

Type of Data Required

In logistic regression, the independent variables may be at any level of measurement from nominal to ratio. Nominal-level variables must be coded prior to entry, as discussed in Chapter 12 on multiple regression. The dependent variable is categorical, and to date, most statistical software programs handle only dichotomous dependent variables.

Issues Related to Power

Computer software and books such as Cohen (1987) do not cover logistic regression. As more people use the technique, it is reasonable that authors will add calculations of effect and sample sizes to their materials.

Computer Analysis

We have a dichotomous outcome variable called DEPRESS. There are two groups: those who rated themselves as rarely depressed and those who rated themselves as sometimes to routinely depressed. There are three predictor variables:

1. SMOKE5—smoking history: never smoked = 0, quit smoking = 1, and still smoking = 2
2. QOL14—quality of life in past month scored on a 6-point scale: 1 = very dissatisfied to 6 = couldn't be more satisfied
3. IPPATOT—total score on the Inventory of Positive Psychological Attitudes (Kass et al., 1991): high score = positive attitudes; potential range of scores, 30 to 210

See Figure 13-2 for the printout. In dependent variable encoding, you can see that the original values and internal values are the same. The dependent variable was depressed (rarely or sometimes to routinely). It was entered as 0 = not depressed, and 1 = sometimes depressed. This is appropriate coding for the logistic regression procedure, so the original (value given by the investigator) and internal (value assigned by the computer) are the same. If the data had been entered as yes = 1 and no = 2, for example, the variable would have been recoded.

Coding

Just as in multiple regression, categorical independent variables are coded. You can use dummy (indicator), effect (deviation), or orthogonal coding. The computer program will produce the dummy or effect coefficients for you. You name the variable and tell it what type of coding you want. You also can specify orthogonal contrasts.

Interaction terms also may be entered into the equation. This is especially important when considering risk factors. Does smoking and drinking coffee increase the odds of a myocardial infarction more than adding up odds of each taken separately?

−2 Log Likelihood

"The probability of the observed results, given the parameter estimates, is known as the *likelihood*. Since the likelihood is a small number, less than 1, it is customary to use −2 times the log of the likelihood (−2 LL) as a measure of how well the estimated model fits the data" (Norusis, 1994, p.10). In regression, we evaluate models with and without particular variables to determine if they are making a significant contribution to the explanatory power. In logistic regression, comparison of observed to predicted values is based on the log likelihood (LL) function. A good model is one that results in a high likelihood of the observed results. This means a small value for −2 LL. The value for −2 LL is 238.85112.

The method is enter, which means that all the variables were entered in one step, not in a stepwise or hierarchical fashion. All three variables were entered on step 1. In the SPSS, program it is possible to use forward stepwise or backward stepwise or to enter variables in some particular order or by subsets.

Assessing the Overall Fit of the Model

To test the null hypothesis that the observed likelihood does not differ from 1, the value of −2 *LL* is tested with a chi-square distribution with the degrees of freedom equal to $N − p$, where N = number of cases, and p = number of parameters estimated. We had 177 cases and four parameters estimated (three independent variables and one constant). So our degrees of freedom are $177 − 4 = 173$.

Goodness of Fit Statistic

This statistic compares the observed probabilities to those predicted by the model (like regression in which you compare the scores that would be predicted for each subject given the prediction equation with the scores they actually received). In other words, it examines the residuals. This statistic also has a chi-square distribution, and the same *df* as −2 LL.

When the significance is large for the test of −2 LL or the goodness of fit statistic, you do not reject the null hypothesis that the model fits. In other words, a nonsignificant result indicates that the model fits. A significant result indicates that it does not fit. In SPSS for Windows 7.0, the chi-square values, *df*s, and significance levels for −2 LL and goodness of fit are not included in the output.

Model Chi-Square

The model chi-square is the difference between −2 LL for the model with only a constant and −2 LL for the complete model. In other words, does adding our predictors do anything for the model? It tests the null hypothesis that the coefficients for

(text continues on page 300)

Logistic Regression

Total number of cases: 177 (Unweighted)
Number of selected cases: 177
Number of unselected cases: 0

Number of selected cases: 177
Number rejected because of missing data: 4
Number of cases included in the analysis: 173

Dependent Variable Encoding:

Original   Internal
Value   Value
  .00   0
 1.00   1

Dependent Variable..   DEPRESS   DEPRESSED

Beginning Block Number 0.   Initial Log Likelihood Function

-2 Log Likelihood   238.85112

* Constant is included in the model.

```
Beginning Block Number  1.  Method: Enter

Variable(s) Entered on Step Number
1..      SMOKE5      Smoking History
         QOL14       quality of life in past month
         IPPATOT     Positive Psychological Attitudes

Estimation terminated at iteration number 5 because
Log Likelihood decreased by less than .01 percent.

-2 Log Likelihood       140.219
Goodness of Fit         163.291

                    Chi-Square    df  Significance

Model Chi-Square       98.632     3     .0000
Improvement            98.632     3     .0000

Classification Table for DEPRESS
                              Predicted
                     RARELY   SOME TO ROUTINELY    Percent Correct
                       R      I       S
                   +--------+--------------------+
Observed
  RARELY        R  I   76   I        17         I    81.72%
                   +--------+--------------------+
  SOMETIMES TO  S  I   15   I        65         I    81.25%
  ROUTINELY        +--------+--------------------+
                                        Overall       81.50%
```

FIGURE 13-2

Computer output of logistic regression. (*continued*)

```
        Observed Groups and Predicted Probabilities

 20 +                                                                +
    I                                                                I
    I  R                                                             I
    I  R                                                             I
 15 +  R                                                             +
    I  R                                                             I
    I  R                                                             I
    I  S R                                                          SI
    I  R R                                                          S+
 10 +  R R                                                          SI
    I  R R                                                          SI
    I  R R                                              S   S   S  SI
    I  R R                                              S   S   S  SI
  5 +  RSR          S                              S    S   S   S  S+
    I  RRRR     R        SS              SS         S   S SR S  SS SI
    IRRRRRRRRRRRR  RRRSSR R   R   SRSRSR  S SR S  SS SSSSSSSSSI
    IRRRRRRRRRRRR  RRRSRR R   RRRSRRRRRSRS RR RRSS RSSS SSRSSRSSSI
Predicted ------+---------+---------+---------+---------+--------
 Prob:    0      .25       .5       .75        1
 Group:   RRRRRRRRRRRRRRRRRRRRRRRRRRRRRRRRSSSSSSSSSSSSSSSSSSSSSSSSSSSSS

  Predicted Probability is of Membership for SOMETIMES TO ROUTINELY
  Symbols: R - RARELY
           S - SOMETIMES TO ROUTINELY

  Each Symbol Represents 1.25 Cases.
```

```
------------- Variables in the Equation -------------

Variable          B        S.E.      Wald      df      sig        R

SMOKE5          .8996      .2997     9.0112     1     .0027     .1713
QOL14          -.5716      .2284     6.2626     1     .0123    -.1336
IPPATOT        -.0564      .0101    31.1972     1     .0000    -.3496
Constant      10.5290     1.7028    38.2317     1     .0000


                                 90% CI for Exp(B)
Variable       Exp(B)      Lower     Upper

SMOKE5         2.4586     1.5018    4.0250
QOL14           .5646      .3878     .8221
IPPATOT         .9452      .9296     .9610
```

FIGURE 13-2 (END)

all the independent variables equal 0. This is comparable to the overall F in regression. In our example, we have 3 dfs for the three independent variables. The result is significant ($p = 0.0000$). The null hypothesis is rejected, indicating that the three variables add to the model. The -2 LL was 238.85112 at the beginning step; after adding the variables, it became 140.219. The difference between these two numbers, 98.632, is the model chi-square, or the explanatory power of the three independent variables.

Improvement

Improvement is the change in -2 LL between successive steps of building a model. It tests the null hypothesis that the coefficients for the variables added at the last step are 0. Because we had only one step, these numbers are the same. If we had requested a stepwise solution, these numbers would be different.

Classification Table

In our example, we see that 32 subjects were misclassified. Fifteen people who rated themselves as sometimes to routinely depressed were predicted by the model to be rarely depressed. Seventeen people who rated themselves as rarely depressed were predicted by the model to be sometimes to routinely depressed. The model predicted correctly 81.72% of the rarely depressed group and 81.25% of the sometimes to routinely depressed group; the overall prediction was 81.50% correct.

Diagram of Observed Groups and Predicted Probabilities

The predicted classification is based on the probabilities, that is, greater than or less than 0.5. You cannot tell from the table whether the misclassified individuals had calculated probabilities that were close to the 0.5 level. You can change the rules if there are problems with misclassification in one direction or the other (i.e., you can change from 0.5 to some other value). In the diagram, you can see where the misclassified individuals fell. Note that R stands for the rarely depressed group and S for the sometimes to routinely depressed group. Now look below .5. Any Ss that occur below .5 are misclassified. (Note that each symbol represents 1.25 cases.) Only one is just below the .5 cutoff. Above the .5 location, we see the Rs that have been misclassified. Several of these fall very close to the .5 level.

Variables in the Equation

The b-weights associated with each independent variable and the constant term are given in the first column. The b-weights in multiple regression are used to create a prediction equation; that is, knowing a person's score on each variable, we can use the weights and the constant term to predict the individual's score on some outcome measure. In logistic regression, these weights are used to determine the probability of a subject doing one thing or the other. In our example, this is the probability of being depressed or not. Instead of a score, as with the continuous variables used as dependent variables in regression, we get a probability from 1 to 0. If the probability is greater than 0.5, the individual would be predicted to be sometimes to routinely depressed; if less than 0.5, the individual would be predicted to be rarely depressed. We demonstrate the formula for these calculations after explaining the other columns in this section.

The signs associated with the b-weights indicate the direction of the relationship. Because being depressed is coded 1 and not depressed is coded 0, we would predict that those who smoke more, report lower quality of life, and have less positive psychological attitudes are more likely to be depressed.

The next column contains the standard errors for the predictors and the constant. In general, a statistic is divided by its standard error to give the value that is tested for significance. For large sample sizes, the test that a b coefficient is equal to 0 can be based on the Wald statistic, which has a chi-square distribution. When a variable has 1 df, the Wald statistic is simply the square of the result of dividing the b value by its standard error. For example, the coefficient for SMOKE5 is 0.8996. Dividing that by the standard error of 0.2997 and then squaring the result equals the Wald value of 9.0112. (For categorical variables, the Wald statistic has dfs equal to one less than the number of categories.) The value is significant at the 0.0027 level.

Using the 0.05 level, all three of the coefficients are significant. The Wald statistic has an undesirable property. When the absolute value of the regression coefficient becomes large, the estimated standard error is too large. This produces a Wald statistic that is too small, leading to nonsignificant results, even when the null hypothesis should be rejected. When you have a large coefficient, you should not rely on the Wald statistic for hypothesis testing. Instead, you should build a model with and without that variable and base your hypothesis test on the difference between the two likelihood-ratio chi-squares (Norusis, 1994).

As with multiple regression, the contribution of individual variables in logistic regression is difficult to determine. The contribution of each variable depends on the other variables in the model. This is a problem when independent variables are highly correlated.

The R statistic represents the partial correlation (i.e., the correlation of one independent variable with the dependent variable with the other variables held constant). R can range in value from -1 to $+1$. A positive value indicates that as the variable increases in value, so does the likelihood of the event occurring. If R is negative, the opposite is true. In our example, IPPATOT has the highest partial correlation with the dependent variable. After controlling for smoking history and quality of life, the correlation between positive psychological attitudes and depression is $-.3496$. Squaring that indicates that 12.2% of the variance in depression is explained by positive psychological attitudes.

Exp (B) is the odds ratio. Mathematically, this is e (the base of the natural logarithm, 2.718) raised to the power of b. In this example, 2.718 raised to the power of 0.8996 (b for SMOKE5) is 2.4586. Remember that the odds ratio is the ratio of one probability to the other. In this example, it is the probability of being depressed over the probability of not being depressed. In linear regression, b indicates the amount of change in the dependent variable for a one-unit change in the independent variable. To understand logistic coefficients, we need to think in terms of the odds of an event occurring. The logistic coefficient (b) is the change in the log odds associated with a one-unit change in the independent variable with the other variables held constant. Thus, if SMOKE5 went up 1 point, the log odds would go up 2.4586.

Example

The following example helps clarify the relationships expressed in this table of variables in the equation. The probability of an event is determined by the following formula:

$$\frac{1}{1 + e^{-z}}$$

e = base of the natural logarithm, 2.718

z = constant + b_1X_1 + b_2X_2 + b_3X_3 + . . .

In our example:

$$z = 10.5290 + .8996(\text{SMOKES}) - .5716(\text{QOL14}) - .0564(\text{IPPATOT})$$

Ratings of two individuals:

	Jane	*Susan*
Smoking history	2	1
Quality of life	4	4
Total IPPA	180	180

Looking at the ratings, we see that Jane and Susan have different scores on smoking history. Jane is still smoking (2) and Susan has quit smoking (1). On the other two variables, they have the same scores. What is the probability of each of these being in the depressed group, given the data collected?

First, the z-scores for each individual are calculated as:

$$\text{Jane} \quad z = 10.529 + .8996(2) - .5716(4) - .0564(180)$$
$$z = -0.1102$$

$$\text{Susan} \quad z = 10.529 + .8996(1) - .5716(4) - .0564(180)$$
$$z = -1.0098$$

The formulas for determining the estimated probabilities of these individuals being in the depressed group are:

$$\text{Jane} \quad \frac{1}{1 + 2.718^{-(-0.1102)}}$$

$$\text{Susan} \quad \frac{1}{1 + 2.718^{-(-1.0098)}}$$

Jane   1/2.1165 = .4725

Susan   1/3.7451 = .2670

Because both probabilities are less than 0.5, we would predict that both of these women would fall into the rarely depressed group. As we pointed out, the odds of an event are the probability of occurrence over the probability of nonoccurrence. Thus, for our subjects, the odds of falling into the depressed group are:

$$\text{Jane} \quad \frac{0.4725}{1 - 0.4725} = .8957$$

$$\text{Susan} \quad \frac{0.2670}{1 - 0.2670} = .3643$$

and the odds ratio is:

$$\frac{.8957}{.3643} = 2.4586$$

We would say that the odds for Jane falling into the depressed group are 2½ times higher than for Susan. The only difference in their scores on the three predictor variables was that Jane scored 2 on SMOKE5 and Susan scored 1. Look again at the odds ratio for SMOKE5. It is 2.4586, the same as the odds ratio for Jane and Susan. What we have demonstrated is that a 1-point increase on a variable results in an increase in odds as listed in Exp(B), the odds ratio.

The clearest use of the odds ratio is when the independent variable is categorical. In our example, we have three categories, never smoked, quit smoking, and still smoking, and we demonstrated what moving from one category to the next does in terms of the odds ratio. It is not as interesting when the change is just 1 point on a scale. For example, our IPPATOT variable is scored from 30 to 210. A 1-point increase in that scale is not of any practical interest. You can calculate the odds for some more meaningful change by multiplying the b value by the change you want and then performing an exponentiation on that number.

For IPPATOT, if 30 points were of interest, $0.0564 \times 30 = 1.692$. Raising 2.718 to the power of $1.692 = 5.43$, so for every 30-point decrease (due to negative sign) in IPPATOT, the odds go up 5.4 times of being in the depressed group.

Because the odds ratio is usually the parameter of interest in a logistic regression due to its ease of interpretation, be aware that as a point estimate, the distribution is skewed, because it is bounded away from zero. If the sample size is large enough, this is not a problem. Confidence intervals often are used to demonstrate more clearly the odds ratio. These interval estimates are provided in some software packages. (An exponentiation is performed on the usual formula; that is, you raise 2.718 to a power derived from the b-weight $\pm 1.96 \times$ the standard error.) Note in our example that the odds ratios are not right in the middle of the confidence intervals.

Example From the Literature

Logistic regression was used to determine the probability of having a premature or LBW infant based on predictors, including maternal education, race, weight gain, and mother's age at birth (Ketterlinus, Henderson, & Lamb, 1990). Using the results of this analysis, the investigators constructed a table listing the estimated probabilities. This is a good example of the use of the multivariate approach, because the probabilities have been calculated for all the possible combinations across the variables (Table 13-7). A practitioner, making note of a client's demographics, could determine the probabilities from this table. For example, a 16-year-old African-American woman with 12 years of education and light weight gain would have a 0.27 probability of having a premature birth and a 0.23 probability of having an LBW infant.

SUMMARY

Logistic regression is now more commonly reported when the outcome measure is categorical. As with all methods of regression, it is of utmost importance to select variables for inclusion in the model based on clear scientific rationale. You can use a stepwise method (forward or backward) in which variables are selected strictly on statistic criteria. An alternative selection method is *best subsets*. Stepwise, best subsets, and other mechanical selection procedures have been criticized because they are based solely on correlations derived from variables measured with some error. Following the fit of the model, the importance of each variable included in the model should be verified (Norusis, 1994). This should include the examination of the Wald statistic for each variable and a comparison of each estimated coefficient with the coefficient from the univariate model containing only that variable. Variables that do not contribute to the model based on these criteria should be eliminated and a new model fit. The new model should be compared to the old model through the likelihood ratio test. Once you have obtained a model that you believe contains the essential variables, you should consider whether to add interaction terms.

As with regression, residuals may be examined to evaluate the model. The residuals in logistic regression are the differences between the observed and predicted probabilities of an event. They should be normally distributed with a mean of 0 and a standard deviation of 1.

Deviance compares the predicted probability of being in the correct group based on the model to the perfect prediction of 1. It can be viewed as a component of -2 LL, which compares a model to the perfect model. Large values for deviance indicate that the model does not fit the case well.

Logistic regression programs are available with most of the software packages for the personal computer; they manage model building with a dichotomous outcome variable very well and provide the additional benefit of odds ratios, which lend interpretability to the data. Programs for managing outcomes with more than two categories are not as widely available.

TABLE 13-7
*Estimated Probabilities of Giving Birth to a Premature or Low
Birth Weight (LBW) Infant by Maternal Race, Education, Age,
Pregravid Weight, and Pregnancy Weight Gain*

Race	Maternal Education (Year)	Age at Birth (Year)	Premature Birth*		LBW	
			Light Weight Gain	Normal Weight Gain	Light Weight Gain	Normal Weight Gain
African-American	0–11	13–15	.47	.41	.29	.13
		16–18	.30	.26	.28	.13
		19–21	.29	.24	.23	.10
		22–30	.29	.24	.33	.16
	12	13–15	.43	.37	.25	.11
		16–18	.27	.22	.23	.10
		19–21	.26	.21	.19	.08
		22–30	.25	.21	.28	.13
	13+	13–15	.39	.33	.20	.09
		16–18	.24	.20	.19	.08
		19–21	.23	.18	.16	.06
		22–30	.22	.18	.23	.10
White	0–11	13–15	.42	.36	.18	.08
		16–18	.26	.22	.17	.07
		19–21	.25	.20	.14	.06
		22–30	.25	.20	.21	.09
	12	13–15	.38	.32	.15	.06
		16–18	.23	.19	.14	.06
		19–21	.22	.18	.11	.05
		22–30	.22	.18	.17	.07
	13+	13–15	.34	.29	.12	.05
		16–18	.20	.17	.11	.05
		19–21	.19	.16	.09	.04
		22–30	.19	.15	.14	.06

Coefficients are adjusted for memory bias.

(From: Ketterlinus, R. D., Henderson, S. H., & Lamb, M. E. [1990]. Maternal age, sociodemographics, prenatal health and behavior: Influences on neonatal risk status. Journal of Adolescent Health Care, 11(5), 428.)

APPLICATION EXERCISES AND RESULTS

EXERCISES

1. Calculate the odds and relative risk of smoking when not on a sports team.

	Smokes	
On a Sports Team	*Yes*	*No*
No	270	500
Yes	50	430

2. Recode the exercise variable into a new variable in which people who exercise rarely or sometimes are scored 0, and those who exercise often or routinely are scored 1. Using the new variable as the outcome measure, determine which of the following variables increases the odds of exercising: education, satisfaction with current weight, health, current quality of life, confidence, and life satisfaction.

RESULTS

1.

	Smokes		
On a Sports Team	*Yes*	*No*	**Row Totals**
No	270	500	770
Yes	50	430	480
	320	*930*	*1250*

Probabilities:

Of smoking when not on team	270/770 = .35
Of not smoking when not on team	500/770 = .65
Of smoking when on team	50/480 = .10
Of not smoking when on team	430/480 = .90

Odds:

Of smoking when not on team	.35/.65 = .54
Of smoking when on team	.10/.90 = .11

Odds ratio:	.54/.11 = 4.91

Risks:

Of smoking when not on team	270/770 = .35
Of smoking when on team	50/408 = .10

Relative risk:	.35/.10 = 3.5

The odds of smoking when not on a team are almost 5 times higher than when on a team. The relative risk of smoking when not on a team is 3.5 times higher.

2. A logistic regression was run to answer the research question. The results are contained in Exercise Figure 13-1. The variables were all entered together. The overall analysis is significant ($p = .0000$). The model was more successful in predicting the rarely/sometimes group (74%) than the often/routinely group (63%). Only two of the variables contributed significantly to the prediction, satisfaction with current weight ($p = .0169$) and health ($p = .0463$). Both variables are measured on a 10-point scale. For every one-point increase in score on satisfaction with current weight, the odds of exercising often or routinely go up 1.2 times. For health, a one-point increase in score increases the odds of exercising 1.3 times.

```
Dependent Variable Encoding:

Original        Internal
Value           Value
     .00        0
   1.00         1

Dependent Variable..   EXER2      Exercise, recoded

Beginning Block Number  0.  Initial Log Likelihood Function

-2 Log Likelihood    222.99686

* Constant is included in the model.


Beginning Block Number  1.  Method: Enter

Variable(s) Entered on Step Number
1..        EDUC       education in years
           SATCURWT   satisfaction with current weight
           HEALTH     overall state of health
           QOLCUR     quality of life in past month
           CONFID     Confidence during stressful situations
           LIFE       Life purpose and satisfaction

Estimation terminated at iteration number 4 because
Log Likelihood decreased by less than .01 percent.

   -2 Log Likelihood      182.486
   Goodness of Fit        154.742

                    Chi-Square    df Significance

   Model Chi-Square      40.511    6      .0000
   Improvement           40.511    6      .0000
```

EXERCISE FIGURE 13-1. Logistic regression, Exercise 2. (*continued*)

Classification Table for EXER2

```
                          Predicted
                 rarely/sometimes  often/routinely   Percent Correct
                        r                 o
Observed              +-------+---------+
  rarely/sometimes  r I  66   I   23    I              74.16%
                     +-------+---------+
  often/routinely   o I  27   I   46    I              63.01%
                     +-------+---------+
                                          Overall      69.14%
```

------------- Variables in the Equation -------------

Variable	B	S.E.	Wald	df	Sig	R
EDUC	.0273	.0511	.2856	1	.5930	.0000
SATCURWT	.1705	.0714	5.7097	1	.0169	.1290
HEALTH	.2370	.1190	3.9689	1	.0463	.0940
QOLCUR	.4071	.2106	3.7355	1	.0533	.0882
CONFID	-.0004	.0203	.0005	1	.9824	.0000
LIFE	.0086	.0187	.2126	1	.6447	.0000
Constant	-6.0672	1.3191	21.1553	1	.0000	

Variable	Exp(B)	90% CI for Exp(B) Lower	Upper
EDUC	1.0277	.9449	1.1177
SATCURWT	1.1859	1.0546	1.3336
HEALTH	1.2674	1.0422	1.5413
QOLCUR	1.5025	1.0625	2.1247
CONFID	.9996	.9667	1.0335
LIFE	1.0086	.9781	1.0401

Observed Groups and Predicted Probabilities

```
        8 +                                                                    +
          I                                                                    I
          I                                                                    I
        6 +                                                                    +
          I                            o                                       I
          I                            o                                       I
F       4 +                   o        o        o      o        o      o       +
R         I                o  o        o   r    o  o   oo ooo   oo ooo   ooo    I
E         I                o  o        o   r    o  o   oo ooo   oo ooo   ooo    I
Q         I          oo    o  or   r   ro  ror  o  r   oooo ooo oooo ooo  oo    I
U         I          oo    o  or   r   ro  ror  o  r   oooo ooo oooo ooo  oo    I
E       2 +  rr  rr  oo rr rror ror ro orrroo oor o r rrrrrrrrroorrrooorrrooooo +
N         I  rr  rr  oo rr rror ror ro orrroo oor o r rrrrrrrrroorrrooorrrooooo I
C         I  r      rr rr rrror r   orrrroroo oooorroo ooorrroo rrorrooorroooooo I
Y         I  r      rr rr rrror r   orrrroroo oooorroo ooorrroo rrorrooorroooooo I
          I rrr rr rrrrrrrrrrroorrrrrr oooorroo rrrrrrrrrrorrrrooooo            I
          I rrr rr rrrrrrrrrrroorrrrrr oooorroo rrrrrrrrrrorrrrooooo            I
Predicted ---------+---------+---------+---------+---------+
  Prob:   0       .25       .5       .75        1
  Group:  rrrrrrrrrrrrrrrrrrrrrrrrrrrrrrrooooooooooooooooooooooooooooooooooooooo
```

Predicted Probability is of Membership for often/routinely

Symbols: r - rarely/sometimes
         o - often/routinely

Each Symbol Represents .5 Cases.

EXERCISE FIGURE 13-1. (END)

14

Grouping Techniques

Jane Karpe Dixon

Objectives for Chapter 14

After reading this chapter, you should be able to do the following:

1 ● Identify research situations in which factor analysis would be appropriate.

2 ● Describe the steps involved in carrying out a factor analysis procedure.

3 ● Interpret factor analysis results from a computer printout or published study.

4 ● Appreciate the potential value of confirmatory factor analysis in supplementing the results of exploratory factor analysis.

Factor Analysis

Researchers in the health care fields often focus their attention on multiple variables. This is a direct result of the nature of the problems under study, which are complex in the real world of patient care. For example, with regard to major causes of illness and death in the developed world (e.g., cancer, heart disease, stroke, diabetes, accidents), we have learned to speak of risk factors rather than one single cause. In some cases, a particular disease may exist only in the presence of a particular agent (e.g., clinical mononucleosis with the Epstein-Barr virus). Even then, however, variables describing personal and environmental characteristics are crucial in influencing the course of the illness or even whether symptoms occur. Also, multiple issues affect such nursing concerns as recuperation following surgery and compliance with health care recommendations. In other chapters of this book, we discuss how multivariate strategies can be used to understand the way multiple causes may lead to a single event. Factor analysis is often an early step in the process of achieving a multivariate perspective on a clinical research problem.

This chapter addresses the understanding of *concepts*. Often when labeling variables, a single word or phrase is used to represent a phenomenon with multiple parts. Our language may be overly general, blending together the multiple aspects of the phenomenon of interest. Consider, for example, the term *satisfaction* with care. Superficially, it seems logical to measure this with a single rating. ("Rate your satisfaction with the care you received.") However, such a rating might involve opinions on a variety of matters, such as perceived competence of caregivers, convenience, and pleasantness of the environment. (As an exercise, think of at least two other aspects of satisfaction with care.) It is hard to know which of these influences are reflected in a subject's satisfaction rating and what such a rating really means. Instead of a global rating, should several aspects be measured separately? There are so many potentially important variables, we may be unable to decide which should be measured and which should not. Factor analysis can help us make such decisions.

The amount of information on which our minds can focus simultaneously is limited. As a convenience, we may concentrate on variables thought to be primary. This will reduce the data burden. In some research endeavors, however, such simplicity of questionnaire may not be necessary, because we have techniques for organizing multivariate data—data on many variables. Factor analysis is one of these techniques. Factor analysis can serve the purpose of *data reduction*. In factor analysis, many variables are "reduced" (grouped) into a smaller number of factors. This is analogous to univariate approaches in which a mean, variance, or correlation coefficient is calculated to reduce individual scores on one or two values. In this chapter, the purposes of factor analysis are explained, and the steps used to carry out a factor analysis are introduced. Because factor analysis is a complex technique, almost exclusively carried out by computer, this chapter emphasizes interpretation rather than calculation. Confirmatory factor analysis, an advanced form of factor analysis, is introduced.

For further information regarding factor analysis, the reader may consult Nunnally and Bernstein (1994) or Child (1990).

RESEARCH QUESTIONS

To explicate the types of research questions that can be answered using factor analysis, a hypothetical example of a factor analysis situation may be helpful. Suppose a researcher measures six variables within a sample of adult male participants in a health maintenance organization. Three of these variables are aspects of body size: height, arm length, and leg length. Three are derived from a health history in which the subject is asked to report the number of specific episodes occurring in the last year. These variables are number of sore throats, number of headaches, and number of earaches. A researcher may want to see how these variables group—which ones go together and which ones do not? How strongly does each variable go with its group? All together, how many dimensions are needed to explain relationships among the variables (Nunnally & Bernstein, 1994)? You may begin to explore answers to these questions through careful examination of the patterns of correlations among these variables. In the matrix of correlations for these six variables, we will probably see that the three size variables have high intercorrelations and that the three history variables also have high intercorrelations; that is, a man with longer than average legs also may have longer than average arms. He is also likely to be taller than average. A person reporting frequent sore throats also may report other discomforts. On the other hand, it would be surprising if the size variables and the history variables were highly related.

A simplified representation of a correlation matrix is shown in Table 14-1. If such a matrix is factor analyzed, a factor matrix defining the two groups of variables would be derived, as shown in Table 14-2. Each column in this table reflects one of the variable groupings or factors. The size variables have high values in one column, and the history variables have high values in the other column. This table, indicating the presence of two distinct groups of variables—two factors—summarizes the information contained in the larger correlation matrix. It reduces the data. Much of the information from a 6 × 6 correlation matrix is conveyed in a 6 × 2 factor matrix.

You may object that the groupings derived were already easily apparent from the correlation table and that an advanced statistical technique is not needed to show what is obvious. This is true, but in the usual case, factor analysis does help us know what we would not otherwise know. Suppose that we had a 20 × 20 correlation matrix with widely ranging correlation coefficients, and the groupings among the variables were subtle. The variables would appear in random order, rather than neatly arranged ac-

TABLE 14-1
Six × Six Correlation Matrix: Size and History Variables

	Height	Arm Length	Leg Length	Number of Sore Throats	Number of Headaches	Number of Earaches
Height	—	Hi	Hi	Lo	Lo	Lo
Arm Length		—	Hi	Lo	Lo	Lo
Leg Length			—	Lo	Lo	Lo
Number of Sore Throats				—	Hi	Hi
Number of Headaches					—	Hi
Number of Earaches						—

"Hi" means correlation of high magnitude, regardless of direction (approaching + 1.00 or approaching − 1.00).

"Lo" means correlation of low magnitude (near zero).

TABLE 14-2
Abbreviated Factor Matrix: Size and History Variables

Variables	Factors	
	I	*II*
Height	Hi	Lo
Arm length	Hi	Lo
Leg length	Hi	Lo
Number of sore throats	Lo	Hi
Number of headaches	Lo	Hi
Number of earaches	Lo	Hi

"Hi" means above .40 or below − .40—especially approaching 1.00 or − 1.00.
"Lo" means between− .40 and + .40—especially near zero.

cording to grouping. Then patterns would not be obvious. Factor analysis is a tool through which we may uncover groupings of variables that are *not* obvious.

TYPES OF FACTOR ANALYSIS

Factor analysis is a statistical tool for analyzing scores on large numbers of variables to determine whether there are any identifiable dimensions that can be used to describe many of the variables under study. Sometimes researchers assume that observed covariation between variables is due to some underlying common factors. The collection of intercorrelations is treated mathematically in such a way that underlying traits are identified.

There is some diversity in the purposes for which factor analysis is conducted and the types of procedures used. As implied in the chapter objectives, factor analysis may be exploratory or confirmatory. Exploratory factor analysis is used to summarize data by grouping together variables that are intercorrelated. Most often, this occurs in the early stages of research. Confirmatory factor analysis tests hypotheses about structure of variables. This may follow an exploratory analysis, or it may come directly from theory. Potential purposes of confirmatory factor analysis are explained in more detail later in this chapter.

Another way of thinking about the diversity of types of factor analysis focuses on what exactly is being correlated in the correlation matrix. Most commonly, the correlations are between variables and across subjects. This is called *R*-type. This type of factor analysis dominates the research literature of nursing and other health care professions.

However, it is also possible to construct a correlation matrix based on correlation between subjects and across variables. (That is, a data matrix is transposed so that each row represents a variable, and each column represents a subject prior to calculation of correlations; this can be done easily in some software programs.) A factor analysis performed on such a correlation matrix is *Q*-type. In such an analysis, subjects, rather than variables, are grouped together.

In *P*-type factor analysis, correlations represent relationships across time (repeated measures from a single person). *P*-type factor analysis reveals groupings of variables across time.

This chapter focuses on *R*-type factor analysis, which is the most common in research within the health care professions.

USE OF FACTOR ANALYSIS

The direct purpose of factor analysis is to reduce a set of data so that it may be described and used easily. Other purposes include instrument development and theory construction

Instrument Development

In the research literature of nursing and other health care professions, factor analysis is most often used as a part of the instrument-development process. Factor analysis may be a vital step in creation of a new measurement tool. It is a method for organizing the items into *factors*. A factor is a group of items that may be said to belong together. A person who scores high on one item of a particular factor is likely to score above average on other items of the factor and vice versa. Such an item has high correlations with other items of the same factor and not so high correlations with items of different factors. This principle provides the mathematical basis for assignment of items to factors through the statistical technique of factor analysis.

Factor analysis is often used to test the validity of ideas about items to decide how items should be grouped together into subscales and which items should be dropped from the instrument entirely. The method helps to provide justification for our use of *summated scales* (sets of items summed into scale scores). For example, a researcher may start with 18 items and based on factor analysis decide that these should be organized into two subscales: For each subject, two scores will be calculated. It is also common for some items to be dropped from a scale based on factor analysis results. Factor analysis is an important statistical tool for providing validity evidence concerning the structure of our instruments. In most cases, this is followed by computation of Cronbach's alpha coefficient, which is a measure of internal consistency reliability. Such reliability is an alternative way of looking at the extent to which items go together, similar to the factor analysis itself; however, in computation of reliability, only one set of items is dealt with at a time. Also, reliability computations are useful for further identifying weak items that may be omitted in subsequent analysis. In any case, items that form a strong factor in factor analysis generally yield acceptable alpha coefficients when grouped together in a scale, thus providing evidence of internal consistency reliability and supporting beginning evidence of construct validity for a developing scale.

Theory Development

The building of theory is a principal purpose of research, and factor analysis may support such efforts in a variety of ways: by describing clinical phenomena, exploring relationships, identifying (name) constructs that unite a set of elements, creating units of classification for systems construction, and testing hypotheses. All of these are theory-building functions.

Most basically, approaches to factor analysis may be distinguished as exploratory or confirmatory or in some intermediate position between these poles. Although the emphasis in this chapter is on exploratory approaches (because this is the most reasonable starting point for the beginning user of factor analysis), confirmatory approaches also are addressed; Chapter 16 shows that structural modeling with latent variables incorporates factor analysis into a series of procedures with confirmatory purposes. In a truly exploratory approach, a researcher uses factor analysis to discover a structure that can be meaningfully interpreted. The researcher begins without preconceived expectations about the nature of the structure that will emerge; rather, the structure is allowed to unfold from the data. In a truly confirmatory approach, a hypothesis is developed, and variables relevant to that hypothesis are then identified and (once data are collected) submitted to factor analysis. The researcher asks whether the data fit the hypothesized model better than they fit alternative models. Confirmatory factor analysis has received increasing attention in nursing and other health care research areas in the last decade. More details on this approach appear later in this chapter.

Data Reduction for Subsequent Analysis

Sometimes factor analysis is used solely for data reduction, simply because such reduction may be needed for subsequent analysis. One goal of scientific inquiry is *parsimony*, simplicity of explanation; that is, it is preferable to use one variable, rather than many, to explain a phenomenon. Factor analysis provides a means for creating a single composite variable out of many variables. Often it is used to identify several composite variables, which taken together, summarize the sources of variance contained in all (or most) variables included in a study (or at least of those variables of a particular type). These composite variables are mathematically constructed through a combination of the measured variables. The several composite variables, rather than the larger number of measured variables, are then used in subsequent data analysis. Data reduction of this sort may serve a highly pragmatic function. The researcher may collect a large amount of data, reduce the data through factor analysis, and conduct other analyses (such as regression or analysis of variance) on the reduced data. In these subsequent analyses, the number of variables relative to the number of subjects is kept within reasonable bounds, reliability is augmented, and provided that the meanings of factors are clearly defined and communicated, interpretation of the analysis may be simplified. Often, this is combined with instrument development or theory development.

TYPE OF DATA REQUIRED

Most often, the factor analysis process begins with raw data of subjects by variables and the calculation of Pearson product-moment correlations between these variables on the way to calculating the factor analysis. However, you may also carry out a factor analysis based simply on a correlation matrix available through a published research report. Whatever the actual starting point, the correlation matrix is submitted to factor analysis.

You are already familiar with the correlation matrix, the beginnings of many of our statistical treatments. In such a matrix (as in Fig. 11-3) the two halves are identical; that is, the correlation of X with Y is the same as the correlation of Y with X. We call such a matrix *symmetrical*. Factor analysis may be performed with any symmetrical matrix of correlations.

In the development of a new instrument, however, it is common for some items to be eliminated from consideration prior to conducting factor analysis. This is based on the univariate and multivariate characteristics of each item. This systematic evaluation of individual items is called item analysis. For example, Fleury (1994) created the Index of Readiness to measure readiness to initiate health behavior change. From a sample of cardiac rehabilitation patients, data were collected on 39 Likert type items, but only 20 of these were included in the factor analysis. Others were omitted through the item analysis process. Criteria for inclusion of an item included a standard deviation that was approximately half the mean, indicating an appropriate level of variation among subjects on the variable. Another criterion was moderate correlations with other items (between .30 and .70). In factor analyzing the 20 items, Fleury obtained three factors that she named reevaluation of lifestyle, identification of barriers, and goal commitment.

Criteria used to select some items for factor analysis and eliminate others vary from one study to another; however, they are largely based on understanding of the assumptions and meaning of correlation and the role of factor analysis in summarizing or reducing a correlation matrix.

ASSUMPTIONS

Factor analysis is based on a matrix of correlations between variables, so all data assumptions applicable to calculation and interpretation of correlations apply to factor analysis as well. Data should be interval level or data that the researcher has specifically decided to treat as interval, as typically occurs with Likert-type self-report data. Data should be approximately normally distributed. It is customary to base factor analysis on variables that are measured on a common metric or response format.

A curvilinear relationship between two variables cannot be detected using the Pearson product-moment correlation. Therefore, such a relationship will not be reflected in factor analysis results either. Also, if the correlation matrix is smaller than 10×10, some special considerations may be appropriate.

In general, for meaningful results to be obtained in a factor analysis, correlations between variables should be substantial so that each variable included correlates highly with at least one other variable. Nunnally and Bernstein (1994) recommend inclusion of marker variables with known properties to increase the likelihood that this will occur. Also, all variables included must be reliably measured, and subjects must show some variation in their responses.

SAMPLE SIZE CONSIDERATIONS AND "POWER"

For statistical tests treated earlier in this book, there is a direct relationship between sample size and power of the test to identify statistically significant differences between groups (or relationships between variables), when such differences (or relationships) exist in the population from which the sample is drawn. With a larger sample size, the ability to generalize from the sample to the population is increased. In exploratory models of factor analysis, statistical significance is not tested, and strictly speaking, the concept of "power" does not apply. However, the value of observed sample data in reflecting reality as it exists in the larger population is a major concern in most factor analytic studies, as in most research generally.

In factor analysis, the number of subjects needed is usually assessed in relation to the number of variables being measured. Although factor analysis is especially appropriate when working with a large amount of data, the number of variables that may be included in a factor analysis procedure is limited. It is tied to sample size. Certainly, the number of cases should always exceed the number of variables. A ratio of at least 10 subjects for each variable is desirable to generalize from the sample to a wider population. With smaller ratios, the influence of relationships based on random patterns within the data becomes more pronounced. However, Knapp and Brown (1995) note that ratios as low as three subjects per variable are sometimes acceptable. Another perspective on sample size is that because it is based on correlation, 100 to 200 subjects are enough for most purposes. In any case, sample size may be problematic, and the need for replication of factor studies is increasingly emphasized. An article by Teel and Verran (1991) presents a variety of approaches through which factor solutions obtained in various studies may be compared.

SIX MATRICES

The mathematics of factor analysis is complex. It is based on *matrix algebra*—the branch of mathematics that deals with the manipulation of matrices. However, matrix algebra is beyond the scope of this book, and you do not need an understanding of matrix algebra to conduct a factor analysis. All mathematics can be done by computer.

The process of conducting a factor analysis, as experienced by the clinical researcher working within the structure of a packaged statistical program for the computer, is now presented. This process may involve as many as six matrices. Each matrix is derived from a previous one through the computer program, but the researcher should still *understand* each matrix.

Raw Data Matrix

These are the data that the researcher collects about the study subjects. They are entered into the computer by the researcher in the form of data lines, each containing information about one subject. In such a matrix, each row represents a single subject, and each column represents a variable. You are familiar with this sort of matrix; it is the beginning of any data analysis. A raw data matrix to be factor analyzed would contain many variables. (*Note*: For a *Q*-type analysis, the data matrix would be transposed so that each row is a variable, and each column is a subject.)

Correlation Matrix

You are also familiar with the correlation matrix. When fully depicted, the correlation matrix is a square, symmetrical matrix in which the number of rows and the number of columns each equal the number of variables. Because the correlation matrix is symmetrical (therefore, containing much duplication), it is often depicted in one of several abbreviated forms. The correlation matrix summarizes information in the raw data matrix. It is smaller, with fewer rows and fewer elements than the raw data matrix. This is the beginning of the data reduction process. In some situations, the correlation matrix is altered prior to conducting the factor analysis. This alteration concerns the diagonal that extends from the upper left corner to the lower right corner—the correlation of each variable with itself. Each variable correlates perfectly with itself, so the conventional correlation matrix contains "1.0" as every element in this diagonal. However, in a correlation matrix to be used for a factor analysis, this may not be maintained. Depending on decisions about the factor analysis model to be used, these 1s are sometimes replaced by a number smaller than 1.0 and selected to be specific for each variable, such as an estimate of the common variance with other variables or the reliability of measurement. This is explained below.

Factor Matrix, Unrotated

Based on the correlation matrix, the first of two (or more) factor matrices is calculated. In a factor matrix (Table 14-3), each row represents one variable included in the factor analysis. There are fewer columns, each column representing one factor. In the unrotated factor matrix, the elements within the matrix are the unrotated *factor loadings*—numbers ranging between −1 and +1, which are like correlations of the variable with the factor. The square of a factor loading represents the proportion

TABLE 14-3
Factor Loading Matrix

			Factors		
		I	II	III	h²
	1	.85	.22	.03	.77
	2	.15	•	•	•
Variables	3	.51	•	•	•
	4	.83	•	•	•
	5	.26	•	•	•
Eigenvalues		1.76			
% of variance		.35			

of variance that the item and factor have in common; in other words, this is the proportion of item variance explained by the factor. For example, in Table 14-3, illustrating an unrotated factor matrix, the first variable (1) has a loading of .85 on factor I; approximately 72% of variance is accounted for by this loading ($[.85]^2 = .7225$). Adding the squared loadings across a row, you arrive at the item communality (h^2). This is the portion of item variance accounted for by the various factors. For variable 1 in Table 14-3, the squared factor loadings are totaled as follows: $.85^2 + .22^2 + .03^2 = .77$. The item communality is .77; that is, 77% of item variance is "explained" by the three factors.

If you add the squared loadings contained in a single column, you will obtain the *eigenvalue* for the factor. The eigenvalue represents the total amount of variance explained by a factor. The average of the squared loadings in a column is obtained by dividing the eigenvalue by the number of items in the column (eigenvalue/n). This average represents the percent of interitem variance accounted for by the factor. For the first factor in Table 14-3, the eigenvalue is calculated as follows: $.85^2 + .15^2 + .51^2 + .83^2 + .26^2 = 1.76$. This eigenvalue of 1.76 is divided by 5 (because there are five variables), yielding .352. Thus, approximately 35% of total item variance is accounted for by the first factor. Adding the percent of variance accounted for by each factor tells us how much variance is explained by all the factors.

Factor eigenvalues and variance accounted for are the most important figures contained in the unrotated factor matrix. You may be especially interested in how much variance is accounted for altogether by the important factors; this is simply the sum of variance accounted for by individual factors. Either factor eigenvalues or the variance accounted for by factors may be used to determine the number of potentially interpretable factors contained in the data. Typically, researchers want to interpret the number of factors that each account for at least 5% of variance or the number of factors for which the eigenvalue is 1 or greater. Determination of the appropriate number of factors paves the way for the next matrix of the factor analysis process. However, before moving on to this next matrix, a diversion is needed.

A Note on Extraction Models

For the ambitious reader, further explanation is provided here concerning the choices facing the researcher who is conducting a factor analysis. (If you are a less ambitious reader, you may want to skip this section.) The unrotated factor matrix is obtained through use of an extraction method, and the statistical software packages that are generally used offer a choice of extraction methods. Basically, two general approaches are based on two different assumptions about the data (Ferketich & Muller, 1990).

The distinction has to do with the nature of the variance in the data. One possible assumption is that all measurement error is random. In this case, the mean of deviations (representing the error) is zero. Based on this assumption, a researcher chooses to use the extraction method known as principal components. Using this method of extraction, new variables are exact mathematical transformations of the original data. When this method of extraction is used, *all* variance in the observed variables contributes to the solution. Because each variable correlates perfectly with itself, the 1s (unities) in the diagonal of the correlation matrix are a part of the variance that is analyzed. Using the principal components method, the goal is to convert a set of variables into a new set of variables that is an exact mathematical transformation of the original data.

The other possible assumption to be made is that measurement error consists of a systematic component and a unique component. The systematic component may reflect common variance due to factors that are not directly measured (Ferketich & Muller, 1990). These are called *latent factors*. Based on this assumption, a researcher chooses to use any of a class of extraction methods categorized as "common factor analysis." This includes methods named principal axis, image, alpha, generalized least squares, and unweighted least squares. Because the researcher making this assumption wants to focus on the common variance, it is not appropriate to use the full correlation matrix. Instead, the diagonals are altered so that instead of consisting of unities (1s), an estimate of the communalities (h^2) is used. Such modification of a matrix may seem surprising to someone new to factor analysis. In common factor analyses, the matrix analyzed does not reflect the full variance in the data; rather, the covariance is analyzed.

While some research methodologists place strong emphasis on the distinction between principal components and common factor analysis (Ferketich & Muller, 1990), Nunnally and Bernstein (1994) argue that in a well designed study involving a sufficient number of subjects, choice of extraction model makes little practical difference in the results obtained. They do note, however, that the principal component method will lead to elements of the matrix being a bit larger. This is because approaches to common factor analysis always involve replacing the "ones" in the diagonal of the correlation matrix with numbers that are less than 1. Thus, the factor loadings that emerge are a bit smaller. We have seen that eigenvalues, variance accounted for by factor, and item communalities are all a direct function of the magnitude of the loadings, so it follows that these are smaller also. Thus, the factor solution may *appear* to be less good, but this is simply an artifact of the methods decision. Nunnally and Bernstein (1994) also note that the principal components method is more reliable because with this method, you always obtain a factor solution. In common factor analysis, obtaining a solution may not be a sure thing.

When arguing that despite these specific differences, the results are essentially the same with the two methods, Nunnally and Bernstein (1994) refer to an overall similarity in the groupings of items obtained. However, this perspective is not supported by a set of analyses presented by Youngblut (1993), who reported results obtained by analyzing a dataset using principal components and also by six other specific extraction methods. Youngblut reported that the anticipated two-factor solution emerged only with the principal component method. Undoubtedly, the relative differences and similarities between extraction methods will remain a point of contention among research methodologists. Some researchers routinely run multiple factor analyses of the same dataset but with varying methods to gauge the importance of these distinctions and other decision points in the factor analytic process.

Later in this chapter, we return to the problem of choosing a specific extraction model. Now, we return to discussion of the fourth of six matrices.

Factor Matrix, Rotated

The unrotated factors are created (based on the correlations between variables) so that the amount of variance accounted for by each successive factor is maximized. This means that factors may (in geometric terms) run between independent groups of related variables, rather than accurately reflecting the meaning of a group of variables. The consequence of this is that unrotated factors rarely can be meaningfully interpreted. However, just as you may alter an algebraic equation by performing the same operation on both sides, you may transform or "rotate" a factor matrix into any one of an infinite number of mathematically equivalent matrices. If factor rotation is conducted according to the criterion of *simple structure* as described by Thurstone in 1947, the result is a set of factors that are distinct from one another and that, in most situations, can be meaningfully and creatively interpreted by the researcher. In simple structure, factors are set to maximize the number of loadings of great magnitude (near +1 and −1) and loadings of small magnitude (near 0.00) for each factor; that is, a distinct pattern emerges in the factor matrix so that each factor has certain variables that go with it, while other variables do not. Likewise, as simple structure is approached, each variable is identified with *only one* factor. According to Thurstone (1947), the following occur in a factor matrix:

1. Each row should have at least one loading close to zero.
2. Each column should have at least as many variables with near-zero loadings as there are factors.
3. For pairs of columns (factors), several variables should load on one and not on the other.

The essence of interpreting factor analytic results is the process of identifying, from the rotated factor matrix, which variables go with a factor and then naming the factor based on whatever meanings these variables with high loadings have in common. The criterion for considering a loading high varies from study to study, with some researchers using cutoff points as low as 0.30; others use cutoff points as high as 0.55. In the example given previously, Fleury (1994) used .40 for her criterion in determining whether or not a particular item loaded substantially on a factor.

When naming and describing factors, the researcher uses not only knowledge of the statistical technique and how it works, but also an understanding of the subject matter under study, especially an ability to construct new understandings of that subject matter. By facilitating the organization of individual variables into variable groupings, factor analysis opens the door to new conceptualizations and new ways of thinking, provided that the researcher is ready to discover these in the data. More than any other statistical technique, factor analysis requires the full exercise of creative potential.

Factor Score Matrix

Based on the rotated factor matrix, a score for each subject on each factor may be computed. To calculate such *factor scores,* an individual's score on each variable included in a factor is multiplied by the factor loading for the particular variable. The sum of these products is the individual's factor score. The general formula is:

$$\text{Factor score} = \text{sum of} \left(\begin{array}{c} \text{individual's} \\ \text{score on} \\ \text{variable} \end{array} \right) \times \left(\begin{array}{c} \text{factor loading} \\ \text{of variable} \\ \text{on factor} \end{array} \right)$$

Factor scores can be calculated automatically within factor analysis procedures in statistical packages for the computer. Consider an individual included in the data of Table 14-3 who received scores as follows:

Variable	Scores
1	2
2	4
3	1
4	5
5	2

This person's factor score on factor 1 would be calculated as follows:

$$(.85)(2) + (.15)(4) + (.51)(1) + (.83)(5) + (.26)(2) = 1.7 + .6 + .51 + 4.15 + .52 = 7.48.$$

This factor score, based on the strength of the correlation of each variable with the factor, could be used instead of the individual's unweighted (i.e., summative) score on the factor. The factor score is based on the relative "importance" of each variable to the factor as indicated by that correlation. This individual's unweighted score would be simply the sum of the scores on the five variables (2 + 4 + 1 + 5

TABLE 14-4
Factor Score Matrix

		Factors			
		I	*II*	•	•
Subjects	1	7.48	•	•	•
	2	•	•		
	•	•	•		
	•	•	•		
	•	•	•		
	n	•	•		

+ 2 = 14). It is conventional among researchers to use factor scores when conducting further analysis on the same dataset. This operationalizes the data reduction purpose of factor analysis. An example of such usage is presented later in the chapter.

In contrast, when factor analysis is used primarily for the purpose of instrument development, it is conventional to derive an approach for creation of unweighted scores from the factor results obtained. These are the summative scales (usually subscales) that become a part of the protocol for how the instrument is to be scored and interpreted in future usage.

The factor score matrix has as many rows as subjects, with each column representing one factor. The structure of such a matrix is illustrated in Table 14-4. The factor score matrix is smaller than the raw data matrix because there are fewer factors than variables. The data have been reduced.

Factor Correlation Matrix

Factor rotation is often *orthogonal,* with resulting factors uncorrelated with each other. This is usually desirable for instrument development, in which the researcher seeks to create subscales that are independent of one another. Alternatively, factor rotation also may be *oblique,* with factors that are not totally unrelated to each other. Advocates of oblique rotation assert that in the real world, important factors are likely to be correlated; thus, searching for unrelated factors is unrealistic. Novice factor analysts should probably plan to use an orthogonal, rather than oblique, rotation because it is easier to interpret. The *Varimax* (variance maximized) method, is available on all widely used computer packages. This tends to produce factors that have low loadings with some variables and high loadings with other variables. Other alternatives are *Quartimax,* which is likely to yield a first, very general factor with many high loadings, and *Equamax,* which combines characteristics of *Quartimax* and *Varimax,* balancing the advantages and disadvantages of each.

With orthogonal rotation, one factor loading matrix is produced. It represents regression weights (called a *pattern matrix*) and correlation coefficients (called a *structure matrix*). Because the solution is orthogonal, the regression weights are equal to

TABLE 14-5
Factor Correlation Matrix

	Factor 1	*Factor 2*	*Factor 3*
Factor 1	1.00	0.65	0.30
Factor 2		1.00	0.45
Factor 3			1.00

the correlation coefficients. The loadings are interpreted as were those in the unrotated factor matrix. A squared loading represents the variance accounted for in a variable by a particular factor. The squared loadings may be added across a row to determine total variance accounted for in a variable by all the factors and so on.

Because with oblique rotation there is correlation among the factors, the *factor pattern matrix* (the regression weights) and the *factor structure matrix* (containing correlation coefficients) are not the same. The two matrices are produced and interpreted differently. The pattern matrix is generally considered preferable as a basis for interpreting the meanings of factors. The square of a loading in a factor pattern matrix represents the variance accounted for by a particular variable, but because other factors may share some of this variance (due to intercorrelation among factors in an oblique solution), the total variance in an item accounted for by all the factors *cannot* be determined by adding the squared loadings in a row (h^2).

In oblique rotation, a matrix displaying the correlation of each factor with every other factor is displayed in a factor correlation matrix. The structure of such a matrix is shown in Table 14-5.

STEPS OF A FACTOR ANALYTIC STUDY

The steps of a factor analytic study are as follows:

1. Formulate a research question or hypothesis. If factor analysis is the appropriate statistical technique for answering research questions or testing the hypothesis, proceed with the following steps.
2. Collect data of interest.
3. Calculate and examine univariate data on a variable-by-variable basis, identifying variables that should not be included in the factor analysis because of failure to meet initial assumptions or criteria.
4. Calculate and examine bivariate relationship data—again with an eye toward identifying variables and relationships that should not be included in the factor analysis.
5. "Run" the factor analysis. Unless you have a good reason to do otherwise, use an orthogonal rotation. If you have predicted certain factors, specify in the computer program how many factors you expect; otherwise, let the computer determine the number of factors in the course of the factor analysis, based on eigenvalues

in the unrotated factor matrix. Note the total proportion of interitem variance accounted for by the factor solution and the number of factors involved.

6. Name and interpret factors from the rotated factor loading matrix. (Sometimes researchers experiment with several factor solutions to choose the one that can be most meaningfully interpreted.)

7. If subsequent analyses are planned, use factor analysis results to decide how to combine variables; calculate these new or combined variables for each subject. (Usually, factor scores can be easily calculated on the computer.) Consider the reliabilities of the derived scores. Then conduct the subsequent analyses.

8. Relate findings to the existing literature, and disseminate results through presentation and publication. If appropriate, repeat the analysis with other available populations.

COMBINING FACTOR ANALYSIS WITH OTHER APPROACHES

Factor analysis is often used as an early stage of a multistage analysis, as indicated by steps 7 and 8. Subsequent analyses may be conducted as part of an instrument development and validation process or because of substantive interest. For example, after Fleury (1994) identified three factors of her index of readiness and determined the internal consistency reliability of these as subscales, she correlated these with another instrument, the index of current health behaviors, designed to measure current risk modification efforts. Numerous relationships in the expected direction were found. People higher on reevaluation of lifestyle were making more individual attempts to quit smoking (r = .19), and smoking behaviors were reduced (r =. 35). Likewise, goal commitment correlated with indicators of dietary modification, such as dietary fat reduction (r = .30) and so on. These data were taken as evidence of the concurrent validity of the Fleury's index of readiness.

Such findings may have important substantive and instrument development implications. Generally, factor analysis tends to be most useful when combined with other analyses within a single study.

EXAMPLE OF A COMPUTER PRINTOUT

As an example, an edited computer printout of a principal components analysis is shown in Figure 14-1. The data analyzed are from a 10-item scale designed to measure self-assessed health. Responses were obtained from 310 subjects. The 10 × 10 correlation matrix was submitted to principal components analysis with Equamax rotation using the SPSS computer package. (Equamax rotation was used to balance the need for interpretable factors with the need for simplified, interpretable variables.)

The first four lines reprint the procedure commands needed to implement the computer run. Few command statements are needed because of heavy use of default options. For example, principal components is the default extraction method.

(text continues on page 328)

```
4  0  factor variables=all
5  0             /plot=eigen
6  0             /format=sort
7  0             /rotation=equamax
```

---------------------- F A C T O R   A N A L Y S I S ----------------------

ANALYSIS NUMBER 1 LISTWISE DELETION OF CASES WITH MISSING VALUES

EXTRACTION 1 FOR ANALYSIS 1, PRINCIPAL-COMPONENTS ANALYSIS (PC)

INITIAL STATISTICS:

VARIABLE	COMMUNALITY	*	FACTOR	EIGENVALUE	PCT OF VAR	CUM PCT
		*				
PURPOSE	1.00000	*	1	4.54230	45.4	45.4
ENERGY	1.00000	*	2	1.43410	14.3	59.8
SYMPTOM	1.00000	*	3	.88429	8.8	68.6
CHRONIC	1.00000	*	4	.71156	7.1	75.7
EMOTION	1.00000	*	5	.58654	5.9	81.6
SPORATIC	1.00000	*	6	.45276	4.5	86.1
DISABIL	1.00000	*	7	.38327	3.8	89.9
MAJILL	1.00000	*	8	.36480	3.6	93.6
SOCTIES	1.00000	*	9	.33923	3.4	97.0
ACCEPT	1.00000	*	10	.30113	3.0	100.0

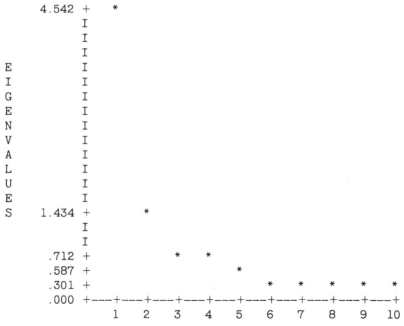

FIGURE 14-1
Computer printout of a principal component analysis.

PC EXTRACTED 2 FACTORS

FACTOR MATRIX:

	FACTOR 1	FACTOR 2
ENERGY	.78644	.00606
EMOTION	.76618	−.27295
PURPOSE	.75584	−.30671
ACCEPT	.74274	−.42868
SOCTIES	.67430	−.55553
CHRONIC	.66493	.47268
SYMPTOM	.66435	.43335
MAJILL	.60852	.21185
DISABIL	.54621	.46797
SPORATIC	.45500	.31310

FINAL STATISTICS:

VARIABLE	COMMUNALITY	*	FACTOR	EIGENVALUE	PCT OF VAR	CUM PCT
		*				
PURPOSE	.66537	*	1	4.54230	45.4	45.4
ENERGY	.61852	*	2	1.43410	14.3	59.8
SYMPTOM	.62915	*				
CHRONIC	.66556	*				
EMOTION	.66153	*				
SPORATIC	.30506	*				
DISABIL	.51734	*				
MAJILL	.41517	*				
SOCTIES	.76329	*				
ACCEPT	.73542	*				

EQAMAX ROTATION 1 FOR EXTRACTION 1 IN ANALYSIS 1-KAISER NORMALIZATION.

EQUAMAX CONVERGED IN 3 ITERATIONS.

ROTATED FACTOR MATRIX:

	FACTOR 1	FACTOR 2
SOCTIES	.87278	.03934
ACCEPT	.83860	.17936
PURPOSE	.76662	.27869
EMOTION	.75167	.31068
ENERGY	.57979	.53138
CHRONIC	.17696	.79639
SYMPTOM	.20288	.76680
DISABIL	.09198	.71336
MAJILL	.30983	.56496
SPORATIC	.12802	.53728

FIGURE 14-1 (CONTINUED)

(Alternatively, any one of six methods of common factor analysis could have been used.)

The table that follows the label "initial statistics" presents two types of information: 1) Because the extraction method was a principal components analysis, the diagonals in the correlation matrix to be analyzed were kept as unities; this is indicated by the repetition of 1.000 in each row for the second column. Had any type of common factor analysis (e.g., principal axis, maximum likelihood) been used instead, communality estimates would have replaced 1's in the diagonal. The multiple R of the regression equation that predicts the variable from other variables would be used as the default communality estimate for each variable. Alternatively, the researcher could use communality estimates obtained in some other way (e.g., item reliabilities) and specify these into the program.

2) Moving toward the right, the next four columns under "initial statistics" contain the information needed relative to general characteristics of the unrotated factors. Note that 10 factors are listed. This is because the number of unrotated factors obtainable equals the number of variables included in a principal components analysis. The purpose of this part of the analysis is, however, to determine how many of the 10 factors should be rotated for conceptual interpretation. Eigenvalues and percent of variance accounted for are given. The first two factors each have an eigenvalue greater than 1, and each of these accounts for 10% of variance or more. The right-hand column gives cumulative percent of variance accounted for; the first two factors together account for 59.8% of the interitem variance.

In this printout, a plot of eigenvalues was requested in line 5 of the procedure commands (/plot = eigen). This provides a graphic representation of the relative values of eigenvalues. Because eigenvalues often are the key criteria for determining number of factors to be rotated, this can be useful as it provides a basis for identifying a logical breaking point between eigenvalues. This approach to determining the number of factors is called the Scree test.

In this analysis, two factors were extracted. These are displayed in the next table labeled, "factor matrix," which contains the unrotated factor matrix. As usual, the first factor is a generalized factor on which all variables load. The second factor, containing positive and negative loadings, has a bipolar quality. Typically, no attempt is made to derive conceptual interpretations of these unrotated factors. Next, the two factors with eigenvalues greater than 1 are rotated, and the final solution is derived.

Under the heading "final statistics," the second column shows final communalities achieved for each variable in the rotated factor matrix. The next column repeats information already given concerning the rotated factors only.

The last table, "rotated factor matrix," represents the culmination of this effort. These rotated factors are to be conceptually interpreted. Note that the items are now listed by strength of loading, rather than by the order in which they were listed previously. This reordering was requested in line 6 of the procedure commands (/format = sort); use of such an option is highly recommended. Otherwise, the researcher must reorder items from highest to lowest.

After inspecting the items that load on a factor and their respective loadings, the investigator gives each factor an appropriate name as a way of capturing its meaning. Note that this analysis results in a clear distribution of the variables between the two factors. There is only one variable with substantial ($>.35$) loadings on both factors. See which one it is.

It is energy with loadings of .58 and .53, respectively. In the naming process, the researcher gives most emphasis to the three or four variables with the highest loadings. In this analysis, factor 1 was named psychological health, and factor 2 was named physiological health. Subjects could receive a score on each of these factors. Most often, a factor analysis includes more variables and more factors than shown here. The researcher who wants to include a tabular presentation of a factor analysis in a research thesis or article should present it in an easily readable format.

Other Options

A factor analysis may be more complicated than the one shown here—not simply because of the inclusion of more variables and more factors. Rather than principal components analysis, any of a variety of extraction methods representing common factor analysis may be used. Principal axis factoring differs from principal components mainly in that the correlation matrix diagonals are squared multiple correlations, rather than 1s, in the first step. Following this initial step, communalities are estimated from the factor matrix, and factoring is repeated with these communalities in the diagonal. Each such step is one iteration. This is repeated until the estimated communalities and calculated communalities are approximately the same.

Another important method of extraction within the class of common factor analysis is alpha factoring, which is designed to maximize the alpha reliability of the factors. It is assumed that the particular variables measured are a sample of the universe of variables represented by the factor. You want to generalize not to the population of cases from which research subjects were drawn, but to the universe of variables from which the measured variables were sampled. Ferketich and Muller (1990) point out that this method is highly appropriate for instrument development efforts, particularly the early stages.

Other extraction methods available in the common statistical packages are image factoring, unweighted least squares, and generalized least squares. However, these may be less important to the sort of applications discussed here. Finally, the maximum likelihood method of extraction is an available option. This method lays the groundwork for a confirmatory factor analysis process, and it is discussed later in this chapter.

PRESENTATION IN THE LITERATURE

The printout described previously was central to the analysis of a recently published study (Dixon, Dixon, & Hickey, 1993), so it may be useful to take a look at the presentation of data in the research report. The study combined the various purposes of factor analysis. Needs for instrument development, theory building, and data reduction each played a role in the conceptualization and planning of the approach taken when looking at this data. The World Health Organization (1958, p. 459) definition of health indicates that it involves a synthesis of various components. "Health is a state of complete physical, mental and social well-being and not merely the absence of disease and infirmity." Factor analysis is an effective tool for exploring the meaning of multivariate phenomena and for illuminating how the various parts relate to the whole and to the other parts.

As part of a larger study, health self-assessment data were elicited on one general item (called Global Health Assessment) and for 10 specific items thought to represent aspects of health. The specific items relate to purposefulness in living, energy level, symptomatic conditions, chronic conditions, emotional experience, sporadic illness, physical disability, major illnesses, social ties, and acceptance of life. Each item was rated on a six-point scale with 1 representing the most negative response and 6 representing the most positive response. Subjects, drawn from master's-level graduates of a school of nursing, consisted of 310 women who were in their sixth or seventh decade of life and who had received their master's degree between 1941 and 1965.

In this study, health self-assessments were obtained as part of a larger study on the relationships between social involvement, self-fulfillment, and health among professional women in this age group. Instrumentation was created specifically for this study, and the reported factor analysis was initiated in the spirit of instrument development. However, as the results began to inspire significant theoretical interest, theory development became an important goal of this line of analysis. In pursuit of this theoretical interest, factor analytic results were used to create predictor variables for subsequent regression analysis. Thus, the data reduction purpose of factor analysis was invoked as well.

Prior to presentation of the table that displays rotated factor loadings, we first presented descriptive univariate and some bivariate data about the items. This is displayed in Table 14-6, which appeared in the published article. This table includes means and standard deviation of each of the 10 specific items and correlations of each item with two other variables—the Global Health Assessment and illness index, which was based on self-report of most significant illness experienced at various times of life (Dixon, Dixon, Spinner, Sexton, & Perry, 1991). An initial look at the data on an item-by-item basis is an important preliminary step in the factor analysis process, so inclusion in a research report is appropriate. Means were generally high, indicating positive self-reports of health. However, the item energy level had the lowest mean, the largest standard deviation, and the highest correlation with Global Health Assessment.

The 10 × 10 matrix of intercorrelations between the items was calculated and carefully studied. However, it was not included in the published article due to space constraints. All 45 correlations computed were positive and significant to the .01 probability level; they ranged from .65 to .14.

The rotated factor matrix, with two factors, was presented in its simplest possible form. This is displayed in Table 14-7. Only the rotated factor loadings are given in the table. Other information about the factors—the eigenvalues, variance accounted for by each factor, and cumulative variance accounted for by all factors—

TABLE 14-6
*Means, Standard Deviations, and Correlations
With Global Health Self-Assessment and Illness Score
of Elements of Health Items*

			Correlations	
Element of Health Items	*M*	*SD*	*Global Health Self-Assessment*	*Illnesses Index*
Major illnesses	5.6	.96	.29**	−.38**
Physical disability	5.4	1.06	.41**	−.21**
Social ties	5.3	.93	.30**	−.12*
Purposefulness in living	5.3	.92	.59**	−.18**
Acceptance of life	5.2	.94	.48**	−.13†
Sporadic illnesses	5.2	1.01	.24**	−.04
Chronic conditions	5.1	1.09	.57**	−.45**
Emotional experience	5.1	1.07	.41**	−.17**
Symptomatic complaints	5.0	1.04	.59**	−.28**
Energy level	4.8	1.16	.69**	−.22**

*p < .05.

†p < .01.

**p < .001.

(From Dixon, J. K., Dixon, J. P., & Hickey, M. [1993]. Energy as a central factor in the self-assessment of health. Advances in Nursing Science, *15[4], 1–12.)*

TABLE 14-7
Rotated Factor Loadings of Elements of Health Items

	Factor Loadings	
Element of Health Item	*Factor 1*	*Factor 2*
Social ties	.87	.04
Acceptance of life	.84	.18
Purposefulness in living	.77	.28
Emotional experience	.75	.31
Energy level	.58	.53
Chronic conditions	.18	.80
Symptomatic complaints	.20	.77
Physical disability	.09	.71
Major illnesses	.30	.56
Sporadic illnesses	.13	.54

(From Dixon, J. K., Dixon, J. P., & Hickey, M. [1993]. Energy as a central factor in the self-assessment of health. Advances in Nursing Science, *15[4], 1–12.)*

could also have been included in the table, but they were reported in the text instead. As shown in the computer printout (Fig. 14–1, under "initial statistics"), eigenvalues are 4.5 and 1.4, respectively, with variance accounted for of 45.4% and 14.3%, such that cumulative variance accounted for is 59.8%. (The apparent discrepancy is due to rounding.) Had these figures been incorporated into the table, they would have been inserted below the factor loadings for each of the two columns representing the two rotated factors. Consult Munro, Jacobson, and Brooten (1994) for an example of a published rotated factor loading matrix that includes these additional details about the factors. Additionally, such a table may be extended horizontally to include a column for item communalities. Other points of variation of table presentation are whether or not factor names are included in the tables, the presence or absence of alpha reliabilities, and whether "low" loadings (e.g., below .30) are reported or omitted.

Beyond naming the factors "Psychosocial Health" and "Physiological Health" (as noted previously) based on patterns of item loadings, it was noted that the item energy level was the only variable with a substantial loading on both factors. Loadings were above .50 in both cases. This suggests the possibility of a conceptual link with both sets of items.

Cronbach's alpha coefficients (calculated with energy level omitted due to its relationship to both factors) was .86 for the four-item psychosocial health factor and .75 for the five-item physiological health factor.

As a later step in the analysis of these data, a forward regression analysis was conducted using three predictor variables—psychosocial health, physiological health, and energy level. Again, energy level was kept separate because of its unique status in relating to both factors. The dependent variable in the regression analysis was global health assessment. Energy level entered the equation on the first step, accounting for 48% of variance in the dependent variable. Psychosocial health and physiological health added only 7% to variance accounted for as they were added in subsequent steps. Taken together, these results suggest a special place for energy level in the self-assessment of health. With connection to *both factors* of a two-factor solution, energy seems to be at the core of what people think of when asked to describe their health.

INTRODUCTION TO CONFIRMATORY FACTOR ANALYSIS

The maximum likelihood method of extraction is distinct from those previously described in the inclusion of a test for goodness of fit. That is, the adequacy of the factor model is evaluated using a test of statistical significance. While researchers using other methods of extraction may rely on such statistical criteria as absolute magnitude of eigenvalues, percent of variance accounted for, or Scree test in determining the appropriate number of factors, a researcher using the maximum likelihood technique may determine number of factors through the chi-square statistic. (The generalized least squares method of extraction also allows the calculation of a goodness of fit statistic.)

In this process, the adequacy of the factor model is tested. This is based on the assumption that the sample is from a multivariate normal population. Any factor model is an attempt to summarize or reduce a multivariate dataset. In the maximum likelihood method, the hypothesis tested is that the factor model derived is a good fit with the original data. Because statistical significance would indicate a difference between the factor model and the full data, the researcher hopes to obtain a chi-square that is nonsignificant, indicating that a good fit is obtained. This is a reversal of the usual usage of tests of statistical significance in which the researcher generally hopes to obtain statistical significance, indicating that the data obtained are not consistent with the null hypothesis of no difference (or no relationship).

Initial results can be used to guide continued refinement of the factor model. What do you do if statistical significance is obtained on the chi-square value, indicating significant difference between the factor model and the full data, an inadequate fit? You rerun the analysis, making adjustments in the criteria governing number of factors to be derived. In SPSS, this is done with the CRITERIA command. (To obtain three, rather than two, factors, CRITERIA = FACTORS [3].) In any factor solution, increasing the number of factors will increase the statistical adequacy of factor model; the goal is to obtain the number of factors that is the smallest number necessary to achieve an acceptable fit. So you do not want to accept a solution with any more factors than are necessary. You may repeatedly run analyses, adding a factor with each repetition until the chi-square statistic obtained is nonsignificant. Alternatively, if on the first run the chi-square statistic is nonsignificant, you repeat the analysis with one factor fewer to determine the smallest possible number of factors that will yield a nonsignificant chi-square.

The development of confirmatory factor analysis in recent decades is due largely to the work of K.G. Jöreskog and is based on maximum likelihood techniques. Made accessible to researchers through the LISREL family of computer programs (Jöreskog & Sörbom, 1989), complex forms of confirmatory factor analysis not only guide the researcher as to the appropriate number of factors, but also allow the researcher to specify what variables relate to which factors and to identify relationships between variables that are not captured by the factors. (However, they may conceivably indicate the existence of an additional factor). Modifications are suggested by how much a factor model may be improved, and changing goodness of fit statistics aids in interpretation of the value of the improvement. Remember that the goal of confirmatory factor analysis is to identify latent (unmeasured) variables that underlie the set of variables that are measured. These latent variables are the reason behind the specific measured values obtained. Thus, in figures depicting confirmatory factor models, either hypothesized or obtained, the direction of arrows leads from the latent variable to the measured variable. Two examples of such figures appear later in this section; another may be found in Wineman, Durand, and McCulloch (1994). The nature of these latent variables is confirmed through confirmatory factor analysis; these latent variables may then become the foundation of subsequent analysis, as in structural equation modeling.

Confirmatory factor analysis can be applied to the health care professions research literature in four major ways:

1. Confirmatory factor analysis may directly follow exploratory factor analysis to evaluate, and perhaps modify, the factor structure that is obtained. Using this approach, Wineman and others (1994) divided their sample of a clinical population

residing in the community into two groups. Subjects completed the Ways of Coping Questionnaire (Folkman & Lazarus, 1988), a 66-item instrument with responses on a four-point scale. Data from the group consisting of one third of the subjects ($n = 218$) were used for the exploratory factor analysis. Data from the remaining subjects ($n = 437$) were used in the subsequent confirmatory factor analyses, which was repeated several times before a model with an acceptable fit and acceptable reliabilities was found. All of this followed earlier use of both exploratory and confirmatory factor analysis in which expectations derived from earlier work by the instrument developers were not supported in the data of this clinical sample. In another published study, Champion (1995) reversed the usual ordering of exploratory factor analysis followed by confirmatory factor analysis. She conducted a confirmatory factor analysis first, based on her original hypothesis about her benefits and barriers scale for mammography use. Because the results of this did not seem definitive, an exploratory factor analysis was then undertaken.

2. Confirmatory factor analysis approaches are also appropriate for comparing factors across samples. Data from the first sample are used to generate a measurement model. Then the researcher attempts to fit the data from the second sample to the same model. When recommending this approach, Teel and Verran (1991) assert that "confirmatory factor analysis provides a severe test of factor similarity across different samples." A logical extension of this approach is the use of confirmatory factor analysis to establish measurement equivalence across different samples or across time (Stommel, Wang, Given, & Given, 1992). Does the measure work the same way with various samples? Does it work the same way at different times? Does each factor reflect the same combination of items with one sample and with another? Are the actual factor loadings (unstandardized) the same? Do the factors relate to each other in the same way within one sample and another? Taken together, these characteristics may be called factorial invariance. Through use of confirmatory factor analysis techniques, Stommel et al. (1992) demonstrated that the caregiver reaction assessment was factorially invariant across different patient groups and across repeated measurement occasions. It was equivalent among caregivers of people with cancer and caregivers of people with Alzheimer's disease, and it was stable over time.

3. Confirmatory factor analysis has been recommended for studies using the multi-trait-multimethod approach to construct validity. This is because of its ability to handle systematically hypotheses that posit that some sources of variation are due to content distinctions between variables; however, this is crossed with other sources of variation due to method distinctions in the same variables. (Consult Figueredo, Ferketich, & Knapp [1991] for elaboration of this recommendation.)

4. Confirmatory factor analysis is used as the first step of structural equation modeling—establishing the measurement model so that the latent (i.e., unmeasured) variables are identified. This is discussed further in Chapter 16. An example of this usage may be seen in a study of the impact of emotions on the interrelationship between creative intelligence and conventional skills (Dixon, Hickey, & Dixon, 1992).

In exploratory analysis, it is assumed that all observed variables are related to (i.e., affected by) all of the common factors. In confirmatory approaches, you may develop specific expectations so that each variable is assumed to relate to some common factors but not to others (Long, 1983). Hypotheses about the relationships in the data may be specific. However, as pointed out by Goodwin and Goodwin (1991), "the exploratory–confirmatory distinction is often tenuous" (p. 239); exploratory techniques often are used by researchers with well-specified expectations, and confirmatory techniques may be applied in a highly exploratory manner.

Example From the Literature

The process of confirmatory factor analysis is illustrated with an example from the literature. The published study selected for this section is atypical. It is distinctive in displaying factor models as they emerged before modifications were made and after these modifications. Thus, it provides a special look at the way initial results guide the researcher's decisions about how the factor model should be modified. Such modification decisions are central to the value of confirmatory factor analysis.

Gulick (1989) examined the structure of the multiple sclerosis-related symptoms checklist, consisting of 26 signs and symptoms thought to be characteristic of multiple sclerosis. Subjects provided self-report data indicating the frequency with which they experienced each symptom. A six-point scale ranged from never (0) to always (5). Data from 491 subjects who completed the third year of a longitudinal study were first submitted to a principal components analysis with Varimax rotation. This was an exploratory factor analysis. A five-factor solution incorporating 22 of the 26 items and accounting for 59.3% of interitem variation was derived. The factor loading matrix is represented in Table 14-8. (Note that the format of this published factor loading matrix is in some ways different from the format of the other published factor loading matrix displayed in Table 14-7.)

Based on these results, a graphic model was constructed, which was evaluated in a confirmatory factor analysis. This is reprinted in Figure 14-2 with circles used to illustrate the latent variables (the factors) and rectangular boxes used to represent measured variables. Arrows from the latent variables to the measured variables represent the assumption that the latent characteristics form the foundation of the obtained measurement. The numbers accompanying these arrows are the factor loadings obtained, and correlations obtained between factors also are shown. The three numbers in the lower left corner of the figure provide an evaluation of the model. The coefficient of determination may be thought of as a reliability. This is not problematic. However, the chi-square value (984.87) is statistically significant, and the goodness of fit ratio of 0.801 is not high enough. Ideally, this should be 0.9 or higher. The relationships between measured variables have not been fully captured by this model.

Modification indices obtained in the computer printout suggested a number of modifications. In all, seven changes were made. One of these involved associating an observed variable (falling) with a second factor (elimination). The other six in-

TABLE 14-8
Factor Loading Matrix of Exploratory Factor Analysis

MS-Related Symptom	Varimax Rotated Factor Analysis				
	Skeletal	Elimination	Emotions	Kinesthetic	Head
X_1 Arm weakness	.511	.040	.065	.218	.308
X_2 Leg weakness	.693	.104	−.009	.186	.122
X_3 Spasms	.583	.079	.141	.358	.113
X_4 Tremors	.482	.022	.191	.231	.222
X_5 Knee locking	.721	.022	.085	.220	.023
X_6 Balance problems	.719	.132	.048	−.048	.020
X_7 Falling	.657	.293	.176	−.130	.079
X_8 Urine frequency: day	.046	.772	.001	.272	.101
X_9 Urine frequency: night	−.006	.786	−.022	.281	.105
X_{10} Trouble making bathroom: day	.247	.802	.125	−.025	.047
X_{11} Trouble making bathroom: night	.235	.811	.144	−.022	−.014
X_{12} Loneliness	.110	.041	.835	.056	.112
X_{13} Depression	.140	.110	.877	.096	.143
X_{14} Anxiety	.081	.040	.821	.196	.152
X_{15} Pain	.216	.074	.302	.542	.062
X_{16} Burning	.203	.173	.142	.642	.021
X_{17} Numbness	.122	.076	.024	.785	.147
X_{18} Pins and needles	.068	.096	.009	.754	.112
X_{19} Double vision	.133	−.040	.033	.112	.744
X_{20} Blurred vision	.140	.031	.045	.108	.793
X_{21} Difficulty swallowing	.174	.138	.192	.094	.590
X_{22} Forgetfulness	−.010	.149	.391	−.002	.557
Percent of explained variance	26.600	1.220	8.600	7.500	6.300
Eigenvalue (principal component method)	3.184	2.702	2.372	2.233	2.064
Theta reliability coefficient	.800	.840	.867	.736	.687

Note: Item-factor loadings are underlined.

(From Gulick, E. E. [1989]. Model confirmation of the MS-related symptom checklist. Nursing Research, 38, 147–153.)

volved the pairing of measured variables due to relationships between their residual variances. That is, there was a relationship between arm weakness and leg weakness, over and above their common connection with the latent variable, skeletal. The modified model is displayed in Figure 14-3. The researcher points out that the chi-square value decreased by more than half (= 405.08), and the goodness of fit index also improved (0.910), suggesting a satisfactory model. Although the chi-square val-

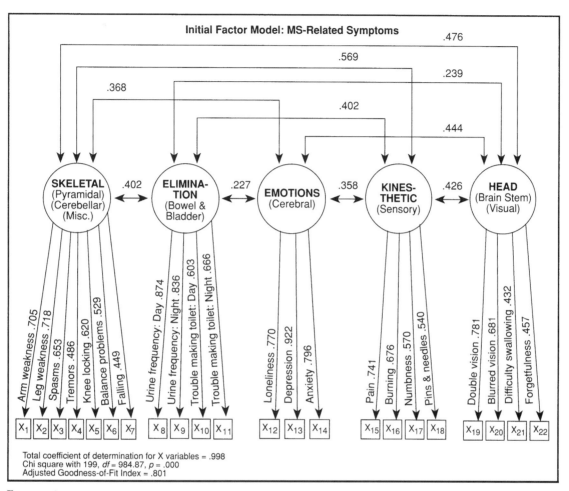

FIGURE 14-2

Graphic depiction of initial model by confirmatory factor analysis. (From Gulick, E. E. [1989]. Model confirmation of the MS-related symptom checklist. *Nursing Research, 38,* 147–153.)

ue remains statistically significant in the modified model, the author points out its sensitivity to sample size, and she suggests an alternative criterion—the ratio of chi-square to *df.* The ratio of 2.11 to 1 obtained is within acceptable range.

The use of confirmatory factor analysis by nonstatisticians is a relatively new development in the research literature, but clearly this is a trend for the future. Structural equation modeling, described in Chapter 16, builds further on the application of maximum likelihood methods in the discovery of causal patterns between latent variables.

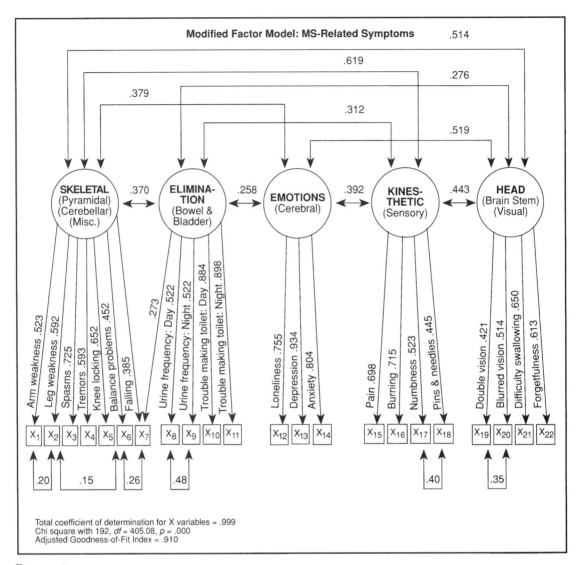

FIGURE 14-3
Graphic depiction of improved model by confirmatory factor analysis. (Gulick, E. E. [1989].
Model confirmation of the MS-related symptom checklist. *Nursing Research, 38,* 147–153.)

SUMMARY

The factor analysis techniques presented in this chapter are distinct from many other statistical techniques in the tremendous potential for researcher creativity to shape
understanding of the results obtained. Through application of statistical techniques,
you arrive at numbers that indicate groupings in the data. Most often, these are group-

ings of variables. These groups must then be named or described by the researcher, a creative process in which clinical wisdom, knowledge of the literature, and research sophistication must be integrated. This creative process is the key element on which the value of the factor analysis must rest. A factor analysis solution is well suited to inform the creative process. However, factor loadings and goodness of fit indices are only as valuable as the interpretation of the factors is insightful.

APPLICATION EXERCISES AND RESULTS

EXERCISES

1. Factor analyze the 30 items in the IPPA scale. According to the developers of the scale, LIFE consists of the following 17 questions: items 1, 3, 4, 6, 8, 9, 11, 12, 13, 19, 20, 21, 23, 25, 27, 28, 30. CONFIDENCE consists of 13 questions: items 2, 5, 7, 10, 14, 15, 16, 17, 18, 22, 24, 26, 29. See how your results compare.

RESULTS

1. We ran a principal components factor analysis with Varimax rotation. That resulted in five factors. We then forced the number of factors to two and reran the analysis. The results of our second analysis are contained in Exercise Figure 14-1 (see pp. 340–341). You may have selected different rotation and extraction methods and can compare your results with ours. To save space, we have printed only final statistics, rotated matrix, and scree plot.

   The first factor accounted for 47% of the variance, and the second factor accounted for 7%. The first factor contains 15 of the 17 questions associated with the life purpose and satisfaction scale. Two items from the self-confidence scale (items 22 and 29) also loaded on this scale. Both of these items had slightly smaller but still substantial loadings on factor 2. The second factor contains 11 of the 13 self-confidence items plus two items from the life satisfaction scale (items 19 and 30). Thus, this analysis generally supported the structure proposed by the authors of the scale. The scree plot also indicates that the two-factor solution is appropriate, although some might argue that the substantial overlap between factors indicates a unidimensional scale.

Final Statistics:

Variable	Communality	*	Factor	Eigenvalue	Pct of Var	Cum Pct
		*				
IPA1	.49947	*	1	14.17350	47.2	47.2
IPA2	.50709	*	2	2.02289	6.7	54.0

Rotated Factor Matrix:

	Factor 1	Factor 2
IPA25	.75237	.29631
IPA3	.73670	.31654
IPA21	.73282	.36816
IPA8	.72056	.14925
IPA4	.71460	.18759
IPA23	.71264	.39076

IPA20	.70750	.33570
IPA9	.69620	.42021
IPA1	.66488	.23960
IPA13	.65303	.22556
IPA28	.61171	.42299
IPA12	.59196	.44027
IPA22	.58208	.55720
IPA11	.58012	.34977
IPA6	.56984	.12015
IPA29	.44964	.44493
IPA27	.43792	.39919
IPA26	.18550	.78995
IPA15	.22535	.74984
IPA2	.12487	.70107
IPA14	.25826	.66036
IPA10	.21394	.65655
IPA5	.30299	.65455
IPA24	.32284	.64966
IPA7	.31561	.64708
IPA18	.32685	.64534
IPA19	.30981	.63809
IPA17	.44150	.61184
IPA30	.53243	.57745
IPA16	.33764	.53125

Factor Scree Plot

EXERCISE FIGURE 14-1. Factor analysis of IPPA items.

15

Path Analysis

ANNE E. NORRIS[1]

OBJECTIVES FOR CHAPTER 15

After reading this chapter, you should be able to do the following:

1 ● State the three conditions necessary for causality.

2 ● Draw a recursive path model.

3 ● Identify which independent variables are theorized to have indirect effects in addition to direct effects on the dependent variable.

4 ● Identify the appropriate regression analyses needed to calculate the path coefficients in a model.

5 ● Calculate the direct and indirect effects of an independent variable in a model.

THE RESEARCH QUESTION

Path analysis is used to answer questions regarding the relationships between a set of independent variables and a dependent variable. Path analysis is based on simple regression techniques, but by looking at these relationships, it takes the researcher a step beyond the traditional regression analysis discussed in Chapter 12. Path analysis moves beyond testing whether a set of independent variables predicts a phenomenon to examining the relationships among those variables. Asher (1983) argues that by taking this step beyond regression analysis, we achieve a richer understanding of our phenomena. For example, Robinson (1995) used path analysis to

[1]*Acknowledgments: The author wishes to thank Dr. Karen Aroian and Ms. Gina Ankner, MS, RN, for their careful review and critique of this chapter.*

examine how social support, income and education, spiritual beliefs, and coping influenced the grief response of widows (Fig. 15-1).

Path models are considered a type of "causal model," and path analysis is referred to as a causal modeling technique. Path models depict theorized, directional relationships among a set of variables. For example, in Robinson's (1995) model depicted in Figure 15-1, social support, income and education, and spiritual beliefs are depicted as influencing or "causing" the widow's total combined coping.

Path analysis is literally an analysis of the paths or lines in a model that represent the influence of one variable on another. It is used to answer research questions about the effect of an independent (X_1) variable on the dependent variable (Y) in the model. As you will learn in this chapter, independent variables may have both direct ($X_1 \rightarrow Y$) and indirect effects. Indirect effects arise when the independent variable is theorized to influence other independent variables (e.g., X_2, X_3) in the model (e.g., $X_1 \rightarrow X_2 \rightarrow Y$). In Robinson's (1995) path model, social support, income and education, and spiritual beliefs influence coping, which in turn influences the widow's grief response. Thus, the diagram indicates that these variables have indirect effects on the dependent variable (grief response) through their influence on coping. The direct lines between these three variables and the dependent variable, grief response, indicate that these variables have direct effects on the dependent variable as well.

By analyzing the paths, path analysis provides information about the consisten-

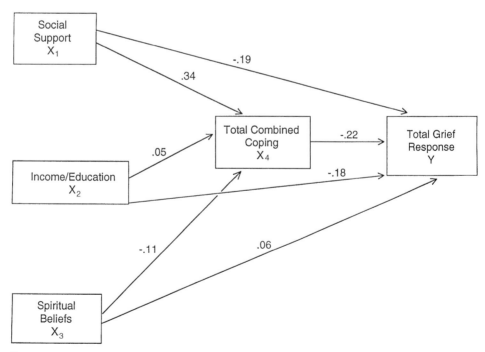

FIGURE 15-1
Robinson's (1995) path model.

cy between data and a theorized path model. If the data do not fit the theorized relationships in the model, this suggests the model (and the theory that generated it) may warrant revision. On the other hand, data that are consistent with the model are supportive, but not definitive. Such data merely indicate that the model (and the theory) was not disconfirmed.

Ideally the path model should be drawn before the data are collected. However, in secondary data analysis, the model is drawn after the data are collected but before the analysis is conducted. In primary and secondary data analysis, the model may also be drawn after completing a regression analysis because the researcher wants to examine the relationships between the independent variables. In either case, Asher (1983) recommends working with a model that is based on an a priori theoretical or substantive understanding of the relationships between variables in the model. Although it is important to modify a model in response to statistical results, the path analysis should not become a "mindless" attempt to find a model that best fits the data. Such attempts result in models that may not replicate and may have questionable theoretical value.

TYPE OF DATA REQUIRED

Path analysis requires the same type of data as needed for linear multiple regression. In other words, you need a dependent variable that is continuous and normally distributed. Ideally, the independent variables are also continuous. Some researchers use the coding techniques (dummy, effect, orthogonal) discussed in Chapter 12 to include categorical variables, but by doing so, they violate a statistical assumption underlying path analysis (see Assumptions) and jeopardize the validity of their findings. In addition, the researcher should strive to have a large enough dataset to follow Nunnally and Bernstein's (1987) recommendation of 30 subjects per independent variable in the model to increase the likelihood that findings can be replicated and are not mere artifact.

Although path analysis is considered a causal modeling technique, it can be performed with either cross-sectional or longitudinal data. For example, Robinson's (1995) data are cross-sectional. Hence, it is important to understand some of the theoretical assumptions underlying path analysis, namely those pertaining to causation.

ASSUMPTIONS

There are two types of assumptions that must be considered with path analysis: theoretical and statistical.

Theoretical Assumptions

In the strictest sense, causation is investigated with experimental designs in which the independent variable is manipulated, the subsequent effects of this are measured, and variables that could confound or influence the effect of the independent variable are controlled for (e.g., subjects are randomized to condition). However, path analysis typically involves testing a causal or path model with data that do not result from an experimental design. For example, path analysis can be done with survey data, data produced by a review of medical records, and so forth. Given this, many researchers have reservations about using such models to imply causation (Pedhazur, 1982). Hence, while the notion of causation is implicit, careful terminology is used. For example, independent variables may be called predictor variables but are described as "influencing" rather than causing the dependent variable.

Nevertheless, theoretical assumptions of causation are implicit in path analysis, and such assumptions are strengthened when three conditions of causation are met (Kenny, 1979). First, there must be an observed and measurable relationship between X_1 and Y. In other words, X_1 and Y must be correlated.

Second, X_1 should precede Y in time. That is, it must be possible to temporally order X_1 and Y, such that X_1 occurred first. This condition may seem easy to meet, but it can be quite complicated. Consider a cross-sectional dataset concerning a health behavior, such as engaging in regular exercise, and predictors of this behavior, such as education and beliefs about exercise. For education, the matter is straightforward. It is safe to assume that education temporally precedes current exercise. For beliefs, it is less clear. Do we assume that beliefs about exercise were present first? This would be consistent with hypothesizing that these beliefs lead to engaging in regular exercise. On the other hand, could the exercise have occurred before the beliefs developed or were fully formed? This would be consistent with hypothesizing that engaging in regular exercise changes or alters beliefs about exercise. The researcher must take a stand on the hypothesized causal direction. Otherwise the model would be nonrecursive, and nonrecursive path models cannot be tested with cross-sectional data. This example illustrates the problem with using causal modeling techniques to imply causation. It also underscores the importance of theory: We can use theory to resolve the dilemma of whether the belief or the behavior came first. For example, Pender's (1987) Health Promotion Theory and Fishbein and Ajzen's (1975) Theory of Reasoned Action both specify that beliefs guide behavior. Therefore, we can use these theories to guide us in assigning a direction between beliefs and behaviors, such that beliefs are theorized to influence engaging in exercise (Fig. 15-2).

Third, X_1 and Y should have a nonspurious relationship. This means that the observed, measurable, and temporally ordered relationship between X_1 and Y will not disappear when the effects of other variables on this relationship are controlled for.

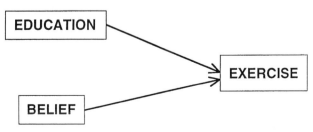

FIGURE 15-2
Education influences exercise. Belief influences exercise.

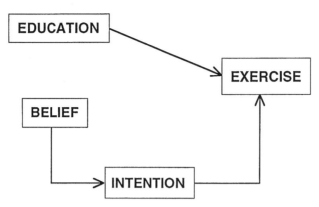

FIGURE 15-3
Intention confounds the relationship between belief and exercise because belief influences intention, which in turn influences exercise.

For example, suppose in our predictors of exercise analysis, we found that the relationship between beliefs and engaging in exercise disappeared when the effects of intention to exercise were statistically controlled for (i.e., we entered intention into a regression analysis predicting exercise behavior first, with belief entered on the second step and found that the beta for belief was no longer significant). This would mean that the earlier relationship between belief and exercise was spurious—it only appeared to exist because belief and exercise were correlated with intention. Another way to say this is that the relationship was confounded by intention. If we found this, we would modify the diagram of our causal model from Figure 15-2 to the one depicted in Figure 15-3.

This third condition of causation seems straightforward. We can use regression to test whether the data meet this assumption, but the problem is that we are only able to do this if we have measured the right confounding variable. It is difficult (perhaps impossible) to identify and rule out all the variables that could confound the observed relationship between X_1 and Y. The solution is to use theory, existing literature, and discussions with colleagues to identify variables that seem clearly likely to confound the relationships in the model and then include measures of such variables in the analysis (Asher, 1983). Unfortunately, in secondary data analysis, the researcher works with an existing dataset and can include only those variables that are contained in the dataset. Thus, such researchers may need to recognize this as a limitation of their results.

Statistical Assumptions

Related to Multiple Regression

The statistical assumptions in path analysis are of two types. You are already familiar with the first one. These are the assumptions of normal distributions, homoscedasticity, and linear relationships discussed in Chapter 12 for multiple regression analysis. These assumptions arise because path analysis consists of a series of regression equations.

Unique to Path Analysis

The second type of assumptions is unique to path analysis. The assumptions are necessitated by the use of path analysis to calculate the direct and indirect effects of variables in the path model. There are four of these assumptions:

1. When two independent variables are correlated with one another and diagrammed as having no other variables influencing them, their relationship cannot be analyzed, and the magnitude of this relationship is represented by the correlation coefficient (Pedhazur, 1982).
2. It is assumed that the flow of causation in the model is unidirectional (Pedhazur, 1982). The model is "recursive." This means that if we start with any independent variable in a model and move our fingers along the straight lines in the direction of the arrows from one variable to the next we will not come back to the independent variable with which we started—we will not find ourselves moving in a circle.
3. It is assumed that the variables in the model are measured on an interval scale (Pedhazur, 1982). However, Asher (1983) argues that this assumption can be somewhat relaxed with ordinal variables, particularly as the number of categories in the ordinal variable increases.
4. All variables in the model are measured without error—measurement error is assumed to be zero (Pedhazur, 1982). This last assumption underscores the importance of having reliable measures of variables in the path model.

POWER

Power analyses in path analysis are the same as those discussed in Chapter 12 for multiple regression, so they are not discussed in detail here. Path analysis involves more than one regression analysis. Hence, the power analysis should be calculated for the regression equation that involves the smallest effect size (or requires the largest number of subjects). This will ensure that you have enough power to detect the significance of important paths in the model.

KEY TERMS

Path analysis brings with it a set of terms common to causal models in general. We have already discussed recursive and nonrecursive models and direct and indirect effects. The next section discusses these terms in more detail and introduces some additional ones.

Recursive and Nonrecursive Models

As discussed previously in this chapter, an assumption in path analysis is that the model is recursive. That is, there is a one-way flow of causation in the model. Another way of thinking about this is that in a recursive model, all the paths between variables are one-way roads. The only exception is when theory and previous research is insufficient to support a direction being assigned to the "road." In this case, a correlational rather than a directional relationship is assumed and indicated by a curved line with an arrow at each end. In a nonrecursive model, at least one of the paths between two variables is a two-way road, or a set of paths within the model is circular. These models do not meet the assumptions necessary for standard path analysis. There is a way to use longitudinal data to translate some theoretical models that are inherently nonrecursive into a recursive form that can then be tested with path analysis (Asher, 1983; Pedhazur, 1982).

Indirect and Direct Effects

An independent variable in a model can be diagrammed as having one of three kinds of effects on the dependent variable, depending on its relationships with other variables in the model: 1) only direct, 2) only indirect, or 3) both direct and indirect. In Figure 15-4, a path model of factors influencing engaging in regular exercise, intention has only a direct effect on the dependent variable. This effect is reflected in the direct line between intention and exercise, which points toward exercise. In this same figure, age and education also have direct effects on exercise, and age and education are correlated.

In Figure 15-5, education has only an indirect effect on exercise through its relationship with intention. There is no direct line between education and exercise as there was in Figure 15-4. However, there is a direct line between education and intention, which points toward intention, and between intention and the dependent variable.

In Figure 15-6, education has direct and indirect effects on the dependent variable. As in Figures 15-4 and 15-5, intention has only a direct effect.

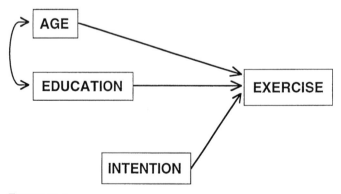

FIGURE 15-4
Age, education, and intention have direct effects.

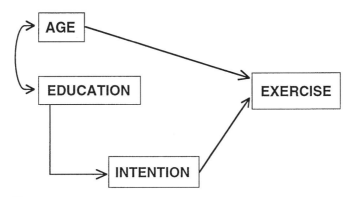

FIGURE 15-5
Education has an indirect effect. Age and intentions have direct effects.

Endogenous and Exogenous Variables

All variables in a path model can be described as endogenous or exogenous. This is an important distinction because to do path analysis, you need to perform a regression analysis for every endogenous variable in the model. Endogenous variables are diagrammed as being influenced by other variables in the model. Variables diagrammed as independent of any influence are the exogenous variables (Bollen, 1989).

Dependent variables are always endogenous, but some independent (or predictor) variables can be endogenous if they are being influenced by other independent variables in the model. Thus, in Figure 15-6, intention is an independent variable and an endogenous variable. This means that to analyze the path model depicted in Figure 15-6, we need two regression analyses, one with exercise regressed onto age, education, and intention and one with intention regressed onto

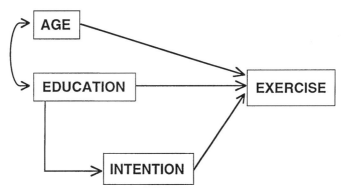

FIGURE 15-6
Education has direct and indirect effects.

education. Age is not included in the equation for intention because it has no direct or indirect effect on this variable.

In the diagrams in this chapter, endogenous and exogenous variables are indicated with a square drawn around them. This square indicates that these variables correspond to a subject's response or score in a particular dataset. Variables demarcated with a square are called measured variables or indicators of specific theoretical constructs. As you will learn in Chapter 16, circles are used to indicate that a variable is an unmeasured, theoretical construct.

Path Coefficients

Path coefficients are produced by the various regression analyses used in the path analysis. They represent the magnitude of the influence of one variable on another in the path model.

The subscripts used in the notation for path coefficients are ordered so that the letter or abbreviation representing the variable being influenced is always listed first, and the one for the variable doing the influencing is listed second. Thus, in Figure 15-4, the path coefficient for the path between intention and exercise is $p_{e,i}$.

Either the standardized (beta) or the nonstandardized (b) regression coefficient can be used as the value for the path coefficient, but the former is more common. Use of the standardized coefficient allows comparison of the magnitude of one path in the model with that of other paths in the model. Thus, the standardized coefficient makes it possible for the reader to determine which independent variable has the greatest direct effect on the dependent variable. In contrast, the nonstandardized coefficient makes it possible to evaluate how the magnitude of a particular path varies in different sample subgroups or study populations. Pedhazur (1982) recommends that both coefficients should be reported, or if only reporting standardized coefficients, then the standard deviations of all the variables should be reported so that interested readers can calculate the nonstandardized value.

Standardized path coefficients may be more common because these coefficients are needed to determine the direct, indirect, and total effect of an independent variable. The determination of these effects is discussed later (see Determining Direct and Indirect Effects and Conducting a Path Analysis).

Identification

Causal models can be overidentified, just identified, or underidentified. Visually, just identified models are easy to recognize because all the variables in the model are interconnected by a path (Pedhazur, 1982). Such models can become overidentified

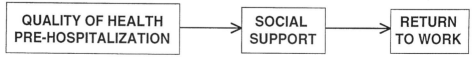

FIGURE 15-7
Overidentified model.

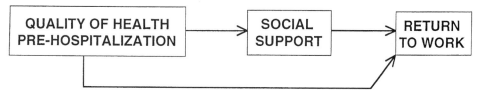

FIGURE 15-8
Just identified model.

through the process of "theory trimming" or the deletion of nonsignificant paths in the model (Heise, 1969). Note how the overidentified model in Figure 15-7 becomes the just identified model in Figure 15-8 with the addition of the direct path between quality of health prehospitalization and return to work ($p_{r,q}$). The just identified model becomes underidentified in Figure 15-9 when the path $p_{s,r}$ is added, and the model becomes nonrecursive. In Figure 15-10, the addition of this same path to the overidentified model (see Fig. 15-7) results in a nonrecursive model that is partially underidentified.

An advantage of overidentified models is that unlike just identified or underidentified models, the model as a whole can be statistically evaluated for its fit to the data. The results of this statistical test can be used to support the validity of the path model, although this is not commonly done in the published literature. A discussion of this statistic is beyond the scope of this chapter, but if you are interested in learning more about it, Pedhazur (1982) is an excellent resource.

DETERMINING DIRECT AND INDIRECT EFFECTS

Being able to determine the direct and indirect effects of an independent variable is an important advantage of path analysis (Asher, 1983). It allows us to know the total effect of an independent variable, which could be important when deciding which independent variables you want to target in an intervention. Being able to determine these effects also allows us to compare them. For example, it is possible for an independent variable to have an indirect effect that is greater than its direct effect or vice versa. It is also possible that the two effects may cancel each other out in the sense that they could be similar in magnitude but opposite in direction (one positive, the other negative).

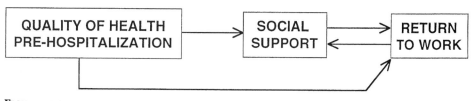

FIGURE 15-9
Underidentified model.

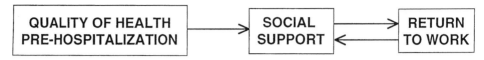

FIGURE 15-10
Partially underidentified model.

Pedhazur (1982) presents a method for using matrix algebra to ease the calculation of direct and indirect effects for more complex models (i.e., models with many variables and many paths). However, for simplicity, an alternative method developed by Wright (1934) is presented in this chapter; it does not require a knowledge of matrix algebra.

Using Wright's (1934) method, it is possible to work directly from the diagram of the path model and identify the simple (direct effect) and compound (more than one path is involved) paths relevant to a particular variable. These compound effects can either be meaningful (indirect) or nonmeaningful (noncausal).

According to Wright (1934), the value of any one compound path is equal to the product of the simple paths that comprise it. Thus, in the hypothetical model depicted in Figure 15-11, the compound path from quality of health prehospitalization to return to work through social support is equal to $p_{s,q}$ multiplied by $p_{r,s}$.

In the hypothetical model depicted in Figure 15-12, there are two possible meaningful compound paths between quality of health prehospitalization and return to work. There is the one we identified previously, $(p_{s,q})(p_{r,s})$, and there is a new one that takes us from quality of health prehospitalization to return to work through social support and adherence. The value of this new compound path is $(p_{s,q})(p_{ad,s})(p_{r,ad})$.

In Figure 15-12, there is also a nonmeaningful compound (or noncausal) path between quality of health prehospitalization and return to work through age. This compound path is equal to $(p_{r,a})(p_{q,a})$. This compound path ignores the direction of the relationships specified by the path model. This is why it is noncausal and considered nonmeaningful. However, it is an important component of the correlation between quality of health prehospitalization and return to work.

Wright (1934) found that when a path model is correctly specified, the correlation between two variables is equal to the sum of the simple (direct effect) and all possible compound paths (indirect effect and noncausal) between these two variables. Measurement error may enter in and cause the correlation to be approximately, rather than exactly, equal to the sum of the direct effect, indirect effect, and non-

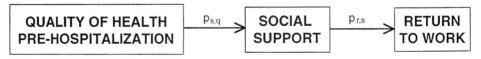

FIGURE 15-11
Model with one compound path from quality of health prehospitalization to return to work through social support.

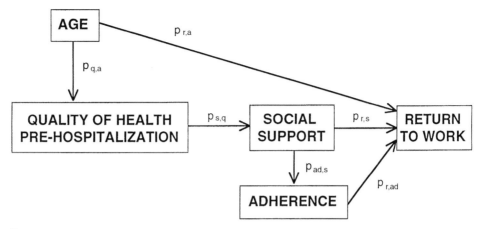

FIGURE 15-12
Model with two meaningful and one nonmeaningful compound paths from quality of health prehospitalization to return to work.

causal component. However, incorrect specification of the model could cause the sum of the direct and indirect effects and noncausal component to be noticeably less than the correlation. This noticeable difference between the sum and the correlation is an indication that the model may need revision (Asher, 1983).

Thus, in Figure 15-12 we could describe the correlation between quality of health prehospitalization and return to work with the following equation:

$$r = (p_{s,q})(p_{r,s}) + (p_{s,q})(p_{ad,s})(p_{r,ad}) + (p_{r,a})(p_{q,a})$$

In this equation, there is no direct effect; $(p_{s,q})(p_{r,s}) + (p_{s,q})(p_{ad,s})(p_{r,ad})$ is the sum of the total indirect effect of the variable, and $(p_{r,a})(p_{q,a})$ is the noncausal component of the correlation.

It is important to identify all the compound paths in a model that are relevant to the correlation between two variables. Otherwise, you might, through error, conclude incorrectly that a path model needs respecification. Wright (1934) has provided three rules that result in the identification of all possible compound paths between two variables. These rules guide the researcher as he or she looks at a diagram of a path model and traces out the possible different compound paths. The goal is for the researcher to identify compound paths that are meaningful (indirect effects) and compound paths that are not meaningful (noncausal) because both are part of the correlation.

Wright's (1934) Three Rules for Identifying All Compound Paths

1. No compound path involves going through the same variable more than once.
2. No compound path involves going forward with the direction of an arrow through a variable and then backward against the direction of a second arrow through a second variable (although it is perfectly acceptable to go backward first and then forward).

3. No compound path involves going through a curved, double-headed arrow line (i.e., a diagrammed relationship between two variables that has been left as a correlation) more than once.

The second rule sounds complicated, but we have already been applying it to identify the nonmeaningful compound path in Figure 15-12 for the variables quality of health prehospitalization and return to work. You may want to review Figure 15-12 and trace this path once more. The third rule hints at the problem with including a correlation in a path model, namely that the correlation may get in the way of determining the indirect effect of an independent variable. For this reason, researchers are encouraged to assign direction to hypothesized relationships between variables whenever possible but not at the expense of theory or logic and reason.

CONDUCTING A PATH ANALYSIS

Conducting a path analysis involves preparation, analysis, and a consideration of the limitations of the analysis. In the next section, we go through the steps needed to conduct a path analysis, using two examples: 1) a computer example of a study of factors influencing individuals' perceptions of their overall state of health and 2) an example from the published literature, Fink's (1995) test of conceptual framework for family well-being.

Computer Example: A Study of Factors Influencing Individuals' Perceptions of Their Overall State of Health

This example is an illustration of how researchers can use path analysis to move a step beyond traditional regression analysis. The researchers start the path analysis after completing a regression analysis in which the factors that influence an individual's perception of health have been identified.

The independent variables in this example are satisfaction with current weight, frequency of exercise, and scores on an inventory of personal attitudes about self, life, and work. Age and education were tested for inclusion as independent variables but were not significant in this final regression model and were dropped. The sample size is 172, and the independent variables are continuous and fairly normally distributed. We are comfortable in continuing with the analysis because we know that multiple regression is somewhat robust (i.e., able to tolerate) to mild to moderate violations of normality, particularly as the sample size increases. The only information we have about measurement error is that the Cronbach's alpha for the inventory of personal attitudes is .86.

Preparation

Draw the Model to be Tested With Path Analysis. This path model is drawn after using regression analysis to identify which variables from a theoretical framework are significantly related to the dependent variable of interest. The results of this regression analysis are depicted in Table 15-1. To draw the model, we also need 1) a table of correlations among the variables in the regression (see Table 15-2); 2) familiarity with the research findings and theory pertinent to this topic; 3) logic and reason to assign, when possible, a temporal order to the independent variables that are correlated with one another and for which research findings and theory are not available; and 4) awareness of the need to maintain a one-way flow of causation to meet assumptions necessary for path analysis.

An examination of the correlations listed in Table 15-2 reveals that all the independent variables are correlated with one another. This means that we must attempt

TABLE 15-1
Regression Results Used to Create Path Model in Computer Example

**** M U L T I P L E   R E G R E S S I O N ****

Listwise Deletion of Missing Data

Equation Number 1   Dependent Variable..   OVERALL STATE OF HEALTH

Block Number   1.   Method: Enter   FREQ EXERCISE   PERSONAL ATT   SATIS

Variable(s) Entered on Step Number
   1..   SATISFACTION WITH CURRENT WEIGHT
   2..   PERSONAL ATTITUDES
   3..   FREQUENCY OF EXERCISE

Multiple R	.66310
R Square	.43970
Adjusted R Square	.42964
Standard Error	1.57202

Analysis of Variance

	DF	Sum of Squares	Mean Square
Regression	3	323.87298	107.95766
Residual	167	412.70012	2.47126
F =	43.68530	Signif F = .0000	

---------------- Variables in the Equation ----------------

Variable	B	SE B	Beta*	T	Sig T	
FREQ EXERCISE	.471076	.138493	.225259	3.401	.0008	*These beta
PERSONAL ATT	.025629	.004108	.391484	6.239	.0000	weights are used
SATIS.	.198391	.048556	.261990	4.086	.0001	for the path coeffi-
(Constant)	1.367691	.607703		2.251	.0257	cients in
						Figure 15-14.

End Block Number   1   All requested variables entered.

TABLE 15-2
Correlations Among Variables in Computer Example

Correlation Coefficients

	HEALTH	FREQ EXER	PERS ATT	SATIS
HEALTH	1.0000	.4845	.5527	.4593
	(172)	(172)	(172)	(171)
	P= .	P= .000	P= .000	P= .000
FREQ EX	.4845	1.0000	.3701	.4087
	(172)	(172)	(172)	(171)
	P= .000	P= .	P= .000	P= .000
PERS ATT	.5527	.3701	1.000	.2689
	(172)	(172)	(173)	(171)
	P= .000	P= .000	P= .	P= .000
SATIS	.4593	.4087	.2689	1.0000
	(171)	(171)	(171)	(171)
	P= .000	P= .000	P= .000	P= .
PERS ATT	.5527	.3701	1.0000	.2689
	(172)	(172)	(173)	(171)
	P= .000	P= .000	P=	P= .000
SATIS	.4593	.4087	.2689	1.0000
	(171)	(171)	(171)	(171)
	P= .000	P= .000	P= .000	P= .

to assign a direction to these relationships. Theories about health behavior hold that attitudes guide behavior (Norris & Ford, 1995). Therefore, we can assign a direction to the relationship between personal attitudes and frequency of exercise, and draw a path ($p_{f,p}$) to represent this (Fig. 15-13). Research on exercise suggests that individuals who exercise moderately and regularly may be more satisfied with their weight (Tucker & Maxwell, 1992), and there is no evidence that individuals in our sample exercise excessively. Consequently, we draw a path ($p_{s,f}$) in Figure 15-13 to represent the influence of frequency of exercise on satisfaction with current weight. Research and theory are not available for assigning a direction to the relationship between personal attitudes and satisfaction with current weight. Here we use logic and reason and awareness of the need to maintain a one-way flow of causation. It is reasonable to hypothesize that a general set of attitudes should influence satisfaction with something specific, such as current weight, so we assign a direction to the path between these two variables ($p_{s,p}$) to represent this. Only one direction can be assigned to this relationship that will ensure the model meets the necessary assumption of one-way flow of causation. If we hypothesized that satisfaction with current weight influenced personal attitudes, the model would have a component that is cir-

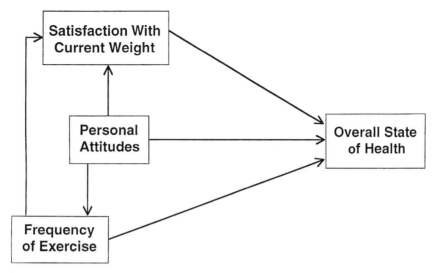

FIGURE 15-13
Diagram of initial path model.

cular or nonrecursive. You can see this if you redraw the model in Figure 15-13 so that it contains the path $p_{p,s}$ in place of $p_{s,p}$.

Identify the Regression Analyses Needed to Calculate the Path Coefficients and Test the Paths in the Model. Now look at the model in Figure 15-13, and count the number of endogenous variables to determine the number of regression analyses needed. You should come up with three endogenous variables: 1) the dependent variable, overall state of health; 2) frequency of exercise, which is endogenous to personal attitudes; and 3) satisfaction with current weight, which is endogenous to frequency of exercise and personal attitudes.

Thus, we need three regression analyses for this model:

1. Overall state of health regressed onto satisfaction with current weight, frequency of exercise, and scores on an inventory of personal attitudes about self, life, and work
2. Frequency of exercise regressed onto personal attitudes
3. Satisfaction with current weight regressed onto frequency of exercise and personal attitudes

The second regression analysis is nothing more than the correlation between frequency of exercise and personal attitudes. The path between an endogenous and exogenous variable is always equal to the correlation between these two variables whenever there is an endogenous variable with only one variable exogenous to it and the exogenous variable is fully exogenous and has no other variables influencing it.

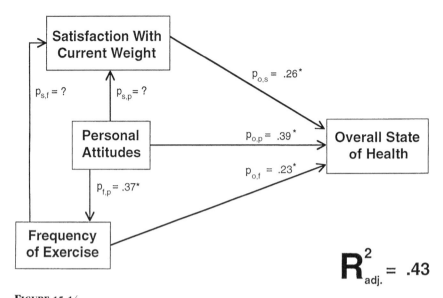

FIGURE 15-14

Diagram of model prior to running third regression analysis to test paths to endogenous variables. (*Path coefficient is significant at $p < .05$.)

Analysis

Calculating the Path Coefficients. We know what many of these coefficients are from our prior work. Figure 15-14 shows what we know using information from Tables 15-1 and 15-2. We are using the betas or the standardized coefficients for our diagram because we are not looking at group differences.

To calculate the remaining coefficients, we run the third regression analysis identified in our previous preparation—the one with satisfaction with current weight as the dependent variable. The results of this third regression analysis are presented in Table 15-3.

From the results depicted in Table 15-3, we see that the path ($p_{s,p}$) between personal attitudes and satisfaction with current weight could be dropped from the model because the beta weight for personal attitudes is not significant ($p > .06$). It makes sense to drop this path because we did not have strong theoretical support for including it. Also if we drop it, our model becomes overidentified, which is advantageous should we choose to test the overall fit of this model to our data.

We still use the beta weight in Table 15-3 associated with personal attitudes for the path between frequency of exercise and satisfaction with current weight because personal attitudes may influence satisfaction with weight *indirectly* through its effect on frequency of exercise. The regression analysis we have just run controls for this indirect effect. Figure 15-15 depicts our final path model. We need to refer to this model to complete the second step of the analysis.

TABLE 15-3
Regression Results for Paths to Endogenous Independent Variable in Computer Example

**** MULTIPLE REGRESSION ****

Listwise Deletion of Missing Data

Equation Number 1   Dependent Variable..   SATISFACTION WITH CURRENT WEIGHT

Block Number 1. Method: Enter   EXERCISE   PERSONAL ATT

Variable(s) Entered on Step Number
  1..   PERSONAL ATTITUDES
  2..   EXERCISE

Multiple R	.42894
R Square	.18399
Adjusted R Square	.17428
Standard Error	2.49784

Analysis of Variance

	DF	Sum of Squares	Mean Square
Regression	2	236.33938	118.16969
Residual	168	1048.18693	6.23921
F =	18.93985	Signif F = .0000	

---------------- Variables in the Equation ----------------

Variable	B	SE B	Beta	T	Sig T	
FREQ EXERCISE	.989635	.206385	.358345*	4.795	.0000	[†]Not significant,
PERSONAL ATT	.012065	.006461	.139557	1.867	.0636[†]	so path ($p_{s,p}$) is
(Constant)	1.688235	.956774		1.765	.0795	deleted from final
						model.

*Used for $p_{s,f}$
in Figure 15-15

End Block Number   1   All requested variables entered.

Determining the Direct, Indirect, and Total Effects of the Independent Variables. Now we construct Table 15-4 to help us use Wright's (1934) work about the components of a correlation. We fill in Table 15-4 using the correlation values from Table 15-2 for the leftmost column and the beta weights from Table 15-1 for the simple paths column. These beta weights are the direct effects of the independent variable on overall state of health.

Figure 15-15 is used to identify the paths that need to be multiplied to determine the values for the compound paths. Wright's (1934) rules are used to trace the paths

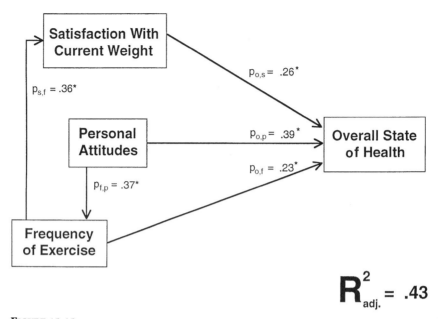

FIGURE 15-15
Final path analysis results for computer example. (*Path coefficient is significant at $p < .05$.)

needed to calculate these compound paths. For example, rule 2 tells us that the co-efficients for $p_{s,f}$ and $p_{o,f}$ should be multiplied to determine the noncausal compo-nent of $r_{s,o}$ and that we do not need to worry about adding the product of $p_{s,f}$ and $p_{f,p}$ because including the latter set of paths would violate rule 2. Note that the com-pound paths are sorted into indirect effects, which are the sums of products for mean-ingful compound paths, and noncausal components, which are the sums of prod-ucts for compound paths that are meaningless.

TABLE 15-4
Table Used to Determine Direct and Indirect Effects of Independent Variables in Figure 15-15

r	= Direct	+ (Indirect)	+ (Noncausal)
r	= Simple	+ Compound + . . . + compound	+ Compound + . . . + compound
$r_{f,o}$	= $P_{o,f}$	+ $(p_{s,f})(p_{o,s})$	+ $(p_{f,p})(p_{o,p})$
.48	= .23	+ (.36)(.26)	+ (.37)(.39)
$r_{p,o}$	= $P_{o,p}$	+ $(p_{f,p})(p_{o,f})$ + $(p_{f,p})(p_{s,f})(p_{o,s})$	+ None
.55	= .39	+ (.37)(.23) + (.37)(.36)(.26)	+ 0
$r_{s,o}$	= $P_{o,s}$	+ None	+ $(p_{s,f})(p_{o,f})$ + $(p_{o,p})(p_{f,p})(p_{s,f})$
.46	= .26	+ 0	+ (.36)(.23) + (.39)(.37)(.36)

TABLE 15-5
Table of Direct Effects, Indirect Effects, and Noncausal Components
Associated With Each Independent Variable in Figure 15-10

	Direct + Indirect	Total Effect	Total Effect + Noncausal
Frequency of exercise (r = .48)	.23 + .09	.32	.46
Personal attitudes (r = .55)	.39 + .12	.51	.51
Satisfaction with current weight (r = .46)	.26 + 0	.26	.39

Table 15-5 contains the value of the direct and indirect effects as determined by using Wright's (1934) formula for the components of a correlation coefficient and his rules for calculating compound paths. Personal attitudes appear to have the greatest effect (.51) on the overall state of health. Also, the sums of the total effect and non-causal component are fairly close to the respective correlation coefficients (within .07) for all three independent variables. This suggests that our model may be well specified. However, we could be underestimating the noncausal component for satisfaction with current weight and the indirect effect of personal attitudes by deleting the path between personal attitudes and satisfaction with current weight ($p_{s,p}$). One way to decide would be to add this path back into the model, add the additional compound paths this change would generate, redetermine the indirect effects, and sum the resulting new values for the total effects and noncausal components. How does this alter our results overall? Does adding this path appreciably change our estimates of the indirect effects of the independent variables? Do the resulting sums of the total effect and the noncausal component suggest that model specification is appreciably improved or worsened?

Consideration of the Analysis' Limitations

Now that we have a final path model, it is important to review the assumptions underlying path analysis to be aware of the limitations of the analysis we have just conducted. First, we need to consider whether any of the relationships in the model may be spurious (i.e., violate the third condition of causation). Are there potentially confounding variables that we should have included?

Second, do we know if we can assume that there is no measurement error in our measures? What evidence do we have to support the reliability of our measures?

Finally, we should remind ourselves of the need to replicate this model with longitudinal data. In this example, we are forced to make assumptions regarding the directions between the variables in our model because we are working with cross-sectional data. Having a positive perception of their overall state of health may cause individuals to exercise more, but we have no way of knowing this. Path analysis does not allow us to evaluate the correctness of the directions we have assigned. Rather, we have assumed that these are the correct directions. Path analysis can tell us only that given our assumptions, this particular path is or is not statistically significant.

Example of Published Path Analysis

This example illustrates Fink's (1995) use of path analysis to test a conceptual framework for family well-being in families providing care to an elderly parent. The seven independent variables are socioeconomic status, family resources (two types), family demands (three types), and family strains. The sample size is 65, and the data are cross-sectional.

All variables are continuous. A review of the means and the standard deviations of the family variables (Table 15-6) suggests that these variables are fairly normally distributed. Socioeconomic status (SES) appears to be fairly normally distributed (range = 13–66; M = 46.31, SD = 11.51). Reliability of the measures is quite good. Six of the eight measures have coefficient alphas > .80. The other two measures, family well-being (alpha = .79) and family strains (alpha = .74), are good to acceptable.

Preparation

Draw the Model to be Tested With Path Analysis. Fink (1995) was interested in testing the overidentified model depicted in Figure 15-16. In addition to specifying the direction of the relationships between variables in the model, Fink proposed that coefficients would be negative or positive in their influence. Family demand variables were predicted to only have an indirect effect on family well-being

TABLE 15-6
Description of Study Variables

Variable	M	(SD)	Potential Range	Actual Range
Family social support	97.13	(12.11)	35–140	70–125
Internal family system resources	44.70	(6.90)	0–60	29.5–57.5
Family life changes	3.99	(2.31)	0–10	0–9
Amount of help	14.85	(12.04)	0–80	1–55
Caregiver's appraisal	28.11	(12.83)	0–88	5–59
Family strains	4.26	(2.55)	0–10	0–10
Family well-being	0.00	(5.05)	NA	−13.82–9.36

(Fink, S. V. [1995]. The influence of family resources and family demands on the strains and well-being of caregiving families. Nursing Research, 44, 143.)

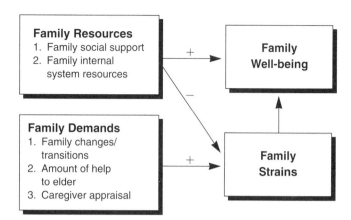

FIGURE 15-16
Theoretical model tested by Fink (1995).

through their influence on family strains. SES was added to this theoretical model prior to the path analysis to control for SES differences on the theorized relationships.

Identify the Regression Analyses Needed to Calculate the Path Coefficients and Test the Paths in the Model. The model in Figure 15-16 specifies two endogenous variables: the dependent variable, family well-being; and independent variable, family strains. Fink (1995) wants to control for the effect of SES on the theorized relationships in Figure 15-16. Thus, SES is added as a predictor variable to both of the regression analyses conducted in the path analysis:

- Family well-being regressed onto family strains, resource variables (social support, internal system resources), and SES
- Family strains regressed onto resource (social support, internal system resources) and demand (life changes, amount of help to elder, caregiver's appraisal) variables and SES

Analysis

Calculating the Path Coefficients. The path coefficients calculated in the regression equations are provided in Figure 15-17. Note that Fink (1995) elected to retain all the paths in the model, although some were not statistically significant. The adjusted R^2 values provided in Figure 15-17 refer to each of the regression equations used to calculate the paths in the model.

Determining the Direct, Indirect, and Total Effects of the Independent Variables. Fink (1995) chose not to calculate any indirect effects because the path between family strains and family well-being was not significant. The substantive direct effects (i.e., path coefficients in Figure 15-17 that are .20 or greater in magnitude) obtained are consistent with the directions theorized in the model depicted in Figure 15-16.

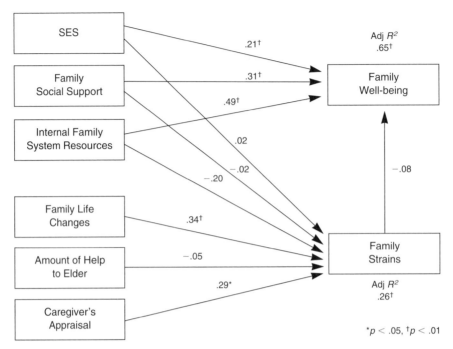

FIGURE 15-17
Results of Fink's (1995) path analysis. (Note: SES has been added to the original theoretical model indicated in Figure 15-16.)

Consideration of the Analysis' Limitations

Fink's (1995) analysis generally appears to meet the theoretical and statistical assumptions for path analysis. For example, by including SES in her analyses, she helps rule out a potentially confounding variable and make the case that the relationships in the model are nonspurious. Her measures are reliable, which argues against measurement error, and her model has a one-way flow of causation.

The only apparent limitations are the cross-sectional nature of her data and the sample size. Hence as she points out, the "findings must be considered tentative given the small sample size and the cross-sectional design" (p. 145).

SUMMARY

Path analysis is a data analysis technique that can be used to inform our understanding of phenomena. It is useful because at the very least, it challenges us to think of the effects of independent variables in more complex ways (Asher, 1983). Although on the surface it may appear complex, path analysis is a relatively simple data analytic technique. It is nothing more than a series of regression analyses and some hand calculations. The difficulty is in thinking through the relationships among a set of variables.

Path analysis, like any statistic, is just a tool in the hands of the researcher. The validity of the model testing and theory building it produces depends on the quality of the data and the thinking that accompanies the use of the statistic.

APPLICATION EXERCISES AND RESULTS

EXERCISES

1. Run the regressions necessary for a path analysis of the model contained in Exercise Figure 15-1. Add the betas to the diagram. Delete any paths that have significance levels less than .05. Rerun regressions if necessary, and add new betas to the model.

RESULTS

1. We ran three regressions to obtain the betas necessary for the path analysis. We have included just the tables with the betas in Exercise Figure 15-2. First, we regressed health on exercise, current satisfaction with weight, and current quality of life. Then we regressed current quality of life on current satisfaction with weight and exercise. Finally, we regressed current satisfaction with weight on exercise, although we could simply have used the correlation between the two variables. Adding the betas to the model as path coefficients results in the model in Exercise Figure 15-3.

Note that all of the path coefficients are significant except the path between current quality of life and current satisfaction with weight. Removing that path from the model means that we must rerun the regression with current quality of life as the dependent variable. Now there is only one independent variable, exercise. That output is contained in Exercise Figure 15-4. Again, we could have used the correlation between the two variables. Exercise Figure 15-5 contains the reduced model with the new beta from the regression in Exercise Figure 15-4.

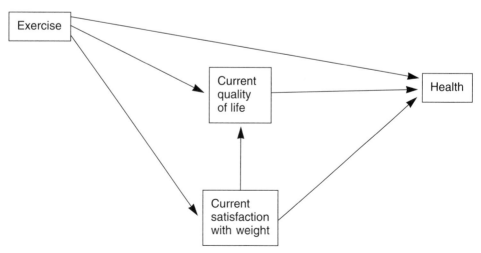

EXERCISE FIGURE 15-1. Model for testing.

Coefficients^a

Model		Unstandardized Coefficients		Standardized Coefficients	t	Sig.
		B	Std. Error	Beta		
1	(Constant)	2.551	.511		4.990	.000
	Exercise	.424	.155	.198	2.731	.007
	Satisfaction with current weight	.230	.050	.297	4.575	.000
	Quality of life in past month	.605	.124	.334	4.870	.000

a. Dependent Variable: overall state of health

Coefficients^a

Model		Unstandardized Coefficients		Standardized Coefficients	t	Sig.
		B	Std. Error	Beta		
1	(Constant)	2.759	.234		11.806	.000
	Exercise	.561	.085	.474	6.568	.000
	Satisfaction with current weight	3.1E-02	.031	.072	.993	.322

a. Dependent Variable: quality of life in past month

Coefficients^a

Model		Unstandardized Coefficients		Standardized Coefficients	t	Sig.
		B	Std. Error	Beta		
1	(Constant)	3.212	.522		6.149	.000
	Exercise	1.136	.192	.410	5.917	.000

a. Dependent Variable: satisfaction with current weight

EXERCISE FIGURE 15-2. Output from three regressions.

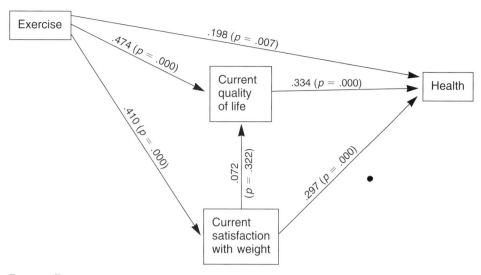

EXERCISE FIGURE 15-3. Betas from initial three regressions.

Coefficients^a

Model		Unstandardized Coefficients		Standardized Coefficients		
		B	Std. Error	Beta	t	Sig.
1	(Constant)	2.857	.211		13.532	.000
	Exercise	.595	.078	.504	7.671	.000

a. Dependent Variable: quality of life in past month

EXERCISE FIGURE 15-4. Regression of quality of life on exercise.

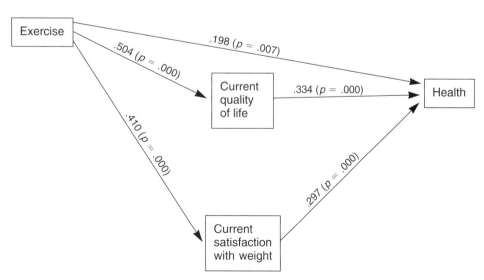

EXERCISE FIGURE 15-5. Reduced model.

Structural Equation Modeling

ANNE E. NORRIS[1]

OBJECTIVES FOR CHAPTER 16

After reading this chapter, you should be able to do the following:

1 ● Describe at least three types of research questions that can be addressed with structural equation modeling (SEM).

2 ● Identify three dataset requirements for conducting SEM.

3 ● Describe the relationship between the measurement model and the theoretical model in SEM.

4 ● Describe the role of theory in the SEM process.

5 ● Critique an SEM analysis on the basis of the model fit statistics and description of the modeling process.

This chapter is an introduction to structural equation modeling (SEM) and assumes an understanding of the concepts and issues discussed in Chapter 15 with respect to path analysis. The purpose of this chapter is to acquaint readers with the possibilities SEM offers and aid them in interpreting SEM results published in the literature. For a more in-depth knowledge of SEM, read one or more of the following: Bollen (1989), Byrne (1994), Hayduk (1987), or Hoyle (1995).

[1]*Acknowledgments: The author wishes to thank Dr. Karen Aroian, Dr. Greg Trompeter, and Ms. Gina Ankner for their careful review and critique of this chapter.*

A GENERAL INTRODUCTION

SEM is a relatively new statistical technique: The first computer program that could perform SEM was not developed until the late 1970s. Like path analysis, SEM is used to test theoretical models. Over the years, SEM has been called covariance structure modeling because covariances are analyzed in SEM; latent variable analysis because SEM analyzes relationships between latent (i.e., unmeasured) variables; and a LISREL analysis because LISREL was the name of the first software available for conducting SEM.

SEM challenges us to think about how we measure theoretical constructs. It allows us to use multiple measures of theoretical constructs, so, for example, researchers do not have to settle for one measure of health. They can use psychological, performance, and physiological measures. Similarly, responses to a health attitudes questionnaire would not have to be totaled and treated as a lump sum to be included in the analysis. With SEM, the individual questionnaire items are treated as different measures of health attitudes.

The measurement of theoretical constructs is critical in SEM. SEM tests two models simultaneously: a measurement model and a theoretical model. Together these two models are called the "full model." The measurement model is a model of how theoretical constructs are measured. The theoretical model is a model of the hypothesized relationships between the theoretical constructs. Valid tests of the theoretical model depend on a "good fit" of the measurement model to the data. The statistics produced in SEM help the researcher determine how good this fit is.

THE RESEARCH QUESTION

SEM allows us to ask old questions in new and more powerful ways and new questions that could not have been addressed without the technology and thinking that underlies SEM. The latter sort of questions are only just beginning to be identified and pursued.

At least three types of "old" questions can be addressed with SEM. First, like path analysis, SEM can be used to test a "causal model." However, unlike path analysis, measurement error is estimated and removed from the relationships between theoretical constructs. Thus, it is possible to get a more precise test of theories. In addition, SEM can be used to analyze nonrecursive models (i.e., models with two-way paths).

Second, SEM provides a new way to examine construct validity. It affords the researcher a level of precision not possible with traditional factor analysis. With SEM, the researcher specifies how many factors or subscales the instrument has and which items are specific to which factor. Correlations between the factors, or lack thereof, can also be specified. For example, Aroian (under review) developed a Demands of Immigration scale. Based on prior research, she hypothesized that there were six dimensions to the demands of immigration and developed items specific to each of these dimensions. She hypothesized that her instrument had six subscales and that each subscale had three items that were unique to it. SEM provided support for this "model" of her instrument (Fig. 16-1) by allowing her to conduct a specific confirmatory factor analysis. Aroian was able to confirm the design of her instrument, which strengthened her argument for its construct validity.

Third, SEM provides a new way to look at group differences. With SEM, it is possible to determine whether the same theoretical model works equally well for explaining the data in different sample subgroups. For example, Norris and Ford (1995) predicted that different theoretical models for explaining condom use were needed for young African-American and Hispanic men and women. They used SEM to compare the models depicted in Figures 16-2 through 16-5. They found that the four models were significantly different: The same model could not be used to explain condom use in all four groups. Moreover, four of the paths that were common to two or more models (e.g., the path age and alcohol use in Figs. 16-2 and 16-3) differed significantly in magnitude as well.

In addition, SEM opens the door to new questions. For example, with SEM, it is possible to first assume that different levels of measurement error are present in data and then test the effect of these different levels on the theoretical relationships spec-

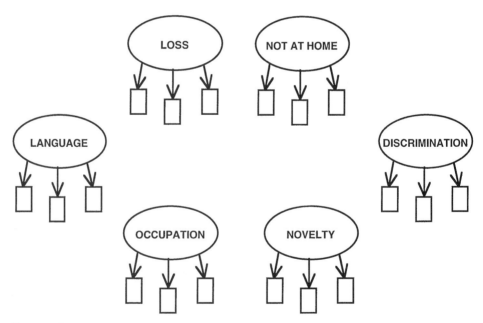

FIGURE 16-1
Aroian's hypothesized factor structure for the Demands of Immigration scale. Correlations among factors are not shown. Each factor is hypothesized to correlate with all other factors. Boxes indicate questionnaire items. Circles represent the factors.

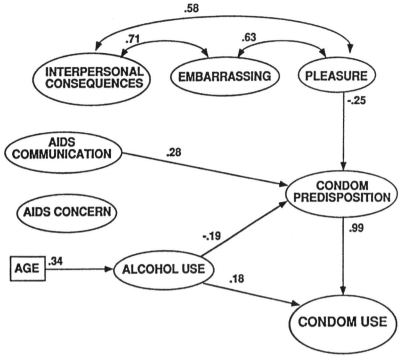

FIGURE 16-2

Model for African-American males. (From Norris, A. E., & Ford, K. [1995]. Condom use by low-income African-American and Hispanic youth with a well-known partner: Integrating the Health Belief Model, Theory of Reasoned Action, and Construct Accessibility Model. Reprinted with permission from *Journal of Applied Social Psychology, 25,* 1818–1821. © V.H. Winston & Son, Inc., 360 South Ocean Blvd., Palm Beach, FL 33480. All rights reserved.)

ified in the model. Thus, conclusions could be made about the robustness of these relationships to problems such as subjects' poor memories, tendency to alter responses to make a better impression, and misreading the question. For example, Rigdon (1994) found that the nonrecursive relationship between stressful life events and depression specified in Ferguson and Horwood's (1984) model became recursive when different assumptions about measurement error were made. (Ferguson and Horwood assumed no measurement error.) Thus, the notion that stressful life events contribute to depression, which in turn contributes to stressful life events (i.e., nonrecursive relationship), is not robust to measurement error. Perhaps, the effect of depression on stressful life events found by Ferguson and Horwood is nothing more than depressed people perceiving their life more negatively? Regardless, Rigdon found that the only relationship that appeared robust was the effect of stressful life events on depression.

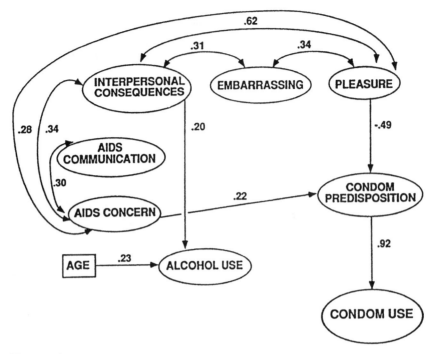

FIGURE 16-3

Model for African-American females. (From Norris, A. E., & Ford, K. [1995]. Condom use by low-income African-American and Hispanic youth with a well-known partner: Integrating the Health Belief Model, Theory of Reasoned Action, and Construct Accessibility Model. Reprinted with permission from *Journal of Applied Social Psychology, 25,* 1818–1821. © V.H. Winston & Son, Inc., 360 South Ocean Blvd., Palm Beach, FL 33480. All rights reserved.)

NINE KEY STRUCTURAL EQUATION MODELING TERMS

Before talking about the type of data and assumptions required for SEM, it is necessary to discuss some of the terms used in SEM. Frequently, different names have evolved to refer to the same term. These different names result from differences in the software used for SEM and in the orientation to SEM. Currently, the two most popular and widely used computer software programs are EQS and LISREL (Byrne, 1995). In this section, names for terms that are unique to these programs are noted.

Indicators, Measured Variables, Proxies, and Manifest Variables

Indicators, measured variables, proxies, and manifest variables are different terms used in SEM to refer to the same thing: measures of a theoretical construct. For simplicity, *indicator* is used in the remainder of this chapter to refer to these measures. Indicators are directly measured by the researcher; they correspond to a specific response to a questionnaire or piece of data in a dataset. In LISREL, the letters X and Y

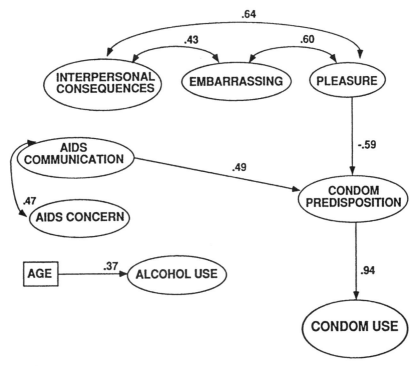

FIGURE 16-4
Model for Hispanic males. (From Norris, A. E., & Ford, K. [1995]. Condom use by low-income African-American and Hispanic youth with a well-known partner: Integrating the Health Belief Model, Theory of Reasoned Action, and Construct Accessibility Model. Reprinted with permission from *Journal of Applied Social Psychology, 25,* 1818–1821. © V.H. Winston & Son, Inc., 360 South Ocean Blvd., Palm Beach, FL 33480. All rights reserved.)

are used to refer to indicators. In EQS, the letter V is used. A universal way of designating a variable as an indicator is to enclose it in a square in the SEM diagram. Hence, we could say that the construct, *health,* in Figure 16-6 has six indicators: psychological well-being, happiness, Karnofsky Performance Status, percent of activities of daily living (ADLs) self-completed, treadmill performance, and resting heart rate.

Measurement Model

The measurement model is a model of how theoretical constructs are measured. For example, Figure 16-6 is a measurement model for the construct *health.* The model, as diagrammed, indicates that we are hypothesizing that well-being and happiness, Karnofsky Performance Status, percent of ADLs self-completed, treadmill performance, and resting heart rate are all indicators for the construct *health.*

Sometimes the focus of the SEM is on the measurement model, such as when SEM is used for confirmatory factor analysis to examine an instrument's construct va-

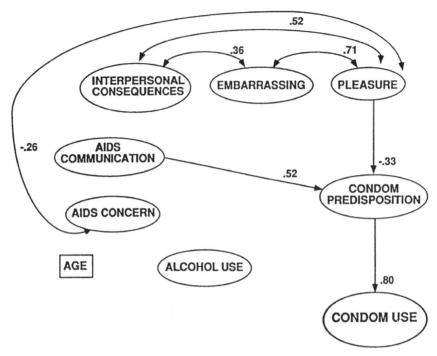

FIGURE 16-5
Model for Hispanic females. (From Norris, A. E., & Ford, K. [1995]. Condom use by low-in-
come African-American and Hispanic youth with a well-known partner: Integrating the
Health Belief Model, Theory of Reasoned Action, and Construct Accessibility Model.
Reprinted with permission from *Journal of Applied Social Psychology, 25,* 1818–1821. © V.H.
Winston & Son, Inc., 360 South Ocean Blvd., Palm Beach, FL 33480. All rights reserved.)

lidity. Other times, the measurement model receives little attention because the researcher is focused on examining relationships between theoretical constructs. However, the validity of any theory testing that SEM provides depends on the fit of the
measurement model to the data. If the measurement model does not fit the data well,
we cannot determine whether a failure to find a hypothesized relationship is due to
a problem with the theory or with measurement.

Theoretical Constructs, Unmeasured Variables, and Latent Variables

In SEM, theoretical constructs are often called unmeasured or latent variables because they are not measured directly by the researcher. To minimize confusion, theoretical constructs are called latent variables for the remainder of the chapter. Latent
variables are free of the random or systematic measurement error inherent in indicator variables (Bollen, 1989). A universal way of identifying a theoretical construct
as a latent variable is to demarcate it with a circle in a diagram of an SEM model.
Thus, the model in Figure 16-6 has one latent variable—health.

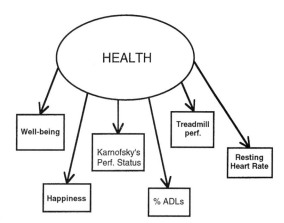

FIGURE 16-6
Measurement model for the construct health.

Figure 16-6 represents health as a single latent variable with psychological, performance, and physiological indicators. Alternatively, we could hypothesize that health is a multidimensional construct with psychological, performance, and physiological indicators measuring its different dimensions. This hypothesis would be consistent with a model for health such as that shown in Figure 16-7. What is advantageous about SEM is that we can test both models (or hypotheses) and see which one fits the data best before testing a larger theoretical model about factors that influence health.

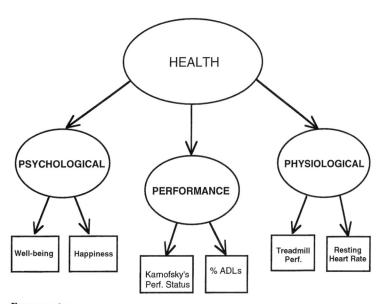

FIGURE 16-7
Measurement model for the health construct as a second order factor.

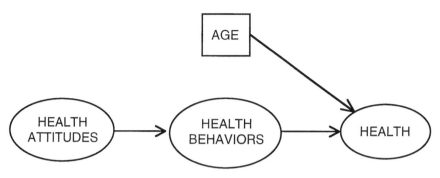

FIGURE 16-8
Hypothetical theoretical model predicting health as a function of age, health attitudes, and health behaviors.

Theoretical Model

The theoretical model is a model of the hypothesized relationships between latent variables. For example, in Figure 16-8, we are hypothesizing that health is influenced by age, health attitudes, and health behaviors. Health attitudes are not diagrammed as having a direct effect on health.

Within the theoretical model, variables are designated as endogenous or exogenous just as they are in path analysis. As you may recall from Chapter 15, endogenous variables are influenced by other variables in the model, whereas exogenous variables are independent of such influences. Thus, in Figure 16-8, health behaviors and health are endogenous variables. In EQS, endogenous and exogenous latent variables are called factors (e.g., F_1, F_2, F_3). In LISREL, Greek letters are used: ξ (xi or ksi) for endogenous and η (eta) for exogenous latent variables.

Coefficients, Parameters, and Parameter Estimates

Researchers refer to path coefficients in the measurement and theoretical model as coefficients, parameters, or parameter estimates. These words are often used interchangeably because they mean the same thing, but for the sake of clarity, the word parameter is used for the rest of the chapter. Unlike EQS, which uses no special notation to denote parameters, the LISREL software uses a system of Greek letters to categorize parameters according to the paths they define. Consequently, researchers (regardless of the software they use) may talk about lambda parameters (λ) when referring to parameters in the measurement model, beta parameters (β) when referring to paths between endogenous variables, or gamma (γ) when referring to paths between one exogenous and one endogenous variable. Researchers further define these parameters by using the same subscript notation discussed in Chapter 15 (e.g., $\gamma_{1,2}$).

Parameters are often called fixed or free. A fixed parameter is not estimated in the SEM analysis. Instead, the researcher assigns it a particular value. For example, researchers typically fix a parameter in the measurement model to be equal to 1.0. This allows a measurement scale (i.e., 0–10 or 1–4) to be determined for the latent variable. Other parameters are fixed to zero to represent the absence of a path between two latent variables or between an indicator and a latent variable.

A free parameter has no value assigned to it. Free parameters are estimated in the SEM analysis: The computer calculates the value as part of the analysis using the covariances of the various indicators.

Both standardized and nonstandardized parameters (i.e., path coefficients) are estimated in SEM. SEM computer programs (e.g., LISREL, EQS) provide significance tests of these parameters as part of the analysis. It is possible to use the standardized parameter estimate and Wright's (1934) method to compute the indirect and total effects of latent variables, just as you would in path analysis (see Chapter 15).

Model Fit Statistics

SEM software programs produce a variety of statistics pertaining to the fit of the model. For example, LISREL produces a goodness of fit index (GFI) and EQS produces a comparative fit index (CFI). Both the GFI and CFI can range from 0 to 1.0. Historically, a good fitting model is one that has a GFI or CFI greater than .90 (Bentler & Bonnett, 1980). However, recent work suggests that even this cutoff may not be high enough in all cases given certain sample sizes, estimation methods, and distributions (Hu & Bentler, 1995).

All SEM programs produce a model chi-square. This chi-square assesses the difference between observed data and a restricted structure resulting from the full (i.e., measurement and theoretical) model (Byrne, 1994). This means that in SEM, the researcher wants the chi-square test to be nonsignificant. The researcher seeks to confirm the null hypothesis (i.e., there is no difference between the data and the model).

A limitation of the model chi-square is that it is greatly influenced by sample size and violations of multivariate normality (Jöreskog & Sörbom, 1988). Bollen and Long (1993) say that any work that uses only the model chi-square to draw conclusions about model fit should be greeted with skepticism.

Two hand-calculated statistics are also used to assess model fit. One of these, Carmine and McIver's (1983) relative chi-square (ratio of chi-square to degrees of freedom), is calculated by dividing the model chi-square by its degrees of freedom. There is no consensus on what value constitutes a good fit (Bollen, 1989), but Carmine and McIver (1983) recommend that relative chi-squares be less than 3.

A second type of hand-calculated statistic, the nested chi-square, is used to determine which of two competing models fits the data significantly better. This is the test we would use to determine which measurement model of health, Figure 16-6 or Figure 16-7, is best. A nested chi-square is calculated by subtracting the chi-square and degrees of freedom for one model from that associated with another competitive model. The significance level associated with this nested chi-square is used to determine whether the fit of one model differs significantly from that of the other. Table 16-1 contains an example of how to calculate the nested chi-square to determine if one measurement model for health fits the data significantly better than the

TABLE 16-1
Example of How to Calculate a Nested Chi-Square

chi-square statistic for model of health depicted in Figure 16-7:	2,006.37, $df = 1,202$
chi-square statistic for model of health depicted in Figure 16-6:	2,021.58, $df = 1,200$
nested chi-square:*	-15.21, $df = \quad 2$

Sign (negative or positive) of the nested chi-square does not matter.

other. The chi-square for Figure 16-7 (second order factor model) is smaller than the one for Figure 16-6. This suggests that the second order factor model fits the data better (remember in SEM we want the chi-square to be nonsignificant). The significance level associated with the nested chi-square confirms this: $\chi^2 = |15.21|$, $df = 2$, $p < .001$.

In general, a variety of fit statistics should be used to evaluate model fit. For example, a researcher may choose to report the CFI, chi-square test, and relative chi-square ratio. A model may be interpreted as fitting the data even when the chi-square is statistically significant if the CFI or GFI is equal to or greater than .90 and the relative chi-square is less than 3.

Identification

Identification of the measurement model and the theoretical model is critical to the estimation of parameters and testing of model fit that occurs in SEM. Just as in path analysis, these models can be overidentified, just identified, or underidentified. In SEM, the computer program cannot generate model fit statistics if the model is just identified. Moreover, if the model is underidentified, the program either will not run or will run only after the computer chooses specific parameters in the model to constrain to be equal to zero. Hence, the measurement and theoretical model being tested must be overidentified. This is not always easy. It is possible for parts or sections of a model to be underidentified. In addition, a model may be overidentified on paper but statistically underidentified in the computer program due to properties of the indicators. A more detailed discussion of how to assess identification in the measurement and theoretical models is beyond the scope of this chapter, but if you are interested in conducting SEM, refer to Bollen (1989) or Hayduk (1987).

Modification Indices

In addition to model fit statistics and parameter estimates, SEM programs provide statistics predicting the potential change in model fit (change in chi-square) associated with adding or deleting parameters. Researchers may use these statistics to guide them in making changes in their model. Two specific types of modification indices produced by EQS are the Lagrange multiplier test (for adding parameters) and Wald test (for deleting nonsignificant parameters). The modification indices produced by LISREL are called "modification indices" and only indicate if specific parameters should be added.

Multiple Group Analysis

Multiple group analysis is a type of analysis in which group differences in measurement and theoretical models are tested. A researcher could use this type of analysis to determine if the factor structure of an instrument is the same in different sample subgroups (e.g., different age, gender, ethnic groups). Group differences in theoretical models are explored when the measurement model is equivalent or at least partially invariant across groups (Byrne, 1994). An equivalent measurement model means that the free parameters are not significantly different across groups. A partially invariant measurement model has at least one free parameter that is equivalent across groups (i.e., the difference is not statistically significant).

It is important to establish that the measurement model is equivalent or partially invariant to avoid having group differences in the theoretical model confounded by measurement differences.

TYPE OF DATA REQUIRED FOR STRUCTURAL EQUATION MODELING

SEM requires data to have three characteristics. First, the data should be continuous and normally distributed. However, new techniques are being developed for categorical data (Muthén, 1993; Von Eye & Clogg, 1994; West, Finch, & Curran, 1995). In addition, special estimation methods and scaled statistics are available that are robust to violations of normality (Byrne, 1994; Hu & Bentler, 1995).

Second, the data should contain multiple indicators of latent variables. At least three indicators of a latent variable are needed for its measurement model to be just identified. Fixing the parameter for one of the three indicators to be equal to 1.0 makes the model overidentified. As noted previously, this is a common practice because it also allows a measurement scale to be determined for the latent variable. Measurement models with less than three indicators can become overidentified if the researcher makes certain assumptions (i.e., fixes certain parameters), such as assuming a measure has no measurement error.

These multiple indicators must capture different aspects or characteristics of a latent variable. Indicators cannot be so redundant (i.e., highly correlated) that one can be used to predict another perfectly or near perfectly. This type of redundancy is called linear dependency. It prevents the model from being statistically identified (Chou & Bentler, 1995). This means that although the model as diagrammed looks identified, high intercorrelations in the data render it statistically underidentified. For example, Aroian only used three of the 11 to 12 items available per subscale from her Demands of Immigration scale in her final SEM analysis. High interitem correlations created "linear dependencies" in her model when all subscale items were used.

Aroian randomly picked items from among the intercorrelated ones to use in the SEM to ensure that her model would be statistically overidentified.

Third, the data should be numerous: SEM requires a large sample size. Assuming the most common method for estimating the parameters in SEM (maximum likelihood [ML]), a typical recommendation is a minimum of 100 to 200 subjects (100–200 per group in a multiple group analysis). However, this size sample may be inadequate if the model is fairly complex (contains several theoretical variables; Bollen, 1989) or the data are not normally distributed (West, et al., 1995). There are no clear rules as to sample size, but Bollen (1989) suggests having at least several subjects per free parameter.

Although SEM is considered a causal modeling technique, it can be performed with either cross-sectional or longitudinal data and is not typically used to analyze data produced from an experimental design. For example, the data used by Norris and Ford (1995) in their multiple group analysis (results depicted in Figures 16-2 through 16-5) are from a survey and are cross-sectional. Thus, it is important to be aware of theoretical assumptions pertaining to causation in SEM.

ASSUMPTIONS

Three types of assumptions must be considered with SEM: theoretical, general statistical, and estimation method specific statistical assumptions.

Theoretical Assumptions

In SEM, the importance of using theory to guide your work cannot be emphasized enough. As in path analysis, theoretical (or causal) assumptions are made in the process of identifying a model to be tested. However, with SEM, assumptions of causation are made regarding measurement of latent variables (e.g., this indicator measures this construct) and relationships between latent variables (e.g., attitudes influence behavior). Assumptions are made when paths are drawn (i.e., parameter does not equal zero) and not drawn (i.e., parameter is equal to zero). For example, in Figure 16-7, there are no paths connecting well-being, happiness, treadmill performance, and resting heart rate with the performance construct. It is assumed that the parameters between these indicators and the performance construct are equal to zero.

As in path analysis, it is important to consider the three conditions of causation: the presence of an observed and measurable relationship between variables, temporal ordering, and nonspuriousness (see Chapter 15 for a discussion of these three conditions). Bollen (1989) and others writing specifically about SEM use the terms association, direction of influence, and isolation to refer to these three conditions of causation. Bollen (1989) talks about meeting a condition of "pseudoisolation" to emphasize the researcher's inability to be absolutely sure that a relationship between two latent variables is nonspurious. Further, he emphasizes the need to recognize the tentativeness of any claims made through SEM about causality and argues for replication as an important check on whether the conditions of association and isolation have been met.

General Statistical Assumptions

There are three types of general statistical assumptions in SEM. Violating these assumptions makes it difficult to identify a model that fits the data well and typically results in poorer fit indices.

The first type of assumptions should already be familiar to you. These are the assumptions of normal distributions, homoscedasticity, and linear relationships discussed in Chapter 12 for regression analysis. These assumptions arise because, like path analysis, SEM involves solving a series of regression equations. Although SEM is somewhat robust to violations of normality, inclusion of categorical variables can bias significance tests of parameters and the model chi-square test by increasing the likelihood that they will be significant (West, et al., 1995). The effect of categorical variables is contingent on their correlation with other variables in the measurement model and must be examined on a case-by-case basis (Bollen, 1989). Variables should be transformed so that their relationships are linear, and a multiple group analysis should be conducted when interactions are predicted. For example, Norris and Ford (1995) used a multiple group analysis to show that different models of condom use were needed for each gender-ethnic subgroup in their sample. Their findings confirmed the effect of a gender-by-ethnicity interaction on condom use.

Second, there are assumptions regarding the error terms in SEM. These assumptions are similar to those made in regression regarding the residuals and are typically met in the course of meeting other SEM assumptions.[2] Although these assumptions are violated when the data are not multivariate normal, they are robust when the sample size is large (Chou & Bentler, 1995).

The third type of assumption pertains to sample size. It is assumed that the sample is "asymptotic"—so large as to approach infinity (Bollen, 1989). Smaller sample sizes (e.g., less than 100 for a *simple* model when ML is used to estimate parameters) increase the probability of rejecting a true model (one that fits the data; West, et al., 1995).

Estimation Method Specific Statistical Assumptions

In addition to general statistical assumptions, distributional assumptions are associated with the method used to estimate the parameters in SEM. This discussion is limited to the ML because it is the most commonly used estimation method (Chou & Bentler, 1995) and performs, on average, better than most other estimation methods even when its assumptions are violated (Bollen, 1989; West, et al., 1995). ML assumes that no single variable or group of variables perfectly explains another in the data set (Bollen, 1989), and indicators have a distribution that is multivariate normal (West,

---

[2]*Specifically, it is assumed that error terms in the model are not correlated with any of the latent variables, independent of one another, and normally distributed (Fox, 1984).*

et al., 1995). This first assumption is why indicators cannot be redundant (i.e., highly intercorrelated). ML is not very robust to violations of this first assumption: Models with variables that correlate at or above .90 cannot be estimated.

Although the multivariate normal assumption is difficult to meet in practice, ML is fairly robust to violation of this assumption (Chou & Bentler, 1995). However, there are two exceptions: (1) when the sample size is small and the model is complex and (2) when categorical or dichotomous variables are used. Special techniques and estimation methods for models with categorical variables are available, although the sample size requirement can become so large that it is not practical (Hoyle & Panter, 1995; Muthén, 1993; Von Eye & Clogg, 1994; West, et al., 1995). In addition, it often makes more theoretical (and statistical) sense to perform a multiple group analysis when dichotomous variables represent group differences such as gender and employment status.

POWER

Power is an important issue in SEM in two respects. First, given the same model, a larger sample is more likely to generate a significant model chi-square and hence rejection of the model regardless of its "truth" (Bollen, 1989; Kaplan, 1995). Even models that fit the data well have small specification errors because it is difficult, if not impossible, to specify a model perfectly. Large sample sizes magnify the effects of these small specification errors, leading to a significant chi-square (i.e., chi-square test is overpowered). Conversely, a small sample size will mask the effect of large specification errors, generating a nonsignificant chi-square and acceptance of a model when it should be rejected.

Second, the probability of committing a Type II error (i.e., accepting a model that should be rejected—accepting the null hypothesis) increases as models are respecified and tested (Kaplan, 1995). However, as demonstrated later in this chapter in the computer examples, respecifying and retesting models is an inherent part of conducting an SEM analysis. Undue inflation of Type II error can be avoided when the SEM analysis is guided by theory, and modifications are selected in model specification that result in the greatest change in model fit (i.e., have the most power). In addition, Chou and Bentler (1995) recommend splitting a dataset in half (when the sample size allows this) and developing a model with one half. The final model can then be retested with the remaining half of the data.

Although power is an important consideration in SEM, evaluating how much power is available in a given SEM analysis is not a simple or straightforward matter. Power is influenced by sample size and misspecification errors (Kaplan, 1995), but misspecification errors are not typically known to the researcher. Different methods of power analysis have been proposed, but a discussion of these and their various shortcomings is beyond the scope of this chapter. Consult Kaplan (1995) and Saris and Satorra (1993) for a discussion of specific methods of power analysis, or MacCallum, Browne, and Sugawara (1996) for a new approach that allows calculation of minimum sample sizes.

CONDUCTING STRUCTURAL EQUATION MODELING

Like path analysis, SEM involves preparation (model specification), analysis (model estimation and testing), and a consideration of the analysis' limitations. Preparation involves drawing a full model (i.e., delineating the measurement model for each latent variable and the hypothesized relationships between these constructs) and fixing parameters to either zero or a nonzero value (e.g., 0.5, 1.0) for identification purposes.

Once the full model has been specified (and the data collected), a computer program (e.g., LISREL, EQS) estimates the parameters and tests the fit of the model to the data. The measurement model is evaluated first, and once the researcher determines that the measurement model fits the data, the theoretical model can be tested.

Fitting the model to the data is rarely accomplished in a single analysis. More often, the computer output suggests that certain parameters are not statistically significant and could be dropped, or additional respecification of the model is needed (i.e., GFI or CFI is less than .90). For example, modification indices (in EQS, the Lagrange multiplier test) may suggest adding parameters to the model. If this makes good theoretical sense, the researcher makes the change, and then the fit of this respecified model is tested. Although it may lead to more model testing, the addition of parameters (i.e., paths to the model) should be made incrementally to observe whether the parameter contributes substantively to the fit of the model (Kaplan & Wenger, 1993).

In the end, the limitations of the SEM analysis help put the results in the proper context. For example, the researcher might consider whether certain assumptions about measurement may have influenced the results in some way. Concern about the validity of the final model can also arise if many models were tested in the process of finding one that fit the data well.

In the remainder of this section, two computer examples of SEM are discussed, and a published example of SEM is summarized and critiqued. The computer examples provide a flavor of the SEM analysis process, and the critique underscores the need to give SEM articles a careful review.

Computer Example 1: Confirmatory Factor Analysis of the Inventory of Personal Attitudes

This example illustrates the use of SEM to evaluate the construct validity of the Inventory of Personal Attitudes. This 30-item instrument measures general attitudes about self, life, and work that may be health promoting. It was designed to have two factors: Life and Confidence. The data are continuous: The response options consist of a seven-point scale. However, responses to some items appear skewed. The sample size is 173. The software we are using is EQS (Bentler, 1992), and the method of estimation is ML.

The measurement model for Inventory of Personal Attitudes is depicted in Figure 16-9. There are two factors (life, confidence) with eight items as indicators for both factors, an additional 11 that are unique to Life, and another 11 that are unique

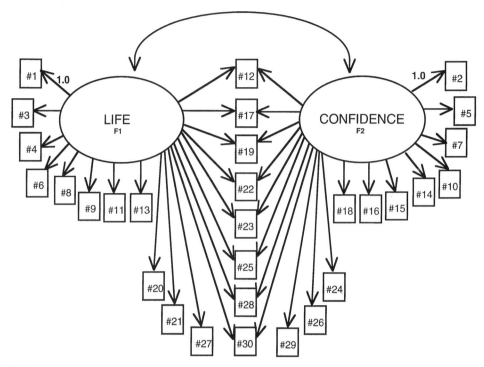

FIGURE 16-9

Measurement model representing the hypothesized factor structure of the Inventory of Personal Attitudes (computer example 1).

to Confidence. Note that each factor has the parameter for one of the unique indicators fixed at 1.0 to allow a measurement scale (i.e., 1–7) to be determined for the factor.

Model fit statistics for the initial model (model specified in Fig. 16-9) are provided in Table 16-2. They indicate that the model does not fit the data very well and needs respecification. The chi-square test is significant, and the CFI (.809) is less than .90. The relative chi-square (1083.163 ÷ 396) is 2.74, which is less than 3.0 and acceptable. Nonetheless, given the other model fit statistics, we turn to the Lagrange multiplier and Wald tests to guide us in respecifying the model.

The probability column listed for the Wald and Lagrange multiplier tests in Table 16-3 represents the significance level for the change in chi-square predicted to result if a specific parameter was dropped or added to the model. F1 refers to the Life factor and F2 refers to the Confidence factor.

For the Wald test, the probability values are all greater than .05. This means that we could drop the parameters listed without significantly worsening the model fit (i.e., increasing the chi-square). For example, the Wald predicts we could drop the parameter V19,F1, which places item 19 on the Life factor (F1) without significantly increasing the chi-square. At this point, we are not so much interested in parsimony

TABLE 16-2
Model Fit Statistics for Computer Example 1

GOODNESS OF FIT SUMMARY

CHI-SQUARE = 1083.163 BASED ON 396 DEGREES OF FREEDOM
PROBABILITY VALUE FOR THE CHI-SQUARE STATISTIC IS LESS THAN 0.001

BENTLER-BONETT NORMED FIT INDEX= 0.731
BENTLER-BONETT NONNORMED FIT INDEX= 0.790
COMPARATIVE FIT INDEX = 0.809

Bentler (1992) recommends the CFI over the other fit indices provided above.

as we are in improving the fit of the model (i.e., obtaining a smaller chi-square), so we move on to the Lagrange multiplier test results.

All of the values in the probability column for the Lagrange multiplier test are less than .05: The Lagrange multiplier test predicts we could significantly improve the model fit by adding certain parameters. It suggests we should add V29,F1 (item

TABLE 16-3
Results of Wald and Lagrange Multiplier Tests
for Initial Model for Computer Example 1

WALD TEST (FOR DROPPING PARAMETERS)
MULTIVARIATE WALD TEST BY SIMULTANEOUS PROCESS

CUMULATIVE MULTIVARIATE STATISTICS

STEP	PARAMETER	CHI-SQUARE	D.F.	PROBABILITY
1	V19,F1	0.195	1	0.659
2	V23,F2	0.604	2	0.739
3	V25,F2	1.180	3	0.758
4	V28,F2	2.074	4	0.722
5	V12,F2	3.887	5	0.566

MULTIVARIATE LAGRANGE MULTIPLIER TEST BY SIMULTANEOUS
PROCESS IN STAGE 1

CUMULATIVE MULTIVARIATE STATISTICS

STEP	PARAMETER	CHI-SQUARE	D.F.	PROBABILITY
1	V29,F1	14.238	1	0.000
2	V16,F1	22.832	2	0.000
3	V8,F2	28.175	3	0.000

29) to the Life factor, V16,F1 (item 16) to the life factor, and V8,F2 (item 8) to the Confidence factor. Our task is to re-examine the instrument to determine whether items 29 and 16 could be indicators for the Life factor in addition to Confidence (the factor for which they are currently indicators) and item 8 could be an indicator for the Confidence factor in addition to Life (the factor for which it is currently an indicator). If so, we should add these parameters and test the re-specified model.

Looking at the instrument, it appears that item 29 (worry about the future) could reflect a life attitude and sense of confidence. The same cannot be said for item 16 (I stand up for myself when I need to) or item 8 (I feel there is a purpose to life). Consequently, we respecify the model with only one change: We make 29 an indicator for both Life and Confidence. We estimate and test this new model but find the model is still a poor fit to the data (CFI = .813; results not shown). The Lagrange multiplier test continues to tell us to add V16,F1 and V8,F1 as it did in the previous analysis, but theoretically this is hard to justify.

We are now at a dead end because adding V29,F1 did not result in a CFI > .90, and additional changes suggested by the Lagrange multiplier test do not make good theoretical sense. We have three options (aside from collecting more data). First, we could test a single factor of the model to see if it fits the data better than a two-factor model.[3] Second, we could drop items with significant skew and kurtosis and rerun the two-factor model; however, this would require dropping one third of the items. Third, we could abandon SEM and use SPSS to do an exploratory factor analysis to see if more than two factors may be present, but problems with non-normality may also threaten the validity of these results.

Let us stop the SEM at this point and consider the limitations of the analysis. Principally, it may not be possible to use SEM to come to any firm conclusions about the construct validity of this inventory. The sample size may not be sufficient to compensate for the non-normality of some of the data. If so, this would make it more difficult to specify a model that fits the data well. Consequently, we are not able to determine whether the model fit statistics reflect problems with the instrument or the need for a larger sample due to problems with non-normality.

Computer Example 2: Testing a Theoretical Model of Condom Use

This example uses SEM to test a theoretical model of condom use for African-American males with a partner that they know well. Specifically, we use SEM to determine which parameters are significant and whether the model as a whole provides a good fit to the data. If additional parameters are added to the model, we need to be able to justify this on theoretical grounds.

The data and model testing results reported here are part of a larger multiple group analysis published by Norris and Ford (1995) in the *Journal of Applied Social Psychology*. The sample size is 203, and the data are cross-sectional. The SEM software is EQS (Bentler, 1992), and the method of estimation is ML. Variables are excluded from the analysis if they have skew or kurtosis > |1.5|.

---

[3]*In fact, I did test this one-factor model, but it did not fit the data any better than the two-factor model. The CFI was .75.*

The theoretical model being tested is depicted in Figure 16-10. This model is an integration of three different health behavior models: Health Belief Model (Janz & Becker, 1984), Theory of Reasoned Action (Fishbein & Ajzen, 1975), and Construct Accessibility Model (Norris & Devine, 1992). The effects of talking about acquired immunodeficiency syndrome (AIDS), age, and alcohol use are also included in response to findings in the literature.

As can be seen in Figure 16-10, the theoretical model contains eight latent variables. Interpersonal consequences, embarrassing, and pleasure are three different types of condom beliefs (i.e., three condom belief factors). Condom predisposition is a new latent variable that combines concepts from the Theory of Reasoned Action (condom attitude, partner norm) and Construct Accessibility Model (state of information in memory). Other latent variables include AIDS communication, AIDS concern (AIDS susceptibility), alcohol use, and condom use. Age is also included; it is demarcated with a square because it has only one indicator and is assumed to be measured without error. This theoretical model is overidentified using criteria described elsewhere (Bollen, 1989; Hayduk, 1987).

The measurement model for the latent variables fits the data well. Separate measurement models were tested for each latent variable: The CFIs for these were > .91, and the relative chi-squares ranged from .20 to 1.80.

Although the model in Figure 16-10 is overidentified on paper, the computer found that the model was statistically underidentified when it estimated and tested

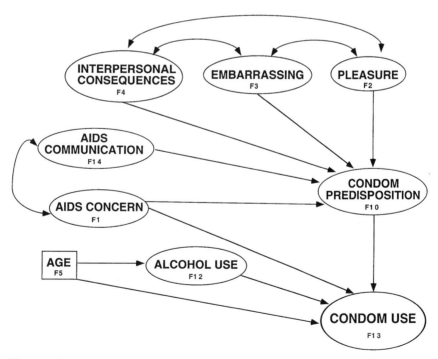

FIGURE 16-10
Initial theoretical model for computer example 2.

TABLE 16-4
Model Fit Statistics for Initial Theoretical Model in Computer Example 2

*** WARNING *** TEST RESULTS MAY NOT BE APPROPRIATE DUE TO CONDITION CODE
PARAMETER   CONDITION CODE
  D10,D10   CONSTRAINED AT LOWER BOUND

GOODNESS OF FIT SUMMARY

CHI-SQUARE =   371.158 BASED ON   242 DEGREES OF FREEDOM
PROBABILITY VALUE FOR THE CHI-SQUARE STATISTIC IS LESS THAN 0.001
THE NORMAL THEORY RLS CHI-SQUARE FOR THIS ML SOLUTION IS   338.987.

BENTLER-BONETT NORMED   FIT INDEX=   0.755
BENTLER-BONETT NONNORMED FIT INDEX=   0.881
COMPARATIVE FIT INDEX   =   0.896

Bentler (1992) recommends the CFI over the other fit indices provided above.

the model. The computer made the model underidentified by constraining the error associated with condom predisposition to be equal to zero. This is indicated by the warning in Table 16-4 that test results may not be appropriate due to condition code and that the parameter D10,D10 (the error term for condom predisposition) is constrained at lower bound.

The computer's constraining of the error term associated with condom predisposition (D10,D10) gives us some direction as to how to respecify the model to improve the likelihood that it can be statistically overidentified. The computer's choice of this particular constraint suggests that there are too many latent variables diagrammed as influencing condom predisposition. How do we know which parameters to drop? The answer is in the Wald test results presented in Table 16-5. Remember, the Wald test predicts whether dropping a particular parameter would significantly worsen the fit of the model. The Wald predicts that four parameters in the model that involve condom predisposition (F10) could be dropped without worsening the fit of the model: F10,F12; F10,F4; F10,F3; and F10,F1. Dropping the paths represented by these four parameters results in the respecified model in Figure 16-11.

We proceed directly to testing the respecified model in Figure 16-11 and ignore results for the Lagrange multiplier test because the constraint imposed by the computer on D10,D10 may affect their validity. The Lagrange multiplier test for this next analysis will tell us whether any of the parameters we have dropped should be added back to the model.

Model fit statistics for this respecified model are provided in Table 16-6. Notice that there is no warning about a condition code: we solved the identification problem. Also, the fit of this new model is acceptable. The model chi-square is significant, but the CFI = .90. The relative chi-square ($375.296 \div 246$) is 1.53. This also argues for the fit of the model because it is less than 3.0.

TABLE 16-5
Results of Wald and Lagrange Multiplier Tests
for Initial Theoretical Model in Computer Example 2

WALD TEST (FOR DROPPING PARAMETERS)
*** WARNING *** TEST RESULTS MAY NOT BE APPROPRIATE DUE TO
CONDITION CODE
MULTIVARIATE WALD TEST BY SIMULTANEOUS PROCESS

CUMULATIVE MULTIVARIATE STATISTICS

STEP	PARAMETER	CHI-SQUARE	D.F.	PROBABILITY
1	F13,F5	0.036	1	0.850
2	F10,F12	0.172	2	0.918
3	F10,F4	0.382	3	0.944
4	F10,F3	0.658	4	0.956
5	D13,D13	1.449	5	0.919
6	F13,F12	2.871	6	0.825
7	F13,F1	4.861	7	0.677
8	F10,F1	7.712	8	0.462

MULTIVARIATE LAGRANGE MULTIPLIER TEST BY SIMULTANEOUS
PROCESS IN STAGE 1

CUMULATIVE MULTIVARIATE STATISTICS

STEP	PARAMETER	CHI-SQUARE	D.F.	PROBABILITY
1	V11,F13	14.847	1	0.000
2	V22,F1	28.271	2	0.000
3	V23,F13	36.500	3	0.000
4	V34,F5	43.684	4	0.000
5	V7,F4	50,027	5	0.000
6	V30,F12	55.977	6	0.000
7	V26,F13	60.882	7	0.000
8	V13,F5	65.656	8	0.000
9	V9,F13	70.214	9	0.000
10	V8,F12	74.643	10	0.000
11	F14,F4	79.050	11	0.000
12	V9,F5	83.102	12	0.000
13	V1,F3	86.974	13	0.000

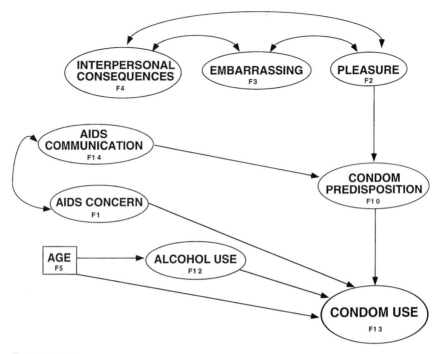

FIGURE 16-11
First respecified model for computer example 2.

TABLE 16-6
*Model Fit Statistics for First Respecified Theoretical Model
in Computer Example 2*

GOODNESS OF FIT SUMMARY

INDEPENDENCE MODEL CHI-SQUARE =   1517.312 ON   276 DEGREES OF FREEDOM

INDEPENDENCE AIC =   965.31161   INDEPENDENCE CAIC =   −200.99448
         MODEL AIC =   −116.70398   MODEL CAIC =   −1156.23766

CHI-SQUARE =   375.296 BASED ON   246 DEGREES OF FREEDOM
PROBABILITY VALUE FOR THE CHI-SQUARE STATISTIC IS LESS THAN 0.001
THE NORMAL THEORY RLS CHI-SQUARE FOR THIS ML SOLUTION IS   342.759.

BENTLER-BONETT NORMED   FIT INDEX=   0.753
BENTLER-BONETT NONNORMED FIT INDEX=   0.883
COMPARATIVE FIT INDEX   =   0.896

Bentler (1992) recommends the CFI over the other fit indices provided above.

TABLE 16-7
Results of Wald and Lagrange Multiplier Tests
for First Respecified Model in Computer Example 2

WALD TEST (FOR DROPPING PARAMETERS)
MULTIVARIATE WALD TEST BY SIMULTANEOUS PROCESS

CUMULATIVE MULTIVARIATE STATISTICS

STEP	PARAMETER	CHI-SQUARE	D.F.	PROBABILITY
1	F13,F5	0.040	1	0.841
2	D13,D13	0.790	2	0.674
3	F13,F12	2.141	3	0.544
4	F13,F1	4.599	4	0.331

MULTIVARIATE LAGRANGE MULTIPLIER TEST BY SIMULTANEOUS
PROCESS IN STAGE 1

CUMULATIVE MULTIVARIATE STATISTICS

STEP	PARAMETER	CHI-SQUARE	D.F.	PROBABILITY
1	V11,F13	12.514	1	0.000
2	V23,F13	23.205	2	0.000
3	V22,F14	32.068	3	0.000
4	V7,F4	39.285	4	0.000
5	V34,F5	46.470	5	0.000
6	V29,F12	52.430	6	0.000
7	V26,F13	58.037	7	0.000
8	V9,F13	62.870	8	0.000
9	V1,F10	67.682	9	0.000
10	V13,F5	72.444	10	0.000
11	V9,F5	76.782	11	0.000
12	V8,F12	80.774	12	0.000

Given acceptable model fit statistics, we want to know if all the paths in this re-specified theoretical model are necessary. Would dropping any of the parameters representing these paths significantly affect the fit of the model? The Wald test results in Table 16-7 indicate that three parameters could be dropped: F13,F5; F13,F12; and F13,F1. These represent the paths from age (F5), alcohol use (F12), and AIDS concern (F1) to condom use (F13). Dropping them results in a second respecified model depicted in Figure 16-12.

Now we turn to the Lagrange multiplier test results in Table 16-7 to determine whether any parameters should be added to the model. None of the parameters listed for this test involve two latent variables (i.e., there are no pairs of F's). This sup-

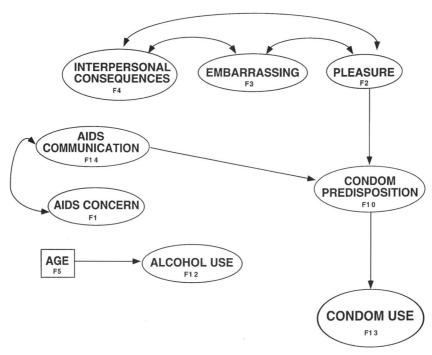

FIGURE 16-12
Second respecified model for computer example 2.

ports our earlier decision to drop the four parameters representing the influence of alcohol use, interpersonal consequences, embarrassing, and AIDS concern on condom use. The pattern of findings from this model testing and estimation argue for assuming these variables have no influence (i.e., these parameters are equal to zero).

The only parameters listed in the Lagrange multiplier test in Table 16-7 are measurement model parameters (e.g., V11, F13). These parameters are ignored because adding them cannot be justified on theoretical grounds. Moreover, the measurement model has already been determined to fit the data well and is not the focus of analysis at this point.

As can be seen in Table 16-8, the fit statistics for the second respecified model (see Fig. 16-12) differ little from those for the first respecified model in Table 16-6. We have simplified our model without sacrificing model fit. In Table 16-9, the Wald test does not suggest dropping any additional paths between the latent variables, and the Lagrange multiplier test does not suggest adding any such paths. Together with the model fit statistics, these two tests argue against any further respecification of the model. Additionally, the Lagrange multiplier test results in the context of these model fit statistics support assuming that the paths from age, alcohol use, and AIDS concern to condom use are equal to zero.

The SEM test of the theoretical model is concluded at this point. We now consider two limitations of the analysis. First, due to sample size constraints, we did not randomly split the dataset in half, develop our model with one half, and then retest

TABLE 16-8
Model Fit Statistics for Second Respecified Theoretical Model in Computer Example 2

GOODNESS OF FIT SUMMARY

INDEPENDENCE MODEL CHI-SQUARE =   1517.312 ON   276 DEGREES OF FREEDOM

INDEPENDENCE AIC =   965.31161   INDEPENDENCE CAIC =   −200.99448
           MODEL AIC = −118.75645   MODEL CAIC = −1170.96737

CHI-SQUARE =   379.244 BASED ON   249 DEGREES OF FREEDOM
PROBABILITY VALUE FOR THE CHI-SQUARE STATISTIC IS LESS THAN 0.001
THE NORMAL THEORY RLS CHI-SQUARE FOR THIS ML SOLUTION IS   349.732.

BENTLER-BONETT NORMED   FIT INDEX=   0.750
BENTLER-BONETT NONNORMED FIT INDEX=   0.884
COMPARATIVE FIT INDEX   =   0.895

Bentler (1992) recommends the CFI over the other fit indices provided above.

it with the remaining half of the data. Thus, it is possible that our findings could re-sult from a Type II error. However, only three models were specified and tested. This limited number argues against our findings being the result of a Type II error. Sec-ond and more serious, the data are cross-sectional, but our model implies causal re-lationships (e.g., talking about AIDS makes people more predisposed to use con-doms). These theoretical relationships need to be validated with longitudinal data.

Summary and Critique of Published SEM Analysis: Predicting Fat in Diets of Marital Partners

Schafer, Keith, and Schafer (1995) used SEM to explain fat consumption by marital partners using the Health Belief Model (Janz & Becker, 1984). The dependent vari-able was percentage of calories from fat (PCF) consumed. Latent variables in the model included threat (susceptibility to the consequences of high-fat diet), cost (neg-ative aspects or personal consequences of changing diet), benefits (benefits of re-ducing fat intake), and self-efficacy (perceived ability to execute successfully be-haviors needed to reduce fat intake). Age and education were also included in the analysis. Each has only one indicator and is assumed to be measured without error.

The sample size was 155 married couples. The data were analyzed with LISREL, and models were run separately for husbands and wives. The method of estimation is ML. The authors do not provide information about the fit of the measurement mod-els in each group.

The theoretical models that resulted from the SEM are depicted in Figures 16-13 and 16-14. The model fits the data better for the husbands (GFI = .91) than for the wives (GFI = .84). The significance of the chi-square tests for each model (husbands, $\chi^2 = 93.8$; wives, $\chi^2 = 151.9$) is not reported. However, given the degrees of free-

TABLE 16-9
Results of Wald and Lagrange Multiplier Tests for Second Respecified Model in Computer Example 2

WALD TEST (FOR DROPPING PARAMETERS)
MULTIVARIATE WALD TEST BY SIMULTANEOUS PROCESS

CUMULATIVE MULTIVARIATE STATISTICS

STEP	PARAMETER	CHI-SQUARE	D.F.	PROBABILITY
1	D13,D13	1.365	1	0.243

MULTIVARIATE LAGRANGE MULTIPLIER TEST BY SIMULTANEOUS
PROCESS IN STAGE 1

CUMULATIVE MULTIVARIATE STATISTICS

STEP	PARAMETER	CHI-SQUARE	D.F.	PROBABILITY
1	V11,F13	12.213	1	0.000
2	V22,F14	23.845	2	0.000
3	V23,F13	32.416	3	0.000
4	V7,F4	39.514	4	0.000
5	V34,F5	46.056	5	0.000
6	V30,F12	52.014	6	0.000
7	V1,F13	57.443	7	0.000
8	V13,F5	62.278	8	0.000
9	V9,F12	66.804	9	0.000
10	V9,F13	71.246	10	0.000
11	V3,F12	75.267	11	0.000

dom (32), we can look up the significance level in a distribution of χ^2 probability table. The significance levels in this table indicate that both model chi-squares are significant ($p < .001$).

The relative chi-square is not reported but is easily calculated by dividing the chi-square by its degrees of freedom (Table 16-10). Doing this, we determine that the relative chi-square for the husband model is 2.93 and 4.75 for the wife model. These fit statistics and the presence of small, nonsignificant parameters argue for respecifying and retesting both models but especially the wife model because it seems to have the poorest fit.

Some interesting gender differences suggest that different theoretical models may be appropriate for each group. For example, note that parameters are significant in the husband model but not the wife model for the path between threat and percent of calories from fat and self-efficacy and percent of calories from fat. Perhaps the model for the wives would have fit the data better if these nonsignificant paths were dropped from the model.

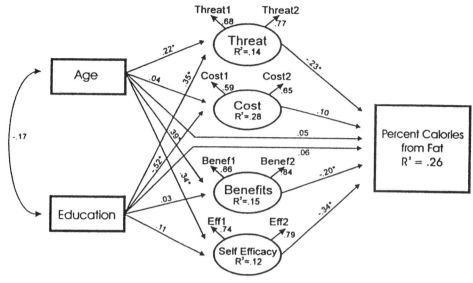

FIGURE 16-13
Path model from Schaefer et al. (1995) for effects of components of the Health Belief Model for percentage of calories from fat. Husbands; $N = 155$. $\chi^2 = 93.8$; GFI = .91. *Significant at the .05 level.

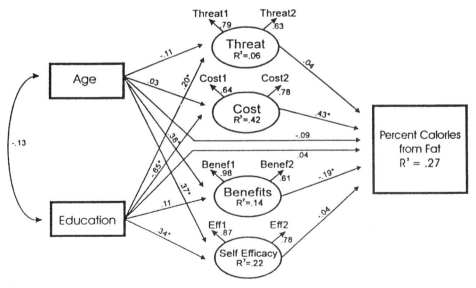

FIGURE 16-14
Path model from Schafer et al. (1995) for effects of components of the Health Belief Model for percentage calories from fat. Wives; $N = 155$. $\chi^2 = 151.9$; GFI = .84. *Significant at the .05 level.

TABLE 16-10
Calculation of Relative Chi-Squares for Summary and Critique
of Schafer et al. (1995)

	Model Chi-Square	*÷ Degrees of Freedom*	*= Relative Chi-Square*
Husband model	93.8	÷ 32	= 2.93
Wife model	151.9	÷ 32	= 4.75

It is unclear why the authors did not perform a multiple group analysis to determine if the measurement models in the two groups were equivalent and if there were statistically significant differences between the two models. It is difficult to determine whether the observed gender differences are meaningful without this additional analysis. It is possible that the gender differences are an artifact of differences in the measurement model. For example, husbands and wives may perceive the cost associated with decreasing fat intake very differently.

It is also unclear why the authors did not respecify and retest their model in each group. For example, the parameters between age and education and percent of calories from fat are nonsignificant and small (−.09–.06) in both groups. This suggests that the effects of age and education on the dependent variable are primarily indirect through their effect on the Health Belief Model variables. The authors could have tested this by respecifying the model with age and education as having only indirect effects and then using a nested chi-square test to see if this new model fit the data better.

In sum, when we consider the limitations of this SEM analysis, we conclude that the authors did not analyze their data sufficiently. As a result, while their data are interesting, it is difficult to make firm conclusions about their findings.

SUMMARY

SEM is a valuable data analytic tool in many respects. For example, SEM affords us greater precision in testing theories and in evaluating construct validity. However, SEM is still just a tool. SEM in and of itself cannot be used to imply causation or ensure construct validity. The use of theory to guide the analysis is essential, but the validity of the result is also influenced by the data and how SEM is used. A beautiful theory can be contradicted by the data, such as when the CFI or GFI is less than .90. Alternatively, the theory can be unnecessarily distorted as a result of Type II error when too many models are run, or problematic data can make the use of SEM unfeasible.

APPLICATION EXERCISES AND RESULTS

There are no computer exercises for this chapter.

Glossary

a: Intercept constant. The point at which the regression line intercepts the Y axis.

Adjusted group means: Group mean scores that have been adjusted for the effect of the covariate on the dependent variable.

Adjusted R^2: R squared adjusted for the number of subjects and variables.

Alpha: The probability of making a type I error.

Analysis of covariance (ANCOVA): A combination of regression and analysis of variance techniques that allows comparison of group means after adjustment for the effect of the covariate.

Analysis of variance (ANOVA): A parametric statistical test that compares between- and within-group variance to measure differences between two or more groups.

A priori contrasts: Planned comparisons based on orthogonal hypotheses.

b: Regression coefficient. In linear regression, it is the rate of change in Y with a one-unit change in X, and it is used to calculate predicted scores. In logistic regression, it is used to calculate probabilities.

Bar graphs: A graph used for nominal or ordinal data. A space separates the bars.

Bartlett's test: A chi-square statistic used to test the significance of lambda.

Beta coefficients: In a regression equation, the weight associated with standardized scores on the variables; a partial correlation coefficient.

Between-group variance: A measure of the deviation of group means from the grand mean.

Biserial correlation: A technique used when one variable is dichotomized and the other is continuous to estimate what the correlation between the two variables would be if the dichotomized variable were continuous.

Blinding: Keeping subjects and observers unaware of treatment assignments.

Box plots: A graphic display that uses descriptive statistics based on percentiles.

Box's M: A measure of the multivariate test for homogeneity of variance. It is very sensitive to departures from normality.

Box's test of equality of covariance matrices: A test of the assumption that the variance–covariance matrices are equal across all levels of the between-subjects factor in a repeated measures analysis of variance.

Canonical coefficient: Equivalent to a *b*-weight in regression; can be used to calculate predicted scores based on actual scores.

Canonical correlation: A measure of the relationship between a set of independent variables and a set of dependent variables.

Canonical variate: A weighted composite of the variables in a set.

Canonical weights: Standard score weights generated in a canonical correlation; like betas in regression; used more for explanation than prediction.

Centroid: The mean of the discriminant scores for a given group.

Chi-square: A statistical test used with categorical (nominal) data. It compares the actual number in each group with the expected number.

Coefficient of determination: The correlation coefficient squared (r^2); a measure of the variance shared by the two variables; a measure of the "meaningfulness" of the relationship.

Common factor analysis: Based on the assumption that there is systematic and random error in measurement. Analysis is based on common variance only.

Compound symmetry: An assumption underlying the repeated measures analysis of variance. The correlations and variances across the measurements are equivalent.

Confidence interval: A range within which the population parameter is estimated to fall based on the statistic and the standard error.

Contingency coefficient: A nonparametric technique to measure the relationship between two nominal-level variables.

Continuity correction (Yates correction): Used in chi-square analysis when the expected frequency in cells in 2 × 2 tables is less than 5.

Continuous variable: Any measure that can assume 11 or more dichotomous levels. With multicategory items, somewhat fewer categories are needed to qualify (Nunnally & Bernstein, 1994, p. 570).

Correlated *t* test (paired *t* test): A parametric test to compare two pairs of scores.

Correlation coefficient: The mathematical relationship between two variables. Values range from −1 to +1.

Correlation matrix: A square symmetric matrix containing correlations between pairs of variables.

Covariate: A continuous variable used to adjust the mean scores of groups. A method for control of extraneous variation.

Cramer's V: Modified phi, used to assess relationship between categorical variables; used with tables larger than 2 × 2.

Cronbach's alpha: A measure of internal consistency reliability.

Cross-validation: Checking the validity of R^2 by calculating it in a second sample.

Communality: The portion of item variance accounted for by the factors.

Degrees of freedom: The freedom of a score's value to vary given what is known about the other scores and the sum of the scores.

Dependent variable: The response or outcome measure.

Deviance: In logistic regression, the comparison between the predicted probability of being in the correct group based on the model to the perfect prediction. Large values indicate poor model fit.

Deviation coding (effect coding): A method of coding nominal-level variables using 1's, −1's, and 0's; reflects the comparison of each group mean with the grand mean.

Discriminant function analysis: A statistical technique that provides a prediction of group membership based on predictor variables.

Discriminant function: The mathematical function that combines information from predictor variables to obtain the maximum discrimination among groups.

Dummy coding (indicator coding): A method of coding nominal-level variables using 1's and 0's; reflects a comparison of the control group mean with other group means.

Effect coding (deviation coding): A method of coding nominal-level variables using 1's, −1's, and 0's; reflects the comparison of each group mean with the grand mean.

Effect size: The impact made by the independent variable on the dependent variable.

Eigenvalue: The amount of variance explained by a factor or discriminant function.

Endogenous variables: Variables that are influenced by other variables in a model.

Epsilon: A correction used in repeated measures analysis of variance when the assumption of compound symmetry has not been met. Epsilon is multiplied by the degrees of freedom, making them smaller, and thus making the test more conservative.

Equamax rotation: Combines the characteristics of Quartimax and Varimax rotation.

Eta: Sometimes called the correlation ratio. It can be used to measure a nonlinear relationship. The range of values is from 0 to 1.

Exogenous variables: Variables that are not influenced by other variables in a model.

Exp(B): The exponent of b or the odds ratio.

F: A measure of the ratio of between to within variance produced by analysis of variance.

Factor: A group of items that "belong" together.

Factor analysis: A statistical tool for analyzing scores on large numbers of variables to determine if any identifiable dimensions can be used to describe many of the variables under study. Intercorrelations are treated mathematically in such a way that underlying traits are identified.

Factor loadings: Correlations of variables with a factor.

Factor matrix: Each row represents one variable; each column represents a factor.

Factor pattern matrix: A matrix produced by oblique rotation in factor analysis. It contains regression weights. It is generally preferable to the structure matrix for interpretation.

Factor scores: Actual scores weighted by factor loadings.

Factor structure matrix: A matrix produced by oblique rotation in factor analysis. It contains correlation coefficients.

Fisher's exact test: An alternative to chi-square for 2×2 tables when sample size and expected frequencies are small.

Fisher's Z_r: Transformation of correlation coefficients into Fisher's Z to create a normal distribution.

Friedman matched samples: A nonparametric analogue of repeated measures analysis of variance.

Goodness of fit statistic: A measure of how well the data fit the model; compares the observed probabilities to those predicted by the model.

Graphs: The visual representations of frequency distributions.

Greenhouse-Geisser: A conservative epsilon value used to alter the degrees of freedom in repeated measures analysis of variance when the assumption of compound symmetry has not been met.

Hierarchical regression: The researcher determines the order of entry of the variables into the equation. Variables may be entered one at a time or in subsets.

Histogram: The appropriate graph for interval and ratio data. There is no space between the bars.

Homogeneity of regression: The direction and strength of the relationship between the covariate and the dependent variable must be similar in each group.

Homogeneity of variance: The variances of the dependent variable do not differ significantly between the groups.

Homoscedasticity: An assumption underlying correlation and regression. For every value of X, the distribution of Y scores must have approximately equal variability.

Hotelling-Lawley trace: The sum of the ratio of the between and within sum of squares for each of the discriminant variables.

Huynh-Feldt: A value for the epsilon correction factor in repeated measures analysis of variance that is less conservative than Greenhouse-Geisser.

Hypothesis: Formal statement of the expected relationships between variables or differences between groups.

Improvement: In logistic regression, the change in $-2LL$ between successive steps of building a model.

Independent variable: The variable that is seen as having an effect on the dependent variable. In experimental designs, the treatment is manipulated.

Indicator: A measured variable in structural equation models; may also be called a manifest variable.

Indicator coding (dummy coding): A method of coding nominal-level variables using 1's and 0's. Reflects a comparison of the control group mean with other group means.

Intercept constant (a): The point at which the regression line intercepts the Y axis.

Interquartile range: The range of values extending from the 25th to the 50th percentile.

Interval-level measurement: A rank order scale in which the distances between the values are equivalent.

Just identified model: All variables in the model are interconnected with each other by a path.

Kendall's Tau: A nonparametric measure of relationship between two ordinal variables.

Kruskal-Wallis H: Nonparametric analogue of analysis of variance; used to compare groups on an outcome measure.

Kurtosis: A measure of whether the curve is normal, flat, or peaked.

Lambda: Wilks' lambda varies from 0 to 1 and represents the error variance. $1 -$ lambda $= R^2$.

Latency effect: Interaction between treatments in repeated measures designs.

Latent variable: A theoretical construct in structural equation models that is not directly measured but represented by measured variables.

Least significant difference test: A post-hoc test that is a modified version of multiple t tests.

Levene's test of equality of error variances: A test of the assumption that the group means have equal variances.

Likelihood: The probability of the observed results given the parameter estimates.

Logistic regression: A technique designed to determine which variables affect the probability of an event.

Lower-bound epsilon: The most conservative approach to "correcting" the degrees of freedom in repeated measures analysis of variance when the assumption of compound symmetry has not been met.

Mann-Whitney U: A nonparametric statistical test to compare two groups. It is analogous to the t test.

Mauchly's test of sphericity: A test of the assumption of compound symmetry in repeated measures analysis of variance.

McNemar: A nonparametric measure of difference between two paired dichotomous measures; used to measure change.

Mean: Arithmetic average.

Measurement: The assignment of numerals to objects or events, according to a set of rules (Stevens, 1946).

Median: The middle value or subject in a set of ordered numbers.

Mixed design: A study that includes between- and within-group factors.

Mode: The most frequently occurring number or category.

Model chi-square: In logistic regression, the difference between minus 2 log likelihood $(-2LL)$ for the model with only a constant and $-2LL$ for the complete model; tests the null hypothesis that the coefficients for all the independent variables equal zero.

Multicollinearity: Interrelatedness of independent variables.

Multiple correlation: The relationship between one dependent variable and a weighted composite of independent variables.

Multiple group comparisons: The two most common are a priori (before the fact) and post-hoc (after the fact) comparisons of group means.

Multivariate analysis of variance: An analysis of variance with more than one dependent variable.

Mutually exclusive: An object or subject is in one, and only one, group in the design.

Nominal: The lowest level of measurement; consists of organizing data into discrete units.

Nonparametric statistics: "Distribution-free" techniques that are not based on assumptions about normality of data.

Nonrecursive model: A model in which causal flow is not unidirectional.

Normal curve: A theoretically perfect frequency polygon in which the mean, median, and mode all coincide in the center, and which takes the form of a symmetrical bell-shaped curve.

Null hypothesis: Proposes that there is no difference between groups or no relationship between variables.

Oblique rotation: The resulting factors are correlated with each other.

Odds ratio: The probability of occurrence over the probability of nonoccurrence.

One-way analysis of variance: Analysis of variance with one factor (independent variable).

One-tailed test of significance: A test used with a directional hypothesis that proposes extreme values are in one tail of the distribution.

Ordinal-level measurement: The rank ordering of data points.

Orthogonal: Independent of each other.

Orthogonal coding: A method of coding orthogonal contrasts between groups. A priori contrasts can be tested through this method of coding.

Orthogonal rotation (Varimax): The resulting factors are not correlated with each other.

Outliers: Values that are extreme relative to the bulk of the distribution.

Overidentified model: A model that contains at least one less path than a just identified model.

Paired *t* test: A parametric test to compare two pairs of scores.

Parameters: Characteristics of the population.

Parametric tests: Statistical tests based on assumptions that the sample is representative of the population and that the scores are normally distributed.

Partial correlation: A measure of the relationship between two variables after statistically controlling for the influence of some other variable(s) on both of the variables being correlated.

Path analysis: A causal model analytic technique using least squares regression.

Path coefficients: The magnitude of the influence of one variable on another in the path model.

Path model: A causal model.

Pearson product moment correlation: A formula used to calculate the correlation between two variables.

Percentile: Describes the relative position of a score.

Phi: A shortcut method of calculating Pearson's correlation coefficient when both variables are dichotomous.

Pillai-Bartlett trace: Represents the sum of the explained variances.

Polygon: A graph for interval or ratio-level variables that is the equivalent of the histogram but appears smoother. It is constructed by joining the midpoints of the top of each bar.

Point-Biserial coefficient: A short-cut method of calculating r when there is one dichotomous and one continuous variable.

Population: All members in a defined group.

Post-hoc tests: Tests of paired comparisons made when the overall test is significant.

Power: The likelihood of rejecting the null hypothesis.

Principal components analysis: A type of analysis that is based on the assumption that all measurement error is random and includes 1's in the diagonal of the correlation matrix that is analyzed.

Quartiles: The first quartile is the 25th percentile, the second is the 50th percentile, the third is the 75th percentile, and the fourth is the 100th percentile.

Quartimax rotation: A method of rotation in factor analysis that tends to produce a first, very general, factor with high loadings.

R: Multiple correlation.

R²: Squared multiple correlation; the amount of variance accounted for in the dependent variable by a combination of independent variables.

R statistic: In logistic regression, represents the partial correlation.

Randomization: Assignment of individuals to groups by chance (i.e., every subject has an equal chance of being assigned to a particular group).

Range: The difference between the maximum and minimum values in a distribution.

Ratio-level measurement: The highest level of measurement. In addition to equal intervals between data points, there is an absolute zero.

Raw data matrix: A matrix containing raw scores for each subject on each variable. The rows represent subjects, and the columns represent variables.

Recursive model: The flow of causation in the model is unidirectional.

Redundancy: In canonical correlation, it is the percent of variance the canonical variates from the independent variables extract from the dependent variables and vice versa.

Regression: A statistical method that makes use of the correlation between two variables and the notion of a straight line to develop a prediction equation.

Regression coefficient (b): The rate of change in Y with a one-unit change in X.

Regression line: The line of best fit formed by the mathematical technique called the method of least squares.

Regression sum of squares: The variance that is accounted for by the variables in the equation.

Relative risk: The risk given one condition versus the risk given another condition.

Repeated measures analysis of variance: A method of analyzing within-cell designs in which subjects are measured more than once on the same variable or where subjects are exposed to all treatments, thus serving as their own controls.

Research problems: Questions that can be answered by collecting facts.

Residual: The difference between the actual and predicted scores; the variance that is not shared by the variables in the correlation; the unexplained or error variance.

Risk: The number of occurrences out of the total.

Roy's greatest characteristic root: An outcome statistic generated by multivariate analysis of variance and based on the first discriminate variate.

Scatter diagram: A graph of pairs of scores for subjects.

Scheffé test: A conservative post-hoc test; may be used with groups of equal or unequal size.

Scree test: A plot of eigenvalues.

Semipartial correlation: The correlation between two variables with the effect of another variable(s) removed from one of the variables being correlated.

Shrinkage formula: An equation that provides an estimate of how much the multiple correlation coefficient is likely to shrink.

Simple structure: A criterion for factor rotation that seeks to maximize high and low loadings to reduce ambiguity.

Skewness: A measure of the shape of an asymmetrical distribution.

Spearman Rho: A shortcut formula for r when you have two sets of ranks.

Standard deviation: A measure of dispersion of scores around the mean. It is the square root of the variance.

Standard scores: z-scores; represent the deviation of scores around the mean in a distribution with a mean of zero and a standard deviation of 1.

Standard regression: All the independent variables are entered together.

Standardized canonical correlations: Similar to beta weights in regression. They are based on the standard scores of the variables and indicate the relative importance of each variable.

Statistics: The field of study that is concerned with obtaining, describing, and interpreting data; the characteristics of samples.

Structural equation modeling: A method of testing theoretical models that analyzes covariances. It tests a measurement model and a theoretical model made up of measured and latent variables.

Tables: When data are organized into values or categories and then described with titles and captions, the result is a statistical table.

Tetrachoric: A coefficient that estimates r from the relationship between two dichotomized variables.

Theoretical model: A model of the hypothesized relationships between latent variables.

Tolerance: A measure of collinearity. The proportion of the variance in a variable that is not accounted for by the other independent variables $(1-R^2)$.

_t_ test: A parametric statistical test for comparing the means of two independent groups.

Tukey's honestly significant difference (HSD): The most conservative post-hoc test.

Tukey's wholly significant difference: A post-hoc test that is intermediate in conservatism between Newman-Keuls and Tukey's HSD.

Two-tailed test of significance: A test used with a nondirectional hypothesis, in which extreme values are assumed to occur in either tail of the distribution.

Type I error: Concluding that a significant difference or relationship exists when it does not.

Type II error: Concluding that there is no significant difference or relationship when there is.

Underidentified model: A nonrecursive model. It contains paths that are not unidirectional.

Valid percent: The percentage with missing data excluded.

Variable: A measured characteristic that can take on different values.

Variance: A measure of the dispersion of scores around the mean. It is equal to the standard deviation squared.

Variance inflation factor: The reciprocal of tolerance.

Varimax rotation: Orthogonal rotation resulting in factors that are not correlated with each other.

Wald statistic: A value tested for significance in logistic regression.

Wilcoxon matched-pairs signed rank test: A nonparametric technique analgous to the paired _t_ test. Used to compare paired measures.

Wilks' lambda: Represents the unexplained or error variance.

Within-groups variance: Variation of scores within the respective groups; represents the error term in analysis of variance.

Within-sample independence: Observations within the sample are independent of each other.

Within-subjects designs: Subjects serve as their own controls. Subjects are measured more than once on the same variable, or subjects are exposed to more than one treatment.

Y': The predicted score in a regression equation.

Zero-order correlation: The measured relationship between two variables.

z-scores: Standardized scores calculated by subtracting the mean from an individual score and dividing the result by the standard deviation; represents the deviation from the mean in a normal distribution.

Stepwise regression: Variables are entered into the equation based on their measured relationship to the dependent variable. Methods include forward entry, backward removal, and a combination of forward and backward called stepwise.

Structure coefficients: The correlations between the dependent and canonical variates. They are generally used for interpretation of results. Values of .30 or greater are considered meaningful.

Student Newman-Keuls: A post-hoc test that is similar to Tukey's HSD, but the critical values do not remain constant.

Sum of squares: The sum of the squared deviations of each of the scores around a respective mean.

Appendices

Percent of Total Area of Normal Curve Between a z-Score and the Mean

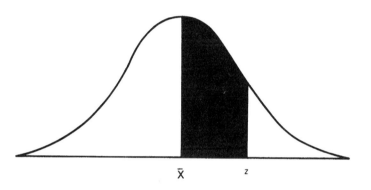

z	0.00	0.01	0.02	0.03	0.04	0.05	0.06	0.07	0.08	0.09
0.0	00.00	00.40	00.80	01.20	01.60	01.99	02.39	02.79	03.19	03.59
0.1	03.98	04.38	04.78	05.17	05.57	05.96	06.36	06.75	07.14	07.53
0.2	07.93	08.32	08.71	09.10	09.48	09.87	10.26	10.64	11.03	11.41
0.3	11.79	12.17	12.55	12.93	13.31	13.68	14.06	14.43	14.80	15.17
0.4	15.54	15.91	16.28	16.64	17.00	17.36	17.72	18.08	18.44	18.79
0.5	19.15	19.50	19.85	20.19	20.54	20.88	21.23	21.57	21.90	22.24
0.6	22.57	22.91	23.24	23.57	23.89	24.22	24.54	24.86	25.17	25.49
0.7	25.80	26.11	26.42	26.73	27.04	27.34	27.64	27.94	28.23	28.52
0.8	28.81	29.10	29.39	29.67	29.95	30.23	30.51	30.78	31.06	31.33
0.9	31.59	31.86	32.12	32.38	32.64	32.90	33.15	33.40	33.65	33.89
1.0	34.13	34.38	34.61	34.85	35.08	35.31	35.54	35.77	35.99	36.21
1.1	36.43	36.65	36.86	37.08	37.29	37.49	37.70	37.90	38.10	38.30
1.2	38.49	38.69	38.88	39.07	39.25	39.44	39.62	39.80	39.97	40.15
1.3	40.32	40.49	40.66	40.82	40.99	41.15	41.31	41.47	41.62	41.77

(continued)

Appendix A (CONTINUED)

z	0.00	0.01	0.02	0.03	0.04	0.05	0.06	0.07	0.08	0.09
1.4	41.92	42.07	42.22	42.36	42.51	42.65	42.79	42.92	43.06	43.19
1.5	43.32	43.45	43.57	43.70	43.83	43.94	44.06	44.18	44.29	44.41
1.6	44.52	44.63	44.74	44.84	44.95	45.05	45.15	45.25	45.35	45.45
1.7	45.54	45.64	45.73	45.82	45.91	45.99	46.08	46.16	46.25	46.33
1.8	46.41	46.49	46.56	46.64	46.71	46.78	46.86	46.93	46.99	47.06
1.9	47.13	47.19	47.26	47.32	47.38	47.44	47.50	47.56	47.61	47.67
2.0	47.72	47.78	47.83	47.88	47.93	47.98	48.03	48.08	48.12	48.17
2.1	48.21	48.26	48.30	48.34	48.38	48.42	48.46	48.50	48.54	48.57
2.2	48.61	48.64	48.68	48.71	48.75	48.78	48.81	48.84	48.87	48.90
2.3	48.93	48.96	48.98	49.01	49.04	49.06	49.09	49.11	49.13	49.16
2.4	49.18	49.20	49.22	49.25	49.27	49.29	49.31	49.32	49.34	49.36
2.5	49.38	49.40	49.41	49.43	49.45	49.46	49.48	49.49	49.51	49.52
2.6	49.53	49.55	49.56	49.57	49.59	49.60	49.61	49.62	49.63	49.64
2.7	49.65	49.66	49.67	49.68	49.69	49.70	49.71	49.72	49.73	49.74
2.8	49.74	49.75	49.76	49.77	49.77	49.78	49.79	49.79	49.80	49.81
2.9	49.81	49.82	49.82	49.83	49.84	49.84	49.85	49.85	49.86	49.86
3.0	49.87									
3.5	49.98									
4.0	49.997									
5.0	49.99997									

(From Hald, A. [1952]. Statistical tables and formulas. *New York: John Wiley & Sons. [Table 1].)*

Distribution of χ² Probability

df	0.20	0.10	0.05	0.02	0.01	0.001
1	1.642	2.706	3.841	5.412	6.635	10.827
2	3.219	4.605	5.991	7.842	9.210	13.815
3	4.642	6.251	7.815	9.837	11.345	16.266
4	5.989	7.779	9.488	11.668	13.277	18.467
5	7.289	9.236	11.070	13.388	15.086	20.515
6	8.558	10.645	12.592	15.033	16.812	22.457
7	9.803	12.017	14.067	16.622	18.475	24.322
8	11.030	13.362	15.507	18.168	20.090	26.125
9	12.242	14.684	16.919	19.679	21.666	27.877
10	13.442	15.987	18.307	21.161	23.209	29.588
11	14.631	17.275	19.675	22.618	24.725	31.264
12	15.812	18.549	21.026	24.054	26.217	32.909
13	16.985	19.812	22.362	25.472	27.688	34.528
14	18.151	21.064	23.685	26.873	29.141	36.123
15	19.311	22.307	24.996	28.259	30.578	37.697
16	20.465	23.542	26.296	29.633	32.000	39.252
17	21.615	24.769	27.587	30.995	33.409	40.790
18	22.760	25.989	28.869	32.346	34.805	42.312
19	23.900	27.204	30.144	33.687	36.191	43.820
20	25.038	28.412	31.410	35.020	37.566	45.315
21	26.171	29.615	32.671	36.343	38.932	46.797
22	27.301	30.813	33.924	37.659	40.289	48.268
23	28.429	32.007	35.172	38.968	41.638	49.728
24	29.553	33.196	36.415	40.270	42.980	51.179
25	30.675	34.382	37.652	41.566	44.314	52.620
26	31.795	35.563	38.885	42.856	45.642	54.052
27	32.912	36.741	40.113	44.140	46.963	55.476

(*continued*)

Appendix B (CONTINUED)

z	0.00	0.01	0.02	0.03	0.04	0.05	0.06	0.07	0.08	0.09
28	34.027		37.916		41.337	45.419		48.278		56.893
29	35.139		39.087		42.557	46.693		49.588		58.302
30	36.250		40.256		43.773	47.962		50.892		59.703

(From Fisher, R. A. [1970]. Statistical methods for research workers [14th ed.]. Darien, CT: Hafner Publishing. [Taken from Table III, pp. 112–113].)

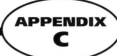

Distribution of t

	Level of Significance for One-Tailed Test					
	0.10	0.05	0.025	0.01	0.005	0.0005
	Level of Significance for Two-Tailed Test					
df	0.20	0.10	0.05	0.02	0.01	0.001
1	3.078	6.314	12.706	31.821	63.657	636.619
2	1.886	2.920	4.303	6.965	9.925	31.598
3	1.638	2.353	3.182	4.541	5.841	12.941
4	1.533	2.132	2.776	3.747	4.604	8.610
5	1.476	2.015	2.571	3.365	4.032	6.859
6	1.440	1.943	2.447	3.143	3.707	5.959
7	1.415	1.895	2.365	2.998	3.499	5.405
8	1.397	1.860	2.306	2.896	3.355	5.041
9	1.383	1.833	2.262	2.821	3.250	4.781
10	1.372	1.812	2.228	2.764	3.169	4.587
11	1.363	1.796	2.201	2.718	3.106	4.437
12	1.356	1.782	2.179	2.681	3.055	4.318
13	1.350	1.771	2.160	2.650	3.012	4.221
14	1.345	1.761	2.145	2.624	2.977	4.140
15	1.341	1.753	2.131	2.602	2.947	4.073
16	1.337	1.746	2.120	2.583	2.921	4.015
17	1.333	1.740	2.110	2.567	2.898	3.965
18	1.330	1.734	2.101	2.552	2.878	3.922
19	1.328	1.729	2.093	2.539	2.861	3.883
20	1.325	1.725	2.086	2.528	2.845	3.850
21	1.323	1.721	2.080	2.518	2.831	3.819
22	1.321	1.717	2.074	2.508	2.819	3.792

(continued)

Appendix C (CONTINUED)

	Level of Significance for One-Tailed Test					
	0.10	0.05	0.025	0.01	0.005	0.0005
	Level of Significance for Two-Tailed Test					
df	0.20	0.10	0.05	0.02	0.01	0.001
23	1.319	1.714	2.069	2.500	2.807	3.767
24	1.318	1.711	2.064	2.492	2.797	3.745
25	1.316	1.708	2.060	3.485	2.787	3.725
26	1.315	1.706	2.056	2.479	2.779	3.707
27	1.314	1.703	2.052	2.473	2.771	3.690
28	1.313	1.701	2.048	2.467	2.763	3.674
29	1.311	1.699	2.045	2.462	2.756	3.659
30	1.310	1.697	2.042	2.457	2.750	3.646
40	1.303	1.684	2.021	2.423	2.704	3.551
60	1.296	1.671	2.000	2.390	2.660	3.460
120	1.289	1.658	1.980	2.358	2.617	3.373
∞	1.282	1.645	1.960	2.326	2.576	3.291

(From Fisher, R. A. [1970]. Statistical methods for research workers (14th ed.). Darien, CT: Hafner Publishing [Table IV, p. 176].)

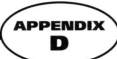

The 5% and 1% Points for the Distribution of F

n_1 Degrees of Freedom (For Greater Mean Square)*

n_2^+	1	2	3	4	5	6	7	8	9	10	11	12	14	16	20	24	30	40	50	75	100	200	500	∞
1	161	200	216	225	230	234	237	239	241	242	243	244	245	246	248	249	250	251	252	253	253	254	254	254
	4,052	**4,999**	**5,403**	**5,625**	**5,764**	**5,859**	**5,928**	**5,981**	**6,022**	**6,056**	**6,082**	**6,106**	**6,142**	**6,169**	**6,208**	**6,234**	**6,258**	**6,286**	**6,302**	**6,323**	**6,334**	**6,352**	**6,361**	**6,366**
2	18.51	19.00	19.16	19.25	19.30	19.33	19.36	19.37	19.38	19.39	19.40	19.41	19.42	19.43	19.44	19.45	19.46	19.47	19.47	19.48	19.49	19.49	19.50	19.50
	98.49	**99.00**	**99.17**	**99.25**	**99.30**	**99.33**	**99.34**	**99.36**	**99.38**	**99.40**	**99.41**	**99.42**	**99.43**	**99.44**	**99.45**	**99.46**	**99.47**	**99.48**	**99.48**	**99.49**	**99.49**	**99.49**	**99.50**	**99.50**
3	10.13	9.55	9.28	9.12	9.01	8.94	8.88	8.84	8.81	8.78	8.76	8.74	8.71	8.69	8.66	8.64	8.62	8.60	8.58	8.57	8.56	8.54	8.54	8.53
	34.12	**30.82**	**29.46**	**28.71**	**28.24**	**27.91**	**27.67**	**27.49**	**27.34**	**27.23**	**27.13**	**27.05**	**26.92**	**26.83**	**26.69**	**26.60**	**26.50**	**26.41**	**26.35**	**26.27**	**26.23**	**26.18**	**26.14**	**26.12**
4	7.71	6.94	6.59	6.39	6.26	6.16	6.09	6.04	6.00	5.96	5.93	5.91	5.87	5.84	5.80	5.77	5.74	5.71	5.70	5.68	5.66	5.65	5.64	5.63
	21.20	**18.00**	**16.69**	**15.98**	**15.52**	**15.21**	**14.98**	**14.80**	**14.66**	**14.54**	**14.45**	**14.37**	**14.24**	**14.15**	**14.02**	**13.93**	**13.83**	**13.74**	**13.69**	**13.61**	**13.57**	**13.52**	**13.48**	**13.46**
5	6.61	5.79	5.41	5.19	5.05	4.95	4.88	4.82	4.78	4.74	4.70	4.68	4.64	4.60	4.56	4.53	4.50	4.46	4.44	4.42	4.40	4.38	4.37	4.36
	16.26	**13.27**	**12.06**	**11.39**	**10.97**	**10.67**	**10.45**	**10.27**	**10.15**	**10.05**	**9.96**	**9.89**	**9.77**	**9.68**	**9.55**	**9.47**	**9.38**	**9.29**	**9.24**	**9.17**	**9.13**	**9.07**	**9.04**	**9.02**
6	5.99	5.14	4.76	4.53	4.39	4.28	4.21	4.15	4.10	4.06	4.03	4.00	3.96	3.92	3.87	3.84	3.81	3.77	3.75	3.72	3.71	3.69	3.68	3.67
	13.74	**10.92**	**9.78**	**9.15**	**8.75**	**8.47**	**8.26**	**8.10**	**7.98**	**7.87**	**7.79**	**7.72**	**7.60**	**7.52**	**7.39**	**7.31**	**7.23**	**7.14**	**7.09**	**7.02**	**6.99**	**6.94**	**6.90**	**6.88**
7	5.59	4.74	4.35	4.12	3.97	3.87	3.79	3.73	3.68	3.63	3.60	3.57	3.52	3.49	3.44	3.41	3.38	3.34	3.32	3.29	3.28	3.25	3.24	3.23
	12.25	**9.55**	**8.45**	**7.85**	**7.46**	**7.19**	**7.00**	**6.84**	**6.71**	**6.62**	**6.54**	**6.47**	**6.35**	**6.27**	**6.15**	**6.07**	**5.98**	**5.90**	**5.85**	**5.78**	**5.75**	**5.70**	**5.65**	**5.65**
8	5.32	4.46	4.07	3.84	3.69	3.58	3.50	3.44	3.39	3.34	3.31	3.28	3.23	3.20	3.15	3.12	3.08	3.05	3.03	3.00	2.98	2.96	2.94	2.93
	11.26	**8.65**	**7.59**	**7.01**	**6.63**	**6.37**	**6.19**	**6.03**	**5.91**	**5.82**	**5.74**	**5.67**	**5.56**	**5.48**	**5.36**	**5.28**	**5.20**	**5.11**	**5.06**	**5.00**	**4.96**	**4.91**	**4.88**	**4.86**
9	5.12	4.26	3.86	3.63	3.48	3.37	3.29	3.23	3.18	3.13	3.10	3.07	3.02	2.98	2.93	2.90	2.86	2.82	2.80	2.77	2.76	2.73	2.72	2.71
	10.56	**8.02**	**6.99**	**6.42**	**6.06**	**5.80**	**5.62**	**5.47**	**5.35**	**5.26**	**5.18**	**5.11**	**5.00**	**4.92**	**4.80**	**4.73**	**4.64**	**4.56**	**4.51**	**4.45**	**4.41**	**4.36**	**4.33**	**4.31**
10	4.96	4.10	3.71	3.48	3.33	3.22	3.14	3.07	3.02	2.97	2.94	2.91	2.86	2.82	2.77	2.74	2.70	2.67	2.64	2.61	2.59	2.56	2.55	2.54
	10.04	**7.56**	**6.55**	**5.99**	**5.64**	**5.39**	**5.21**	**5.06**	**4.95**	**4.85**	**4.78**	**4.71**	**4.60**	**4.52**	**4.41**	**4.33**	**4.25**	**4.17**	**4.12**	**4.05**	**4.01**	**3.96**	**3.93**	**3.91**
11	4.84	3.98	3.59	3.36	3.20	3.09	3.01	2.95	2.90	2.86	2.82	2.79	2.74	2.70	2.65	2.61	2.57	2.53	2.50	2.47	2.45	2.42	2.41	2.40
	9.65	**7.20**	**6.22**	**5.67**	**5.32**	**5.07**	**4.88**	**4.74**	**4.63**	**4.54**	**4.46**	**4.40**	**4.29**	**4.21**	**4.10**	**4.02**	**3.94**	**3.86**	**3.80**	**3.74**	**3.70**	**3.66**	**3.62**	**3.60**
12	4.75	3.88	3.49	3.26	3.11	3.00	2.92	2.85	2.80	2.76	2.72	2.69	2.64	2.60	2.54	2.50	2.46	2.42	2.40	2.36	2.35	2.32	2.31	2.30
	9.33	**6.93**	**5.95**	**5.41**	**5.06**	**4.82**	**4.65**	**4.50**	**4.39**	**4.30**	**4.22**	**4.16**	**4.05**	**3.98**	**3.86**	**3.78**	**3.70**	**3.61**	**3.56**	**3.49**	**3.46**	**3.41**	**3.38**	**3.36**
13	4.67	3.80	3.41	3.18	3.02	2.92	2.84	2.77	2.72	2.67	2.63	2.60	2.55	2.51	2.46	2.42	2.38	2.34	2.32	2.28	2.26	2.24	2.22	2.21
	9.07	**6.70**	**5.74**	**5.20**	**4.86**	**4.62**	**4.44**	**4.30**	**4.19**	**4.10**	**4.02**	**3.96**	**3.85**	**3.78**	**3.67**	**3.59**	**3.51**	**3.42**	**3.37**	**3.30**	**3.27**	**3.21**	**3.18**	**3.16**
14	4.60	3.74	3.34	3.11	2.96	2.85	2.77	2.70	2.65	2.60	2.56	2.53	2.48	2.44	2.39	2.35	2.31	2.27	2.24	2.21	2.19	2.16	2.14	2.13
	8.86	**6.51**	**5.56**	**5.03**	**4.69**	**4.46**	**4.28**	**4.14**	**4.03**	**3.94**	**3.86**	**3.80**	**3.70**	**3.62**	**3.51**	**3.43**	**3.34**	**3.26**	**3.21**	**3.14**	**3.11**	**3.06**	**3.02**	**3.00**
15	4.54	3.68	3.29	3.06	2.90	2.79	2.70	2.64	2.59	2.55	2.51	2.48	2.43	2.39	2.33	2.29	2.25	2.21	2.18	2.15	2.12	2.10	2.08	2.07
	8.68	**6.36**	**5.42**	**4.89**	**4.56**	**4.32**	**4.14**	**4.00**	**3.89**	**3.80**	**3.73**	**3.67**	**3.56**	**3.48**	**3.36**	**3.29**	**3.20**	**3.12**	**3.07**	**3.00**	**2.97**	**2.92**	**2.89**	**2.87**
16	4.49	3.63	3.24	3.01	2.85	2.74	2.66	2.59	2.54	2.49	2.45	2.42	2.37	2.33	2.28	2.24	2.20	2.16	2.13	2.09	2.07	2.04	2.02	2.01
	8.53	**6.23**	**5.29**	**4.77**	**4.44**	**4.20**	**4.03**	**3.89**	**3.78**	**3.69**	**3.61**	**3.55**	**3.45**	**3.37**	**3.25**	**3.18**	**3.10**	**3.01**	**2.96**	**2.89**	**2.86**	**2.80**	**2.77**	**2.75**
17	4.45	3.59	3.20	2.96	2.81	2.70	2.62	2.55	2.50	2.45	2.41	2.38	2.33	2.29	2.23	2.19	2.15	2.11	2.08	2.04	2.02	1.99	1.97	1.96
	8.40	**6.11**	**5.18**	**4.67**	**4.34**	**4.10**	**3.93**	**3.79**	**3.68**	**3.59**	**3.52**	**3.45**	**3.35**	**3.27**	**3.16**	**3.08**	**3.00**	**2.92**	**2.86**	**2.79**	**2.76**	**2.70**	**2.67**	**2.65**
18	4.41	3.55	3.16	2.93	2.77	2.66	2.58	2.51	2.46	2.41	2.37	2.34	2.29	2.25	2.19	2.15	2.11	2.07	2.04	2.00	1.98	1.95	1.93	1.92
	8.28	**6.01**	**5.09**	**4.58**	**4.25**	**4.01**	**3.85**	**3.71**	**3.60**	**3.51**	**3.44**	**3.37**	**3.27**	**3.19**	**3.07**	**3.00**	**2.91**	**2.83**	**2.78**	**2.71**	**2.68**	**2.62**	**2.59**	**2.57**
19	4.38	3.52	3.13	2.90	2.74	2.63	2.55	2.48	2.43	2.38	2.34	2.31	2.26	2.21	2.15	2.11	2.07	2.02	2.00	1.96	1.94	1.91	1.90	1.88
	8.18	**5.93**	**5.01**	**4.50**	**4.17**	**3.94**	**3.77**	**3.63**	**3.52**	**3.43**	**3.36**	**3.30**	**3.19**	**3.12**	**3.00**	**2.92**	**2.84**	**2.76**	**2.70**	**2.63**	**2.60**	**2.54**	**2.51**	**2.49**
20	4.35	3.49	3.10	2.87	2.71	2.60	2.52	2.45	2.40	2.35	2.31	2.28	2.23	2.18	2.12	2.08	2.04	1.99	1.96	1.92	1.90	1.87	1.85	1.84
	8.10	**5.85**	**4.94**	**4.43**	**4.10**	**3.87**	**3.71**	**3.56**	**3.45**	**3.37**	**3.30**	**3.23**	**3.13**	**3.05**	**2.94**	**2.86**	**2.77**	**2.69**	**2.63**	**2.56**	**2.53**	**2.47**	**2.44**	**2.42**
21	4.32	3.47	3.07	2.84	2.68	2.57	2.49	2.42	2.37	2.32	2.28	2.25	2.20	2.15	2.09	2.05	2.00	1.96	1.93	1.89	1.87	1.84	1.82	1.81
	8.02	**5.78**	**4.87**	**4.37**	**4.04**	**3.81**	**3.65**	**3.51**	**3.40**	**3.31**	**3.24**	**3.17**	**3.07**	**2.99**	**2.88**	**2.80**	**2.72**	**2.63**	**2.58**	**2.51**	**2.47**	**2.42**	**2.38**	**2.36**

df																								
22	4.30 **7.94**	3.44 **5.72**	3.05 **4.82**	2.82 **4.31**	2.66 **3.99**	2.55 **3.76**	2.47 **3.59**	2.40 **3.45**	2.35 **3.35**	2.30 **3.26**	2.26 **3.18**	2.23 **3.12**	2.18 **3.02**	2.13 **2.94**	2.07 **2.83**	2.03 **2.75**	1.98 **2.67**	1.93 **2.58**	1.91 **2.53**	1.87 **2.46**	1.84 **2.42**	1.81 **2.37**	1.80 **2.33**	1.78 **2.31**
23	4.28 **7.88**	3.42 **5.66**	3.03 **4.76**	2.80 **4.26**	2.64 **3.94**	2.53 **3.71**	2.45 **3.54**	2.38 **3.41**	2.32 **3.30**	2.28 **3.21**	2.24 **3.14**	2.20 **3.07**	2.14 **2.97**	2.10 **2.89**	2.04 **2.78**	2.00 **2.70**	1.96 **2.62**	1.91 **2.53**	1.88 **2.48**	1.84 **2.41**	1.82 **2.37**	1.79 **2.32**	1.77 **2.28**	1.76 **2.26**
24	4.26 **7.82**	3.40 **5.61**	3.01 **4.72**	2.78 **4.22**	2.62 **3.90**	2.51 **3.67**	2.43 **3.50**	2.36 **3.36**	2.30 **3.25**	2.26 **3.17**	2.22 **3.09**	2.18 **3.03**	2.13 **2.93**	2.09 **2.85**	2.02 **2.74**	1.98 **2.66**	1.94 **2.58**	1.89 **2.49**	1.86 **2.44**	1.82 **2.36**	1.80 **2.33**	1.76 **2.27**	1.74 **2.23**	1.73 **2.21**
25	4.24 **7.77**	3.38 **5.57**	2.99 **4.68**	2.76 **4.18**	2.60 **3.86**	2.49 **3.63**	2.41 **3.46**	2.34 **3.32**	2.28 **3.21**	2.24 **3.13**	2.20 **3.05**	2.16 **2.99**	2.11 **2.89**	2.06 **2.81**	2.00 **2.70**	1.96 **2.62**	1.92 **2.54**	1.87 **2.45**	1.84 **2.40**	1.80 **2.32**	1.77 **2.29**	1.74 **2.23**	1.72 **2.19**	1.71 **2.17**
26	4.22 **7.72**	3.37 **5.53**	2.98 **4.64**	2.74 **4.14**	2.59 **3.82**	2.47 **3.59**	2.39 **3.42**	2.32 **3.29**	2.27 **3.17**	2.22 **3.09**	2.18 **3.02**	2.15 **2.96**	2.10 **2.86**	2.05 **2.77**	1.99 **2.66**	1.95 **2.58**	1.90 **2.50**	1.85 **2.41**	1.82 **2.36**	1.78 **2.28**	1.76 **2.25**	1.72 **2.19**	1.70 **2.15**	1.69 **2.13**
27	4.21 **7.68**	3.35 **5.49**	2.96 **4.60**	2.73 **4.11**	2.57 **3.79**	2.46 **3.56**	2.37 **3.39**	2.30 **3.26**	2.25 **3.14**	2.20 **3.06**	2.16 **2.98**	2.13 **2.93**	2.08 **2.83**	2.03 **2.74**	1.97 **2.63**	1.93 **2.55**	1.88 **2.47**	1.84 **2.38**	1.80 **2.33**	1.76 **2.25**	1.74 **2.21**	1.71 **2.16**	1.68 **2.12**	1.67 **2.10**
28	4.20 **7.64**	3.34 **5.45**	2.95 **4.57**	2.71 **4.07**	2.56 **3.76**	2.44 **3.53**	2.36 **3.36**	2.29 **3.23**	2.24 **3.11**	2.19 **3.03**	2.15 **2.95**	2.12 **2.90**	2.06 **2.80**	2.02 **2.71**	1.96 **2.60**	1.91 **2.52**	1.87 **2.44**	1.81 **2.35**	1.78 **2.30**	1.75 **2.22**	1.72 **2.18**	1.69 **2.13**	1.67 **2.09**	1.65 **2.06**
29	4.18 **7.60**	3.33 **5.42**	2.93 **4.54**	2.70 **4.04**	2.54 **3.73**	2.43 **3.50**	2.35 **3.33**	2.28 **3.20**	2.22 **3.08**	2.18 **3.00**	2.14 **2.92**	2.10 **2.87**	2.05 **2.77**	2.00 **2.68**	1.94 **2.57**	1.90 **2.49**	1.85 **2.41**	1.80 **2.32**	1.77 **2.27**	1.73 **2.19**	1.71 **2.15**	1.68 **2.10**	1.65 **2.06**	1.64 **2.03**
30	4.17 **7.56**	3.32 **5.39**	2.92 **4.51**	2.69 **4.02**	2.53 **3.70**	2.42 **3.47**	2.34 **3.30**	2.27 **3.17**	2.21 **3.06**	2.16 **2.98**	2.12 **2.90**	2.09 **2.84**	2.04 **2.74**	1.99 **2.66**	1.93 **2.55**	1.89 **2.47**	1.84 **2.38**	1.79 **2.29**	1.76 **2.24**	1.72 **2.16**	1.69 **2.13**	1.66 **2.07**	1.64 **2.03**	1.62 **2.01**
32	4.15 **7.50**	3.30 **5.34**	2.90 **4.46**	2.67 **3.97**	2.51 **3.66**	2.40 **3.42**	2.32 **3.25**	2.25 **3.12**	2.19 **3.01**	2.14 **2.94**	2.10 **2.86**	2.07 **2.80**	2.02 **2.70**	1.97 **2.62**	1.91 **2.51**	1.86 **2.42**	1.82 **2.34**	1.76 **2.25**	1.74 **2.20**	1.69 **2.12**	1.67 **2.08**	1.64 **2.02**	1.61 **1.98**	1.59 **1.96**
34	4.13 **7.44**	3.28 **5.29**	2.88 **4.42**	2.65 **3.93**	2.49 **3.61**	2.38 **3.38**	2.30 **3.21**	2.23 **3.08**	2.17 **2.97**	2.12 **2.89**	2.08 **2.82**	2.05 **2.76**	2.00 **2.66**	1.95 **2.58**	1.89 **2.47**	1.84 **2.38**	1.80 **2.30**	1.74 **2.21**	1.71 **2.15**	1.67 **2.08**	1.64 **2.04**	1.61 **1.98**	1.59 **1.94**	1.57 **1.91**
36	4.11 **7.39**	3.26 **5.25**	2.86 **4.38**	2.63 **3.89**	2.48 **3.58**	2.36 **3.35**	2.28 **3.18**	2.21 **3.04**	2.15 **2.94**	2.10 **2.86**	2.06 **2.78**	2.03 **2.72**	1.98 **2.62**	1.93 **2.54**	1.87 **2.43**	1.82 **2.35**	1.78 **2.26**	1.72 **2.17**	1.69 **2.12**	1.65 **2.04**	1.62 **2.00**	1.59 **1.94**	1.56 **1.90**	1.55 **1.87**
38	4.10 **7.35**	3.25 **5.21**	2.85 **4.34**	2.62 **3.86**	2.46 **3.54**	2.35 **3.32**	2.26 **3.15**	2.19 **3.02**	2.14 **2.91**	2.09 **2.82**	2.05 **2.75**	2.02 **2.69**	1.96 **2.59**	1.92 **2.51**	1.85 **2.40**	1.80 **2.32**	1.76 **2.22**	1.71 **2.14**	1.67 **2.08**	1.63 **2.00**	1.60 **1.97**	1.57 **1.90**	1.54 **1.86**	1.53 **1.84**
40	4.08 **7.31**	3.23 **5.18**	2.84 **4.31**	2.61 **3.83**	2.45 **3.51**	2.34 **3.29**	2.25 **3.12**	2.18 **2.99**	2.12 **2.88**	2.07 **2.80**	2.04 **2.73**	2.00 **2.66**	1.95 **2.56**	1.90 **2.49**	1.84 **2.37**	1.79 **2.29**	1.74 **2.20**	1.69 **2.11**	1.66 **2.05**	1.61 **1.97**	1.59 **1.94**	1.55 **1.88**	1.53 **1.84**	1.51 **1.81**
42	4.07 **7.27**	3.22 **5.15**	2.83 **4.29**	2.59 **3.80**	2.44 **3.49**	2.32 **3.26**	2.24 **3.10**	2.17 **2.96**	2.11 **2.86**	2.06 **2.77**	2.02 **2.70**	1.99 **2.64**	1.94 **2.54**	1.89 **2.46**	1.82 **2.35**	1.78 **2.26**	1.73 **2.17**	1.68 **2.08**	1.64 **2.02**	1.60 **1.94**	1.57 **1.91**	1.54 **1.85**	1.51 **1.80**	1.49 **1.78**
44	4.06 **7.24**	3.21 **5.12**	2.82 **4.26**	2.58 **3.78**	2.43 **3.46**	2.31 **3.24**	2.23 **3.07**	2.16 **2.94**	2.10 **2.84**	2.05 **2.75**	2.01 **2.68**	1.98 **2.62**	1.92 **2.52**	1.88 **2.44**	1.81 **2.32**	1.76 **2.24**	1.72 **2.15**	1.66 **2.06**	1.63 **2.00**	1.58 **1.92**	1.56 **1.88**	1.52 **1.82**	1.50 **1.78**	1.48 **1.75**
46	4.05 **7.21**	3.20 **5.10**	2.81 **4.24**	2.57 **3.76**	2.42 **3.44**	2.30 **3.22**	2.22 **3.05**	2.14 **2.92**	2.09 **2.82**	2.04 **2.73**	2.00 **2.66**	1.97 **2.60**	1.91 **2.50**	1.87 **2.42**	1.80 **2.30**	1.75 **2.22**	1.71 **2.13**	1.65 **2.04**	1.62 **1.98**	1.57 **1.90**	1.54 **1.86**	1.51 **1.80**	1.48 **1.76**	1.46 **1.72**
48	4.04 **7.19**	3.19 **5.08**	2.80 **4.22**	2.56 **3.74**	2.41 **3.42**	2.30 **3.20**	2.21 **3.04**	2.14 **2.90**	2.08 **2.80**	2.03 **2.71**	1.99 **2.64**	1.96 **2.58**	1.90 **2.48**	1.86 **2.40**	1.79 **2.28**	1.74 **2.20**	1.70 **2.11**	1.64 **2.02**	1.61 **1.96**	1.56 **1.88**	1.53 **1.84**	1.50 **1.78**	1.47 **1.73**	1.45 **1.70**
50	4.03 **7.17**	3.18 **5.06**	2.79 **4.20**	2.56 **3.72**	2.40 **3.41**	2.29 **3.18**	2.20 **3.02**	2.13 **2.88**	2.07 **2.78**	2.02 **2.70**	1.98 **2.62**	1.95 **2.56**	1.90 **2.46**	1.85 **2.39**	1.78 **2.26**	1.74 **2.18**	1.69 **2.10**	1.63 **2.00**	1.60 **1.94**	1.55 **1.86**	1.52 **1.82**	1.48 **1.76**	1.46 **1.71**	1.44 **1.68**
55	4.02 **7.12**	3.17 **5.01**	2.78 **4.16**	2.54 **3.68**	2.38 **3.37**	2.27 **3.15**	2.18 **2.98**	2.11 **2.85**	2.05 **2.75**	2.00 **2.66**	1.97 **2.59**	1.93 **2.53**	1.88 **2.43**	1.83 **2.35**	1.76 **2.23**	1.72 **2.15**	1.67 **2.06**	1.61 **1.96**	1.58 **1.90**	1.52 **1.82**	1.50 **1.78**	1.46 **1.71**	1.43 **1.66**	1.41 **1.64**
60	4.00 **7.08**	3.15 **4.98**	2.76 **4.13**	2.52 **3.65**	2.37 **3.34**	2.25 **3.12**	2.17 **2.95**	2.10 **2.82**	2.04 **2.72**	1.99 **2.63**	1.95 **2.56**	1.92 **2.50**	1.86 **2.40**	1.81 **2.32**	1.75 **2.20**	1.70 **2.12**	1.65 **2.03**	1.59 **1.93**	1.56 **1.87**	1.50 **1.79**	1.48 **1.74**	1.44 **1.68**	1.41 **1.63**	1.39 **1.60**
65	3.99 **7.04**	3.14 **4.95**	2.75 **4.10**	2.51 **3.62**	2.36 **3.31**	2.24 **3.09**	2.15 **2.93**	2.08 **2.79**	2.02 **2.70**	1.98 **2.61**	1.94 **2.54**	1.90 **2.47**	1.85 **2.37**	1.80 **2.30**	1.73 **2.18**	1.68 **2.09**	1.63 **2.00**	1.57 **1.90**	1.54 **1.84**	1.49 **1.76**	1.46 **1.71**	1.42 **1.64**	1.39 **1.60**	1.37 **1.56**
70	3.98 **7.01**	3.13 **4.92**	2.74 **4.08**	2.50 **3.60**	2.35 **3.29**	2.23 **3.07**	2.14 **2.91**	2.07 **2.77**	2.01 **2.67**	1.97 **2.59**	1.93 **2.51**	1.89 **2.45**	1.84 **2.35**	1.79 **2.28**	1.72 **2.15**	1.67 **2.07**	1.62 **1.98**	1.56 **1.88**	1.53 **1.82**	1.47 **1.74**	1.45 **1.69**	1.40 **1.62**	1.37 **1.56**	1.35 **1.53**

(continued)

415

Appendix D (CONTINUED)

n_1 Degrees of Freedom (For Greater Mean Square)*

n_2^+	1	2	3	4	5	6	7	8	9	10	11	12	14	16	20	24	30	40	50	75	100	200	500	∞
80	3.96	3.11	2.72	2.48	2.33	2.21	2.12	2.05	1.99	1.95	1.91	1.88	1.82	1.77	1.70	1.65	1.60	1.54	1.51	1.45	1.42	1.38	1.35	1.32
	6.96	**4.88**	**4.04**	**3.56**	**3.25**	**3.04**	**2.87**	**2.74**	**2.64**	**2.55**	**2.48**	**2.41**	**2.32**	**2.24**	**2.11**	**2.03**	**1.94**	**1.84**	**1.78**	**1.70**	**1.65**	**1.57**	**1.52**	**1.49**
100	3.94	3.09	2.70	2.46	2.30	2.19	2.10	2.03	1.97	1.92	1.88	1.85	1.79	1.75	1.68	1.63	1.57	1.51	1.48	1.42	1.39	1.34	1.30	1.28
	6.90	**4.82**	**3.98**	**3.51**	**3.20**	**2.99**	**2.82**	**2.69**	**2.59**	**2.51**	**2.43**	**2.36**	**2.26**	**2.19**	**2.06**	**1.98**	**1.89**	**1.79**	**1.73**	**1.64**	**1.59**	**1.51**	**1.46**	**1.43**
125	3.92	3.07	2.68	2.44	2.29	2.17	2.08	2.01	1.95	1.90	1.86	1.83	1.77	1.72	1.65	1.60	1.55	1.49	1.45	1.39	1.36	1.31	1.27	1.25
	6.84	**4.78**	**3.94**	**3.47**	**3.17**	**2.95**	**2.79**	**2.65**	**2.56**	**2.47**	**2.40**	**2.33**	**2.23**	**2.15**	**2.03**	**1.94**	**1.85**	**1.75**	**1.68**	**1.59**	**1.54**	**1.46**	**1.40**	**1.37**
150	3.91	3.06	2.67	2.43	2.27	2.16	2.07	2.00	1.94	1.89	1.85	1.82	1.76	1.71	1.64	1.59	1.54	1.47	1.44	1.37	1.34	1.29	1.25	1.22
	6.81	**4.75**	**3.91**	**3.44**	**3.14**	**2.92**	**2.76**	**2.62**	**2.53**	**2.44**	**2.37**	**2.30**	**2.20**	**2.12**	**2.00**	**1.91**	**1.83**	**1.72**	**1.66**	**1.56**	**1.51**	**1.43**	**1.37**	**1.33**
200	3.89	3.04	2.65	2.41	2.26	2.14	2.05	1.98	1.92	1.87	1.83	1.80	1.74	1.69	1.62	1.57	1.52	1.45	1.42	1.35	1.32	1.26	1.22	1.19
	6.76	**4.71**	**3.88**	**3.41**	**3.11**	**2.90**	**2.73**	**2.60**	**2.50**	**2.41**	**2.34**	**2.28**	**2.17**	**2.09**	**1.97**	**1.88**	**1.79**	**1.69**	**1.62**	**1.53**	**1.48**	**1.39**	**1.33**	**1.28**
400	3.86	3.02	2.62	2.39	2.23	2.12	2.03	1.96	1.90	1.85	1.81	1.78	1.72	1.67	1.60	1.54	1.49	1.42	1.38	1.32	1.28	1.22	1.16	1.13
	6.70	**4.66**	**3.83**	**3.36**	**3.06**	**2.85**	**2.69**	**2.55**	**2.46**	**2.37**	**2.29**	**2.23**	**2.12**	**2.04**	**1.92**	**1.84**	**1.74**	**1.64**	**1.57**	**1.47**	**1.42**	**1.32**	**1.24**	**1.19**
1000	3.85	3.00	2.61	2.38	2.22	2.10	2.02	1.95	1.89	1.84	1.80	1.76	1.70	1.65	1.58	1.53	1.47	1.41	1.36	1.30	1.26	1.19	1.13	1.08
	6.66	**4.62**	**3.80**	**3.34**	**3.04**	**2.82**	**2.66**	**2.53**	**2.43**	**2.34**	**2.26**	**2.20**	**2.09**	**2.01**	**1.89**	**1.81**	**1.71**	**1.61**	**1.54**	**1.44**	**1.38**	**1.28**	**1.19**	**1.11**
∞	3.84	2.99	2.60	2.37	2.21	2.09	2.01	1.94	1.88	1.83	1.79	1.75	1.69	1.64	1.57	1.52	1.46	1.40	1.35	1.28	1.24	1.17	1.11	1.00
	6.64	**4.60**	**3.78**	**3.32**	**3.02**	**2.80**	**2.64**	**2.51**	**2.41**	**2.32**	**2.24**	**2.18**	**2.07**	**1.99**	**1.87**	**1.79**	**1.69**	**1.59**	**1.52**	**1.41**	**1.36**	**1.25**	**1.15**	**1.00**

5% = roman type; 1% = boldface type

*numerator.

+ denominator.

(From Snedecor, G. W. [1938]. Statistical methods. Ames, Iowa: Collegiate Press. [Table 10–3, pp. 184–187].)

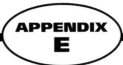

Critical Values of the Correlation Coefficient

	Level of Significance for One-Tailed Test			
	.05	.025	.01	.005
	Level of Significance for Two-Tailed Test			
df	.10	.05	.02	.01
1	.988	.997	.9995	.9999
2	.900	.950	.980	.990
3	.805	.878	.934	.959
4	.729	.811	.882	.917
5	.669	.754	.833	.874
6	.622	.707	.789	.834
7	.582	.666	.750	.798
8	.549	.632	.716	.765
9	.521	.602	.685	.735
10	.497	.576	.658	.708
11	.476	.553	.634	.684
12	.458	.532	.612	.661
13	.441	.514	.592	.641
14	.426	.497	.574	.623
15	.412	.482	.558	.606
16	.400	.468	.542	.590
17	.389	.456	.528	.575
18	.378	.444	.516	.561
19	.369	.433	.503	.549
20	.360	.423	.492	.537
21	.352	.413	.482	.526
22	.344	.404	.472	.515
23	.337	.396	.462	.505

(*continued*)

Appendix E (CONTINUED)

	Level of Significance for One-Tailed Test			
	.05	*.025*	*.01*	*.005*
	Level of Significance for Two-Tailed Test			
df	*.10*	*.05*	*.02*	*.01*
24	.330	.388	.453	.496
25	.323	.381	.445	.487
26	.317	.374	.437	.479
27	.311	.367	.430	.471
28	.306	.361	.423	.463
29	.301	.355	.416	.456
30	.296	.349	.409	.449
35	.275	.325	.381	.418
40	.257	.304	.358	.393
45	.243	.288	.338	.372
50	.231	.273	.322	.354
60	.211	.250	.295	.325
70	.195	.232	.274	.303
80	.183	.217	.256	.283
90	.173	.205	.242	.267
100	.164	.195	.230	.254
125		.174		.228
150		.159		.208
200		.138		.181
300		.113		.148
400		.098		.128
500		.088		.115
1000		.062		.081

(From Fisher, R. A. [1970]. Statistical methods for research workers *[14th ed.]. Darien, CT: Hafner Publishing Co. [Table V.A., p. 211].)*

Transformation of r to z_r

r	z_r	r	z_r	r	z_r	r	z_r	r	z_r
.000	.000	.200	.203	.400	.424	.600	.693	.800	1.099
.005	.005	.205	.208	.405	.430	.605	.701	.805	1.113
.010	.010	.210	.213	.410	.436	.610	.709	.810	1.127
.015	.015	.215	.218	.415	.442	.615	.717	.815	1.142
.020	.020	.220	.224	.420	.448	.620	.725	.820	1.157
.025	.025	.225	.229	.425	.454	.625	.733	.825	1.172
.030	.030	.230	.234	.430	.460	.630	.741.	830	1.188
.035	.035	.235	.239	.435	.466	.635	.750	.835	1.204
.040	.040	.240	.245	.440	.472	.640	.758	.840	1.221
.045	.045	.245	.250	.445	.478	.645	.767	.845	1.238
.050	.050	.250	.255	.450	.485	.650	.775	.850	1.256
.055	.055	.255	.261	.455	.491	.655	.784	.855	1.274
.060	.060	.260	.266	.460	.497	.660	.793	.860	1.293
.065	.065	.265	.721	.465	.504	.665	.802	.865	1.313
.070	.070	.270	.277	.470	.510	.670	.811	.870	1.333
.075	.075	.275	.282	.475	.517	.675	.820	.875	1.354
.080	.080	.280	.288	.480	.523	.680	.829	.880	1.376
.085	.085	.285	.293	.485	.530	.685	.838	.885	1.398
.090	.090	.290	.299	.490	.536	.690	.848	.890	1.422
.095	.095	.295	.304	.495	.543	.695	.858	.895	1.447
.100	.100	.300	.310	.500	.549	.700	.867	.900	1.472
.105	.105	.305	.315	.505	.556	.705	.877	.905	1.499
.110	.110	.310	.321	.510	.563	.710	.887	.910	1.528
.115	.116	.315	.326	.515	.570	.715	.897	.915	1.557
.120	.121	.320	.332	.520	.576	.720	.908	.920	1.589
.125	.126	.325	.337	.525	.583	.725	.918	.925	1.623
.130	.131	.330	.343	.530	.590	.730	.929	.930	1.658
.135	.136	.335	.348	.535	.597	.735	.940	.935	1.697

(*continued*)

Appendix F (CONTINUED)

r	z_r	r	z_r	r	z_r	r	z_r	r	z_r
.140	.141	.340	.354	.540	.604	.740	.950	.940	1.738
.145	.146	.345	.360	.545	.611	.745	.962	.945	1.783
.150	.151	.350	.365	.550	.618	.750	.973	.950	1.832
.155	.156	.355	.371	.555	.626	.755	.984	.955	1.886
.160	.161	.360	.377	.560	.633	.760	.996	.960	1.946
.165	.167	.365	.383	.565	.640	.765	1.008	.965	2.014
.170	.172	.370	.388	.570	.648	.770	1.020	.970	2.092
.175	.177	.375	.394	.575	.655	.775	1.033	.975	2.185
.180	.182	.380	.400	.580	.662	.780	1.045	.980	2.298
.185	.187	.385	.406	.585	.670	.785	1.058	.985	2.443
.190	.192	.390	.412	.590	.678	.790	1.071	.990	2.647
.195	.198	.395	.418	.595	.685	.795	1.085	.995	2.994

(From Hinkle, D. E., Wiersma, W., & Jurs, S. G. [1994]. Applied statistics for the behavioral sciences [3rd ed.]. [Appendix C.6, p. 630]. Boston: Houghton Mifflin. Used by permission.)

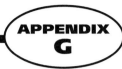

APPENDIX G

Survey for Exercises

BOSTON COLLEGE SCHOOL OF NURSING
A SURVEY FOR NU744

This questionnaire is designed to gather data for use in a course on statistics. The data will be used *only* to help students learn how to use the computer to manage and analyze data. Thank you for your help.

Code Number [   ]

| 1. Gender | Male | 0 |
| | Female | 1 |

2. Age in years [   ]

3. Marital Status	Never married	1
	Married	2
	Living with significant other	3
	Separated	4
	Widowed	5
	Divorced	6

4. Education (in years) [   ]

5. Smoking history	Never smoked	0
	Quit smoking	1
	Still smoking	2

6. Current work status	Unemployed	0
	Part-Time	1
	Full-Time	2

7. Political affiliation	Republican	1
	Democrat	2
	Independent	3

8. Depressed state of mind

Rarely	1
Sometimes	2
Often	3
Routinely	4

9. Exercise

Rarely	1
Sometimes	2
Often	3
Routinely	4

10. Eat 3 regular meals a day

Rarely	1
Sometimes	2
Often	3
Routinely	4

11. How satisfied are you with your current weight? (circle one)

Very Dissatisfied									Very Satisfied
1	2	3	4	5	6	7	8	9	10

12. How satisfied were you with your weight when you were 18?

Very Dissatisfied									Very Satisfied
1	2	3	4	5	6	7	8	9	10

13. Please rate your overall state of health on the following scale (circle one number)

Very Ill									Very Healthy
1	2	3	4	5	6	7	8	9	10

14. How happy, satisfied, or pleased have you been with your quality of life during the past month? (Circle the number for the one answer that comes closest to the way you are feeling.)

extremely happy, could not be more satisfied or pleased	6
very happy most of the time	5
generally satisfied, pleased	4
sometimes fairly satisfied, sometimes fairly unhappy	3
generally dissatisfied, unhappy	2
very dissatisfied, unhappy most of the time	1

15. How happy, satisfied, or pleased were you with your quality of life when you were 18? (Circle the number for the one answer that comes closest to the way you are feeling.)

extremely happy, could not be more satisfied or pleased	6
very happy most of the time	5
generally satisfied, pleased	4
sometimes fairly satisfied, sometimes fairly unhappy	3
generally dissatisfied, unhappy	2
very dissatisfied, unhappy most of the time	1

16. If you were given a tax-free gift of $500,000, and you had only five days to choose one specific way to use it, which of the following would you pick:

1. invest it with a brokerage firm

2. buy a vacation home at a place of my choice.

(continued)

3. pay off my existing mortgage; or, if I don't own a primary residence, buy one of my choice outright.
4. donate the whole amount to a charity of my choice.

17. You are planning your winter vacation. Of the following, which place would you choose to visit:
1. a beachfront condo in Hawaii
2. a chalet in the Swiss Alps
3. a luxury hotel at Disney World in Florida
4. an ocean cruise through the Caribbean Islands

INVENTORY OF PERSONAL ATTITUDES

The following pages contain a series of *statements and their opposites*. Notice that the statements extend from one extreme to the other. Where would you place yourself on this scale? Place a circle on the number that is *most true for you at this time*. Do not put your circles between numbers.

1. During most of the day my energy level is

very high						very low
1	2	3	4	5	6	7

2. When there is a great deal of pressure being placed on me

I remain calm						I get tense
1	2	3	4	5	6	7

3. As a whole, my life seems

dull						vibrant
1	2	3	4	5	6	7

4. My daily activities are

a source of satisfaction						not a source of satisfaction
1	2	3	4	5	6	7

5. I experience anxiety

all the time						never
1	2	3	4	5	6	7

6. I have come to expect that every day will be

new and different						exactly the same
1	2	3	4	5	6	7

7. I am fearful

all the time						never
1	2	3	4	5	6	7

8. When I think deeply about life

I feel there is a purpose to it						I do not feel there is any purpose to it
1	2	3	4	5	6	7

9. I feel that my life so far has

not been productive						been productive
1	2	3	4	5	6	7

10. When I have made a mistake

I feel extreme dislike for myself   I continue to like myself

| 1 | 2 | 3 | 4 | 5 | 6 | 7 |

11. I feel that the work* I am doing

is of no value   is of great value

| 1 | 2 | 3 | 4 | 5 | 6 | 7 |

12. I wish I were different than who I am.

agree strongly   disagree strongly

| 1 | 2 | 3 | 4 | 5 | 6 | 7 |

13. At this time, I have

                                               no clearly defined

clearly defined goals for my life   goals for my life

| 1 | 2 | 3 | 4 | 5 | 6 | 7 |

14. I find myself worrying that something bad is going to happen to me or those I love

all the time   never

| 1 | 2 | 3 | 4 | 5 | 6 | 7 |

15. In a stressful situation,

I can concentrate easily   I cannot concentrate easily

| 1 | 2 | 3 | 4 | 5 | 6 | 7 |

16. When I need to stand up for myself

I cannot do it   I can do it quite easily

| 1 | 2 | 3 | 4 | 5 | 6 | 7 |

17. I feel less than adequate in most situations.

agree strongly   disagree strongly

| 1 | 2 | 3 | 4 | 5 | 6 | 7 |

18. I react to problems and difficulties

with a great deal of frustration   with no frustration

| 1 | 2 | 3 | 4 | 5 | 6 | 7 |

19. When sad things happen to me or other people

I cannot feel positive about life   I continue to feel positive about life

| 1 | 2 | 3 | 4 | 5 | 6 | 7 |

20. When I think about what I have done with my life, I feel

worthwhile   worthless

| 1 | 2 | 3 | 4 | 5 | 6 | 7 |

21. My present life

does not satisfy me   satisfies me

| 1 | 2 | 3 | 4 | 5 | 6 | 7 |

22. In really difficult situations

I feel able to respond in   I feel unable to respond in
positive ways   positive ways

| 1 | 2 | 3 | 4 | 5 | 6 | 7 |

23. I feel joy in my heart

never						all the time
1	2	3	4	5	6	7

24. When I need to relax

I experience a peacefulness free of thoughts and worries						I experience no peace, only thoughts and worries
1	2	3	4	5	6	7

25. I feel trapped by the circumstances of my life.

agree strongly						disagree strongly
1	2	3	4	5	6	7

26. When I am in a frightening situation

I panic						I remain calm
1	2	3	4	5	6	7

27. When I think about my past

I feel no regrets						I feel many regrets
1	2	3	4	5	6	7

28. Deep inside myself

I do not feel loved						I feel loved
1	2	3	4	5	6	7

29. I worry about the future

never						all the time
1	2	3	4	5	6	7

30. When I think about the problems that I have

I do not feel hopeful about solving them						I feel very hopeful about solving them
1	2	3	4	5	6	7

*The definition of work is not limited to income-producing jobs. It includes childcare, housework, studies, and volunteer services.

Bibliography

American Psychological Association (1994). *Publication Manual of the American Psychological Association* (4th ed.). Washington, DC: American Psychological Association.

Anderson, S. E. H. (1995). Personality, appraisal, and adaptational outcomes in HIV seropositive men and women. *Research in Nursing & Health, 18,* 303–312.

Aroian, K. (under review). Development and psychometric evaluation of the Demands of Immigration Scale. *Research in Nursing and Health.*

Asher, A. B. (1983). *Causal modeling* (2nd ed.). Sage University Papers: Quantitative applications in the social sciences series, 3. Newbury Park, CA: Sage Publications.

Barnett, V., & Lewis, T. (1985). *Outliers in statistical data* (2nd ed.). New York: John Wiley & Sons.

Bentler, P. M. (1992). *EQS structural equations program manual.* Los Angeles, CA: BMDP Statistical Software.

Bentler, P. M., & Bonnett, D. G. (1980). Significance tests and goodness of fit in the analysis of covariance structures. *Psychological Bulletin, 88,* 588–606.

Berry, G. (1986). Statistical significance and confidence intervals. *Medical Journal of Australia, 144,* 618–619.

Bollen, K. A. (1989). *Structural equations with latent variables.* New York, NY: John Wiley & Sons.

Bollen, K. A., & Long, J. S. (1993). Introduction. In K. A. Bollen & J. S. Long (Eds.), *Testing structural equation models* (pp. 1–9). Thousand Oaks, CA: SAGE Publications.

Braitman, L. E. (1988). Confidence intervals extract clinically useful information from data. *Annals of Internal Medicine, 108,* 296–298.

Braitman, L. E. (1991). Confidence intervals assess both clinical significance and statistical significance. *Annals of Internal Medicine, 114,* 515–517.

Bray, J. H., & Maxwell, S. E. (1985). *Multivariate analysis of variance.* Series: Quantitative applications in the social sciences 54. Newbury Park, CA: Sage Publications.

Broom, B. L. (1994). Impact of marital quality and psychological well-being on parental sensitivity. *Nursing Research, 43*(3), 138–143.

Brooten, D. *Early hospital discharge and nurse specialist followup.* Program Grant, funded by the National Center for Nursing Research, PO1-NR1859.

Brooten, D. (PI). *Nurse home care for high risk pregnant women: Outcomes and cost.* Grant funded by National Institute for Nursing Research, NR-02867.

Brooten, D., Munro, B. H., Roncoli, M., Arnold, L., Brown, L. P., York, R., Hollingsworth A., Cohen, S. M., & Rubin, M. (1989). Developing a program grant for use in model testing. *Nursing & Health Care, 10,* 314–318.

Brooten, D., Naylor, M., York, R., Brown, L., Roncoli, M., Hollingsworth, A., Cohen, S., Arnold, L., Finkler, S., Munro, B., & Jacobsen, B. (1995). Effects of nurse specialist transitional care on patient outcomes and cost: Results of five randomized trials. *The American Journal of Managed Care, 1*(1), 45–51.

Brown, J. S., Tanner, C. A., & Padrick, K. P. (1984). Nursing's search for scientific knowledge. *Nursing Research, 33,* 26–32.

Burns, N., & Grove, S. K. (1987). *The practice of nursing research: Conduct, critique and utilization.* Philadelphia: W.B. Saunders.

Burroughs, A. K., Asonye, U. O., Anderson-Shanklin, G. C., & Vidyasagar, D. (1978). The effect of nonnutritive sucking on transcutaneous oxygen tension in noncrying, preterm neonates. *Research in Nursing and Health, 1,* 69–75.

Byrne, B. B. (1994). *Structural equation modeling with EQS and EQS/Windows: Basic concepts, applications, and programming.* Thousand Oaks, CA: SAGE Publications.

Byrne, B. B. (1995). One application of structural equation modeling from two perspectives: Exploring the EQS and LISREL strategies. In R. H. Hoyle *Structural equation modeling: Concepts, issues, and applications* (pp. 138–157). Thousand Oaks, CA: SAGE Publications.

Carmines, E. G., & McIver, J. P. (1983). An introduction of the analysis of models with unobserved variables. *Political Methodology, 9,* 51–102.

Carnap, R. (1953). What is probability? *Scientific American, 189,* 128–138.

Champion, V. (1995). Development of a benefits and barriers scale for mammography utilization. *Cancer Nursing, 18*(1), 53–59.

Champion, V., & Scott, C. (1993). Effects of a procedural/belief intervention on breast self-examination performance. *Research in Nursing & Health, 16*(3), 163–170.

Chatfield, C. (1988). *Problem solving: A statistician's guide.* London: Chapman and Hall.

Child, D. (1990). *The essentials of factor analysis* (2nd ed.). London: Holt, Rinehart, & Winston.

Chou, C-P., & Bentler, P. M. (1995). Estimates and tests in structural equation modeling. In R. H. Hoyle (Ed.), *Structural equation modeling: Concepts, issues, and applications* (pp. 37–55). Thousand Oaks, CA: SAGE Publications.

Cleveland, W. S. (1985). *The elements of graphing data.* Belmont, CA: Wadsworth.

Clinton, J. (1982). Ethnicity: The development of an empirical construct for cross-cultural health research. *Western Journal of Nursing Research, 4*(3), 281–300.

Cohen, J. (1983). The cost of dichotomization. *Applied Psychological Measurement, 7,* 249–253.

Cohen, J. (1987). *Statistical power analysis for the behavioral sciences* (rev. ed.) Hillsdale, NJ: Lawrence Erlbaum Associates.

Cohen, J. (1990). Things I have learned (so far). *American Psychologist, 45,* 1304–1312.

Cole, F. L., & Slocumb, E. M. (1995). Factors influencing safer sexual behaviors in heterosexual late adolescent and young adult collegiate males. *Image, 27*(3), 217–223.

Confidence Interval Analysis (CIA). IBM compatible microcomputer program available from Annals of Internal Medicine, Sixth Street at Race, Philadelphia, PA 19106-1657.

Craney, J. M., Hart, E. K., & Munro, B. H. (1992). A comparison of two techniques of care for indwelling arterial introducers after coronary angioplasty. *Journal of Cardiovascular Nursing, 7*(1), 50–55.

Daniel, W. W. (1987). *Biostatistics: A foundation for analysis in the health sciences* (4th ed.). New York: John Wiley & Sons.

Derdiarian, A. K., & Lewis, S. (1986). The D-L test of agreement: A stronger measure of interrater reliability. *Nursing Research, 35,* 375–378.

Dixon, J. K., Dixon, J. P., & Hickey, M. (1993). Energy as a central factor in the self-assessment of health. *Advances in Nursing Science, 15*(4), 1–12.

Dixon, J. K., Dixon, J. P., Spinner, J., Sexton, D., & Perry, C. K. (1991). Psychometric and descriptive perspectives of illness impact over the lifespan. *Nursing Research, 40,* 51–56.

Dixon, J. P., Hickey, M., & Dixon, J. K. (1992). A causal model of the way emotions intervene between creative intelligence and conventional skills. *New Ideas in Psychology, 10,* 233–251.

Duffy, M. E. (1993). Determinants of health-promoting lifestyles in older persons. *Image, 25*(1), 23–28.

Duncan, O. D. (1966). Path analysis: Sociological examples. *American Journal of Sociology, 72,* 1–16.

Edwards, J. N., Herman, J., Wallace, B. K., Pavy, M. D., & Harrison-Pavy, J. (1991). Comparison of patient-controlled and nurse-controlled antiemetic therapy in patients receiving chemotherapy. *Research in Nursing & Health, 14*(4), 249–257.

Ehrenberg, A. S. C. (1977). Rudiments of numeracy. *Journal of the Royal Statistical Society A, 140*(part 3), 277–297.

Evans, L. (PI). *Reducing restraints in nursing homes: A clinical trial.* Funded by the National Institute for Nursing Research, RO1-AG-08324.

Ferguson, D. A., & Horwood, L. J. (1984). Life events and depression in women: A structural equation model. *Psychological Medicine, 14,* 881–889.

Ferketich, S., & Muller, M. (1990). Factor analysis revisited. *Nursing Research, 39,* 59–62.

Figueredo, A. J., Ferketich, S. L., & Knapp, T. R. (1991). More on MTMM: The role of confirmatory factor analysis. *Research in Nursing and Health, 14,* 387–391.

Fink, S. V. (1995). The influence of family resources and family demands on the strains and well-being of caregiving families. *Nursing Research, 44,* 139–146.

Finn, J. D., & Mattsson, I. (1978). *Multivariate analysis in educational research—Applications of the multivariance program.* Chicago: National Educational Resources.

Fishbein, M., & Ajzen, I. (1975). *Belief, attitude, intention, and behavior: An introduction to theory and research.* Reading, MA: Addison-Wesley.

Fisher, R. A. (1970). *Statistical methods for research workers* (14th ed.). Darien, CT: Hafner Publishing.

Fletcher, R. H., & Fletcher, S. W. (1979). Clinical research in general medical journals: A 30-year perspective. *New England Journal of Medicine, 301,* 180–183.

Fleury, J. (1994). The index of readiness: Development and psychometric analysis. *Journal of Nursing Measurement, 2*(2), 143–154.

Folkman, S., & Lazarus, R. S. (1988). *Manual for the ways of coping questionnaire.* Palo Alto, CA: Consulting Psychologists Press.

Fox, J. (1984). *Linear statistical models and related methods with applications to social research.* New York: John Wiley & Sons.

Freedman, D., Pisani, R., Purves, R., & Adhikari, A. (1991). *Statistics* (2nd ed.). New York: W. W. Norton.

Freund, J. E. (1988). *Modern elementary statistics* (7th ed.). Englewood Cliffs, NJ: Prentice-Hall.

Friedman, M. M., & King, K. B. (1994). The relationship of emotional and tangible support to psychological well-being among older women with heart failure. *Research in Nursing & Health, 17,* 433–440.

Gardner, P. L. (1975). Scales and statistics. *Review of Educational Research, 45,* 43–57.

Glass, G. V., & Stanley, J. C. (1970). *Statistical methods in education and psychology.* Englewood Cliffs, NJ: Prentice-Hall.

Goodwin, L. D., & Goodwin, W. L. (1991). Estimating construct validity. *Research in Nursing and Health, 14,* 235–243.

Gould, S. J. (1985). The median isn't the message. *Discover, 6,* 40–42.

Gulick, E. E. (1989). Model confirmation of the MS-related symptom checklist. *Nursing Research, 38,* 147–153.

Hackett, T. P., & Cassem, N. H. (1969). Factors contributing to delay in responding to the signs and symptoms of acute myocardial infarction. *American Journal of Cardiology, 24,* 651–658.

Hald, A. (1952). *Statistical tables and formulas.* New York: John Wiley & Sons.

Hanley, J. A., & Lippman-Hand, A. (1983). If nothing goes wrong, is everything all right? Interpreting zero numerators. *Journal of the American Medical Association, 249,* 1743–1745.

Hayduk, L. A. (1987). *Structural equation modeling with LISREL: Essentials and advances.* Baltimore, MD: The Johns Hopkins University Press.

Hahn, G. J., & Meeker, W. Q. (1991). *Statistical intervals—A guide for practitioners.* New York: John Wiley & Sons.

Hald, A. (1952). *Statistical tables and formulas.* New York: John Wiley & Sons.

Heise, D. R. (1969). Problems in path analysis and causal inference. In E. F. Borgatta & G. W. Bohrnstedt (Eds.), *Sociology methodology 1969.* San Francisco, CA: Jossey-Bass.

Hildebrand, D. K. (1986). *Statistical thinking for behavioral scientists.* Boston: Duxbury Press.

Hinkle, D. E., Wiersma, W., & Jurs, S. G. (1994). *Applied statistics for the behavioral sciences* (3rd ed.). Boston: Houghton Mifflin.

Holm, K., & Christman, N. J. (1985). Post hoc tests following analysis of variance. *Research in Nursing and Health, 8,* 207–210.

Hoshowsky, V. M., & Schramm, C. A. (1994). Intraoperative pressure sore prevention: An analysis of bedding materials. *Research in Nursing & Health, 17,* 333–339.

Hosmer, D. W., & Lemeshow, S. (1989). *Applied logistic regression.* New York: John Wiley & Sons.

Hoyle, R. H. (Ed.) (1995). *Structural equation modeling: Concepts, issues, and applications.* Thousand Oaks, CA: SAGE Publications.

Hoyle, R. H., & Panter, A. T. (1995). Writing about structural equation models. In R. H. Hoyle (Ed.), *Structural equation modeling: Concepts, issues, and applications* (pp. 158–176). Thousand Oaks, CA: SAGE Publications.

Hu, L-T., & Bentler, P. M. (1995). Evaluating model fit. In R. H. Hoyle (Ed.), *Structural equation modeling: Concepts, issues, and applications* (pp. 76–99). Thousand Oaks, CA: SAGE Publications.

Jacobsen, B. S. (1981). Know thy data. *Nursing Research, 30,* 254–255.

Jacobsen, B. S., & Lowery, B. J. (1992). Further analysis of the psychometric properties of the Levine Denial of Illness Scale. *Psychosomatic Medicine, 54,* 372–381.

Jacobsen, B. S., & Meininger, J. C. (1985). The designs and methods of published nursing research: 1956–1983. *Nursing Research, 34,* 306–312.

Jacobsen, B. S., Munro, B. H., & Brooten, D. A. (1996). Comparison of original and revised scoring systems for the Multiple Affect Adjective Checklist, *Nursing Research, 45*(1), 57–60.

Janz, N., & Becker, M. (1984). The Health Belief Model: A decade later. *Health Education Quarterly, 11,* 1–47.

Jöreskog, K. G. (1993). Testing structural equation models. In K. A. Bollen & J. S. Long (Eds.), *Testing structural equation models* (pp. 294–316). Thousand Oaks, CA: SAGE Publications.

Jöreskog, K. G., & Sörbom, D. (1988). *LISREL 7: A guide to the program and applications.* Chicago: SPSS.

Jöreskog, K. G., & Sörbom, D. (1989). *LISREL 7: A guide to the program and applications* (2nd ed.). Chicago: SPSS.

Kalisch, B. J., Kalisch, P. A., & McHugh, M. L. (1982). The nurse as a sex object in motion pictures, 1930–1980. *Research in Nursing and Health, 5*(3), 147–154.

Kaplan, D. (1995). Statistical power in structural equation modeling. In R. H. Hoyle (Ed.), *Structural equation modeling: Concepts, issues, and applications.* Thousand Oaks, CA: Sage Publications.

Kaplan, D., & Wenger, R. N. (1993). Asymptotic independence and separability in covariance structure models. *Multivariate Behavioral Research, 28,* 483–498.

Kass, J. D., Friedman, R., Leserman, J., Caudill, M., Zuttermeister, P. C., & Benson, H. (1991). An inventory of positive psychological attitudes with potential relevance to health outcomes: Validation and preliminary testing. *Behavioral Medicine, Fall,* 121–129.

Kenny, D. (1979). *Correlation and causality.* New York: John Wiley & Sons.

Ketterlinus, R. D., Henderson, S. H., & Lamb, M. E. (1990). Maternal age, sociodemographics, prenatal health and behavior: Influences on neonatal risk status. *Journal of Adolescent Health Care, 11*(5), 423–431.

Klockars, A. J., & Sax, G. (1986). *Multiple Comparisons Series: Quantitative Applications in the Social Sciences,* 61. Newbury Park, CA: Sage Publications.

Knapp, T. R. (1990). Treating ordinal scales as interval scales: An attempt to resolve the controversy. *Nursing Research, 39,* 121–123.

Knapp, T. R., & Brown, J. K. (1995). Ten measurement commandments that often should be broken. *Research in Nursing & Health, 18,* 465–469.

Koopmans, L. H. (1987). *Introduction to contemporary statistics* (2nd ed.). Boston: Duxbury Press.

Kotz, S., & Stroup, D. F. (1983). *Educated guessing: How to cope in an uncertain world.* New York: Marcel Dekker.

LaMonica, E. L., Oberst, M. T., Madea, A. R., & Wolf, R. M. (1986). Development of a patient satisfaction scale. *Research in Nursing & Health, 9,* 43–50.

Last, J. M. (Ed.) (1983). *A dictionary of epidemiology.* New York: Oxford.

Lauter, E., Lauter, H., & Schmidtke, D. (1978). Properties and comparison of procedures of discriminant analysis. *Biometrika Journal, 20*(4), 407–424.

Lee, H. J. (1991). Relationship of hardiness and current life events to perceived health in rural adults. *Research in Nursing and Health, 14*(5), 351–359.

Lentner, C. (Ed.) (1982). *Geigy scientific tables,* Vol. 2 (pp. 89–102). Basel: CIBA-Geigy.

Lewis-Beck, M. S. (1980). Applied regression: An introduction. In *Quantitative applications in the social sciences,* 22. Newbury Park, CA: Sage Publications.

Long, J. S. (1983). Confirmatory factor analysis. *Quantitative applications in the social sciences,* 33. Newbury Park, CA: Sage Publications.

Lowery, B. J., Jacobsen, B. S., & Ducette, J. (1992). Causal attributions, control, and adjustment to breast cancer. *Psychosocial Oncology, 10*(4).

Lybrand, M., Medoff-Cooper, B., & Munro, B. H. (1990). Periodic comparisons of specific gravity using urine from a diaper and collecting bag. *The American Journal of Maternal/Child Nursing (MCN), 15*(4), 238–239.

MacCallum, R. C., Browne, M. W., & Sugawara, H. M. (1996). Power analysis and determination of sample size for covariance structure modeling. *Psychological Methods, 1,* 130–149.

McCain, G. C. (1992). Facilitating inactive awake states in preterm infants: A study of three interventions. *Nursing Research, 41*(3), 157–160.

McGovern, P. G., Pankow, J. S., Shahar, E., Doliszny, K. M., Folsom, A. R., Blackburn, H., & Luepker, R. V. (1996). Recent trends in acute coronary heart disease. *New England Journal of Medicine, 34*(14), 887.

Meininger, J. C. (1985). The validity of Type A behavior scales for employed women. *Journal of Chronic Diseases, 38,* 375–383.

Moore, D. S. (1991). *Statistics: Concepts and controversies* (3rd ed.). New York: W. H. Freeman.

Munro, B. H. (1990). Testing for interactions: The analysis of variance model. *Clinical Nurse Specialist, 4*(3), 128–129.

Munro, B. H., Jacobsen, B. S., & Brooten, D. A. (1994). Re-examination of the Psychometric characteristics of the La Monica-Oberst Patient Satisfaction Scale. *Research in Nursing & Health, 17,* 119–125..

Muthén, B. O. (1993). Goodness of fit with categorical and other non-normal variables. In K. A. Bollen & J. S. Long (Eds.). *Testing structural equation models* (pp. 205–234). Thousand Oaks, CA: SAGE Publications.

Naylor, M. (PI) *Comprehensive discharge planning for the elderly.* Grant funded by the National Institute for Nursing Research, NR-02095-07.

Norris, A. E., & Devine, P. G. (1992). Linking pregnancy concerns to pregnancy risk avoidant action: The role of construct accessibility. *Personality and Social Psychology Bulletin, 18,* 118–192.

Norris, A. E., & Ford, K. (1995). Condom use by low-income African American and Hispanic youth with a well-known partner: Integrating the Health Belief Model, Theory of Reasoned Action, and Construct Accessibility Model. *Journal of Applied Social Psychology, 25,* 1801–1830.

Norusis, M. J. (1994). *SPSS for Windows 6.1 advanced statistics.* Chicago,IL: SPSS.

Norusis, M. J. (1996a). *SPSS Base 7.0 applications guide.* Chicago, IL: SPSS.

Norusis, M. J. (1996b). *SPSS Base 7.0 for Windows User's Guide.* Chicago, IL: SPSS.

Nunnally, J. C., & Bernstein, I. H. (1994). *Psychometric theory* (3rd ed.). New York: McGraw-Hill.

Olson, C. L. (1974). Comparative robustness of six tests of multivariate analysis of variance. *Journal of the American Statistical Association, 69,* 894–908.

Ott, L., & Mendenhall, W. (1990). *Understanding statistics* (5th ed.). Boston: PWS-Kent Publishing.

Pedhazur, E. J. (1982). *Multiple regression in behavioral research, explanation and prediction* (2nd ed.). New York: Holt, Rinehart & Winston.

Pedhazur, E. J., & Schmelkin, L. P. (1991). *Measurement, design, and analysis an integrated approach.* Hillsdale, NJ: Lawrence Erlbaum Assoc.

Pender, N. J. (1987). *Health promotion in nursing practice* (2nd ed.). Norwalk, CT: Appleton & Lange.

Picot, S. J. (1995). Rewards, costs, and coping of African American Caregivers. *Nursing Research, 44*(3), 147–152.

Pollock, S. E., Christian, B. J., & Sands, D. (1990). Responses to chronic illness: Analysis of psychological and physiological adaptation. *Nursing Research, 39*(5), 300–304.

Powell, R. W., McSweeney, M. B., & Wilson, C. E. (1983). X-ray calcifications as the only basis for breast biopsy. *Annals of Surgery, 197,* 555–559.

Quayhagen, M. P., Quayhagen, M., Corbeil, R. R., Roth, P. A., & Rodgers, J. A. (1995). A dyadic remediation program for care recipients with dementia. *Nursing Research, 44*(3), 153–159.

Remington, R. D., & Schork, M. A. (1970). *Statistics with application to the biological and health sciences.* Englewood Cliffs, NJ: Prentice-Hall.

Riegelman, R. K. (1981). *Studying a study and testing a test: How to read the medical literature.* Boston: Little, Brown, & Company.

Rigdon, E. E. (1994). Demonstrating the effects of unmodeled random measurement error. *Structural Equation Modeling, 1,* 375–380.

Robinson, J. H. (1995). Grief responses, coping processes, and social support of widows: Research with Roy's model. *Nursing Science Quarterly, 8,* 158–164.

Rothman, K. J. (1986). *Modern epidemiology.* Boston: Little, Brown, & Company.

Saris, W. E., & Satorra, A. (1993). Power evaluations in structural equation models. In K. A. Bollen & J. S. Long (Eds.), *Testing structural equation models* (pp. 181–204). Thousand Oaks, CA: SAGE Publications.

Schafer, R. B., Keith, P. M., & Schafer, E. (1995). Predicting fat in diets of marital partners using the Health Belief Model. *Journal of Behavioral Medicine, 18,* 419–432.

Schmid, C. F. (1983). *Statistical graphics: Design principles and practices.* New York: John Wiley & Son.

Schroeder, M. A. (1990). Diagnosing and dealing with multicollinearity. *Western Journal of Nursing Research, 12*(2), 175–187.

Skinner, B. F. (1972). *Cumulative record: A selection of papers* (3rd ed.). New York: Appleton-Century-Crofts, Meredith Corporation.

Snedecor, G. W. (1938). *Statistical methods.* Ames, IA: Collegiate Press.

Spielberger, C. D. (1983). *Manual for the State-Trait anxiety inventory.* Palo Alto, CA: Consulting Psychologists Press.

SPSS, Inc. (1996). *SPSS Advanced Statistics 7.0 Update.* Chicago, IL: SPSS.

Stevens, S. S. (1946). On the theory of scales of measurement. *Science, 102,* 677–680.

Stevens, S. S. (1968). Measurement, statistics, and the schemapiric view. *Science, 161,* 849–856.

Stommel, M., Wang, S., Given, C. W., & Given, B. (1992). Confirmatory factor analysis (CFA) as a method to assess measurement equivalence. *Research in Nursing & Health, 15,* 399–405.

Sulzbach, L. M., Munro, B. H., & Hirshfeld, Jr., J. W. (1995). A randomized clinical trial of the effect of bed position after PTCA. *American Journal of Critical Care, 4*(3), 221–226.

Tabachnick, B. G., & Fidell, L. S. (1996). *Using multivariate statistics* (3rd ed.). New York: HarperCollins College Publishers.

Tappen, R. M. (1994). The effect of skill training on functional abilities of nursing home residents with dementia. *Research in Nursing & Health, 17,* 159–165.

Teel, C., & Verran, J. A. (1991). Focus on psychometrics: Factor comparisons across studies. *Research in Nursing and Health, 14,* 67–72.

Thorndike, R. M. (1988). Correlational procedures. In J. P. Keeves (Ed.), *Educational research, methodology, and measurement: An international handbook.* New York: Pergamon Press.

Thurstone, L. L. (1947). *Multiple-factor analysis.* Chicago: University of Chicago Press.

Toothaker, L. E. (1993). *Multiple comparison procedures.* Series: Quantitative Applications in the Social Sciences, #89, Newbury Park, CA: Sage Publications.

Tucker, L. A., & Maxwell, K. (1992). Effects of weight training on the emotional well-being and body image of females: predictors of greatest benefit. *American Journal of Health Promotion, 6,* 338–344.

Tufte, E. R. (1983). *The visual display of quantitative information.* Cheshire, CT: Graphics Press.

Tukey, J. W. (1977). *Exploratory data analysis.* Reading, MA: Addison-Wesley.

Tulman, L. R., & Jacobsen, B. S. (1989). Goldilocks and variability. *Nursing Research, 38,* 377–379.

Verran, J. A., & Ferketich, S. L. (1987). Testing linear model assumptions: Residual analysis. *Nursing Research, 36*(2), 127–129.

Vessey, J. A., Carlson, K. L., & McGill, J. (1994). Use of distraction with children during an acute pain experience. *Nursing Research, 43*(6), 369–372.

Von Eye, A., & Clogg, C. (Eds.) (1994). *Latent variables analysis: applications for developmental research.* Thousand Oaks, CA: SAGE Publications.

Wainer, H., & Thissen, D. (1981). Graphical data analysis. *Annual Review of Psychology, 32,* 191–241.

Watters, N. E., & Kristiansen, C. M. (1995). Two evaluations of combined mother-infant versus separate postnatal nursing care. *Research in Nursing & Health, 18,* 17–26.

Weisberg, H. F. (1992). *Central tendency and variability,* Series: Quantitative Applications in the Social Sciences, No. 83. Newbury Park, CA: Sage Publications.

West, S. G., Finch, J. F., & Curran, P. J. (1995). Structural equation models with non-normal variables: Problems and remedies. In R. H. Hoyle (Ed.), *Structural equation modeling: Concepts, issues, and applications* (pp. 56–75). Thousand Oaks, CA: SAGE Publications.

Wikoff, R. L., & Miller, P. (1991). Canonical analysis in nursing research. Methodology Corner. *Nursing Research, 40*(6), 367–370.

Williams, M. A., Oberst, M. T., & Bjorklund, B. C. (1994). Early outcomes after hip fracture among women discharged home and to nursing homes. *Research in Nursing & Health, 17*(3), 175–183.

Wineman, N. M., Durand, J., & McCulloch, B. J. (1994). Examination of the factor structure of the ways of coping questionnaire with clinical populations. *Nursing Research, 43*(5), 268–273.

Winer, B. J. (1971). *Statistical principles in experimental design* (2nd ed.). New York: McGraw-Hill.

Winkelstein, M. L., & Feldman, R. H. L. (1993). Psychosocial predictors of consumption of sweets following smoking cessation. *Research in Nursing & Health, 16,* 97–105.

Wonnacott, R. J., & Wonnacott, T. H. (1985). *Introductory statistics* (4th ed.). New York: John Wiley & Son.

Wright, S. (1934). The method of path coefficients. *Annals of Mathematical Statistics, 5,* 161–215.

Wu, Y. B., & Slakter, M. J. (1990). Increasing the precision of data analysis: Planned comparisons versus omnibus tests. Methodology Corner. *Nursing Research, 39*(4), 251–253.

Youngblut, J. M. (1993). Comparison of factor analysis options using the home/ employment orientation scale. *Nursing Research, 42*(2), 122–124.

Youngblut, J. M., Loveland-Cherry, C. J., & Horan, M. (1994). Maternal employment effects on family and preterm infants at 18 months. *Nursing Research, 43*(6), 331–337.

Yoder, M. E. (1994). Preferred learning style and educational technology. *Nursing & Health Care, 15*(3), 128–132.

Index

Page numbers followed by *f* refer to figures; page numbers followed by *t* refer to tables.

A

Addition rule, in probability, 67–68
ANCOVA. *See* Covariance, analysis of
ANOVA
    multifactorial. *See* Variance, multifactorial analysis
        of one-way. *See* Variance, one-way analy-
        sis of
A priori contrasts, in one-way analysis of variance,
    154–155, 155*f*–157*f*
Assumption of homoscedasticity, 247, 271*t*–272*t*,
    271–272
Assumptions, testing of, by analyzing residuals,
    270*f*–271*f*, 270–273

B

Backward solution, in selection of variables, in re-
    gression, 267
Bar graphs, 10–11, 11*f*–12*f*
Bell-shaped curve, 53–55, 54*f*
Between-group variation, 142, 142*f*
    sum of squares for, 145–148, 146*t*–147*t*
Between-subjects effects, in repeated measures
    analysis of variance, 206, 208*f*–209*f*
Boston College School of Nursing survey, 421*t*–425*t*

Box plots, 46, 47*f*–48*f*
Box's Test of Equality of Covariance Matrices, 206,
    208*f*
b-weights, in logistic regression, 300–301

C

Canonical correlation, 274–281, 276*f*–279*f*
    computer-assisted, 275, 276*f*–279*f*
    example of, 279, 280*t*, 281
Canonical variates, 274
Canonical weights, 274
Causation
    in path analysis, 345–346
    in structural equation modeling, 380
Central limit theorem, 58–60
Central tendency, measures of, 31–36, 32*t*, 35*f*
    comparison of, 34, 35*f*
    mean as, 31–33, 32*t*
    median as, 33, 35*f*
    mode as, 34, 35*f*
Chi-square, 100–109, 101*t*, 103*f*–105*f*, 107*t*–108*t*
    assumptions underlying, 101–102
    calculation of, 108
    computer analysis using, 103*f*–104*f*, 103–104
        output from, 104*f*–105*f*, 104–107

Chi-square (*continued*)
  continuity correction in, 105*f,* 106
  Cramer's V in, 105*f,* 107
  data required for, 101, 101*t*
  degrees of freedom in, 105*f,* 106
  Fisher's exact test in, 105*f,* 106
  likelihood ratio in, 105*f,* 106
  linear-by-linear association in, 106–107
  in logistic regression, 295, 300
  nested, 377, 378*t*
  phi in, 105*f,* 107
  power analysis in, 107, 107*t*
  power in, 102
  relative, 377, 396*t*
  research questions for, 100
  sample size for, 102
  Yates' correction in, 105*f,* 106
CI. *See* Confidence interval (CI)
Cluster bar graphs, 10, 12*f*
Coding, 259–265, 260*t*–264*t*
  contrasts in, 263, 263*t*
  dummy, 260*t,* 260–261
  effect, 261*t,* 261–262
  of interactions, 264*f,* 264*t,* 264–265
  for logistic regression, 294–295
  orthogonal, 262*t,* 262–263, 263*t*
Coefficient of determination, 235–236
Coefficients
  correlation. *See* Correlation coefficient (*r*)
  in discriminant function analysis, 289
  in structural equation modeling, 376–377
Collinearity, in regression, 268, 269*f*
Comparative fit index, in structural equation model-
    ing, 377
Compound paths, identification of, in path analysis,
    353–354
Compound symmetry, in repeated measures analy-
    sis of variance, 207
Conditional probability, 65, 66*t*
Confidence intervals (CIs), 73–75
  in correlation coefficient, 236–237
  of differences between percentages, 90–93, 92*f*
  hypothesis testing and, 92
  information provided by, 94–96
  interpretation of, 93–94
  for percentages, 85–86
    assumptions underlying, 86–87
  and random sampling, 88
  in regression, 254

and tests of significance, 75–77, 77*f*
  value of, 77
Confirmatory factor analysis, 332–337, 336*t,*
    337*f*–338*f*
  in structural equation modeling, 383–386, 384*f,*
    385*t*
Consistency, checks on, 77
Continuity correction, in chi-square, 105*f,* 106
Contrasts, in coding, 263, 263*t*
Control, partial correlation for, 239–240
Correlated *t* tests, 131, 132*f*
Correlation
  among variables, in path analysis, 356*t*
  assumptions underlying, 226–227, 227*f*
  canonical, 274–281, 276*f*–279*f*
    computer-assisted, 275, 276*f*–279*f*
    example of, 279, 280*t,* 281
  data required for, 225–226, 226*t*
  example of, 242, 243*t*
  linear and nonlinear relationships in, 227*f*
  multiple, 241–242
  partial, 239–240
  power in, 227–228
  research questions for, 224–225
  semipartial, 240–241
Correlation coefficient (*r*), 228*t,* 228–237, 229*f*–235*f,*
    231*t*–234*t*
  analysis of, computer-assisted, 229, 230*f,* 231
  confidence intervals in, 236–237
  critical values of, 417*t*–418*t*
  estimation of, 238–239
  meaningfulness of, 235–236
  no relationship in, 233, 233*f,* 234*t*
  in regression, 257, 257*f*
  relationships measured with, 231*t,* 231–233,
    232*f*–233*f,* 233*t*–234*t*
    perfect negative, 233, 233*f,* 233*t*
    perfect positive, 231*t,* 231–232, 232*f*
  short-cut versions of, 237–238
  significance of, 235
  strength of, 234–235
Correlation matrix
  in factor analysis, 318
  6 x 6, 312, 312*t*
Correlation ratio (eta), 239
Covariance, analysis of, 188–198
  assumptions underlying, 190–192, 191*f*–192*f*
  computer-assisted, 193–194, 195*f*–197*f*
  data required for, 190

example of, 198, 198*t*
and one-time analysis of variance, 192–193
power of, 193
research questions for, 189–190
Cramer's V, in chi-square, 105*f*, 107
Curves, normal, 53–55, 54*f*
tests of significance using, 71, 72*f*
between *z* scores and mean, 407*f*–408*f*

D

Data
organization of, 3–21
transformation of, for correction of failures in
normality, 58
Data reduction, in factor analysis, 315–316
Degrees of freedom (*df*), 72–73
in chi-square, 105*f*, 106
in one-way analysis of variance, 148–149
in regression, 255
Dependence, vs. independence, in probability, 67
Dependent variable
in multivariate analysis of variance, 170
in one-way analysis of variance, 140
in t tests, 125
Descriptive statistics
graphs using, 43–46, 44*f*–45*f*
measurement of variability/scatter as, 36*f*, 36–41,
37*t*–38*t*, 40*t*
measures of central tendency as, 31–36, 32*t*, 35*f*
measures of kurtosis/peakedness as, 42–43
measures of skewness/symmetry as, 41*f*, 41–42
outliers in, 46, 47*f*–48*f*
rounding of, for tables, 43
df. See Degrees of freedom (*df*)
Dichotomized variables, estimation of correlation
coefficient with, 238–239
Differences among means, Tukey's test of, 116*t*
Discriminant function analysis, 288–289, 290*f*, 291
Dummy coding, 260*t*, 260–261

E

Effect coding, 261*t*, 261–262
Effect sizes, 69, 107, 107*t*

Eigenvalue, in factor analysis, 319
Endogenous variables, in path analysis, 349*f*,
349–350
Equamax, 323
Estimates, 73–78, 77*f*
confidence intervals in, 73–75
point, 73–75
Eta (correlation ratio), 239
Exogenous variables, in path analysis, 349*f*,
349–350
Extraction models, in unrotated factor matrix,
320–321

F

F, distribution of, 255, 413*t*–416*t*
Factor analysis, 310–338
assumptions underlying, 316–317
computer-assisted, 325, 326*f*–327*f*, 328–329
confirmatory, 332–337, 336*t*, 337*f*–338*f*
in structural equation modeling, 383–386, 384*f*,
385*t*
data reduction in, 315–316
data required for, 316
eigenvalue in, 319
instrument development in, 314–315
matrices in, 317–324, 319*t*, 323*t*–324*t*
correlation, 318
factor correlation, 323–324, 324*t*
factor score, 322–324, 323*t*–324*t*
raw data, 318
rotated factor, 321–322
unrotated factor, 318–321, 319*t*
with other statistical methods, 325
power in, 317
presentation of data from, 329–332, 331*t*
research questions for, 311–313, 312*t*–313*t*
sample size for, 317
steps in, 324
theory development in, 315
types of, 313–314
Factor correlation matrix, in factor analysis,
323–324, 324*t*
Factor score matrix, in factor analysis, 322–324,
323*t*–324*t*
False null hypothesis, 69
Fisher's exact test, in chi-square, 105*f*, 106

Fisher's measure of kurtosis, 42–43

Fisher's measure of skewness, 42

Fixed parameters, in structural equation modeling, 376–377

Forward solution, in selection of variables, in regression, 266–267

Free parameters, in structural equation modeling, 377

Frequency distribution
in histograms, 17, 19*f*
in tables, 6–8, 7*t*–10*t*

Frequency probability, 62–64, 64*t*

Friedman matched samples, 113–116, 114*f*

G

Goodness of fit
in logistic regression, 295
in structural equation modeling, 377, 386–393, 387*f*–390*f*, 388*t*–393*t*

Graphs, 9–21, 11*f*–20*f*
advantages of, 9
bar, 10–11, 11*f*–12*f*
construction of, guidelines for, 19–21
histogram, 11–14, 13*f*–15*f*
line, 43, 44*f*–45*f*
polygons, 14, 16, 16*f*–17*f*
using descriptive statistics, 43–46, 44*f*–45*f*

Greater mean square, 255

Groups, homogeneity of regression across, 191–192, 192*f*

H

Histograms, 11–14, 13*f*–15*f*
frequency distribution in, 17, 19*f*
produced by SPSS, 18*f*
use of, 16–19, 18*f*–20*f*

Homogeneity of regression across groups, 191–192, 192*f*

Homoscedasticity, assumption of, 247, 271*t*–272*t*, 271–272

Hotelling-Lawley trace, 171

Hypothesis, null, 68
false, 69

Hypothesis testing, 68–73, 71*f*–72*f*
and confidence intervals, 92
degrees of freedom in, 72–73
one-tailed, 70–72, 71*f*–72*f*
power of, 70
two-tailed, 70–72, 71*f*–72*f*
types of error in, 68–70

I

Identification
in path analysis, 350*f*–352*f*, 350–351
in structural equation modeling, 378

Independence, vs. dependence, in probability, 67

Independent variable
direct and indirect effects of, in path analysis, 351–354, 352*f*–353*f*, 359–361, 360*f*, 360*t*–361*t*
in *t* tests, 125

Indicators, in structural equation modeling, 372

Inferential statistics, 73

Interactions, coding of, 264*f*, 264*t*, 264–265

Interpercentile measures, 39–40, 40*t*

Interquantile range (IQR), 39

Interval variables, 4–5
histograms for, 11–14, 13*f*–15*f*
polygons for, 14, 16, 16*f*–17*f*
in tables, 6

IQR (interquantile range), 39

J

Just identified model, in path analysis, 350–351, 351*f*

K

Kendall's tau, 238

Kruskal-Wallis, 109–111, 111*f*, 113

Kurtosis, measures of, 42–43

L

Lagrange multiplier test, in structural equation modeling, 384–385, 385*t*, 389*t*, 391*t*, 394*t*
Lesser mean square, 255
Levene's Test for Equality of Error Variances, 128, 129*f*, 135*f*
  in repeated measures analysis of variance, 206, 208*f*
Likelihood ratio, in chi-square, 105*f*, 106
Linear-by-linear association chi-square, 106–107
Linear regression, 249–254, 250*f*–251*f*, 253*f*
Line graphs, 43, 44*f*–45*f*
Logistic regression, 287–304. *See also* Regression, logistic
-2 log likelihood, in coding for logistic regression, 295

M

Manifest variables, in structural equation modeling, 372–373
Mann-Whitney U, 109–111, 111*f*–112*f*, 113*t*
MANOVA. *See* Variance, multivariate analysis of
Matrices, in factor analysis, 317–324, 319*t*, 323*t*–324*t*. *See also* Factor analysis, matrices in
Mauchly's test of sphericity, in repeated measures analysis of variance, 207, 209*f*
McNemar test, 109, 110*f*
Mean, 31–33, 32*t*
  in central limit theorem, 58–60
  differences among, Tukey's test of, 116*t*
  multiple comparisons among, in regression, 265
  standard error of, 59–60
  trimmed, 48–49
  winsorized, 49
  and *z* scores, normal curve between, 407*f*–408*f*
Mean squares, 255
Measured variables, in structural equation modeling, 372–373
Measurement scales, 3–6
  choice of, 5–6
  interval, 4–5
  nominal, 4
  ordinal, 4
  ratio, 5
Median, 33, 35*f*

Method of least squares, 252
Mixed design, in repeated measures analysis of variance, 205
Mode, 34, 35*f*
Model fit statistics, in structural equation modeling, 377–378, 378*t*
Modification indices, in structural equation modeling, 378–379
Multicollinearity, in regression, 268, 269*f*
Multiple group analysis, in structural equation modeling, 379
Multiple regression, 254–255
Multiplication rule, in probability, 66–67
Mutually exclusive events, 67

N

Negative relationship, 233, 233*f*, 233*t*
Nested chi-square, 377, 378*t*
Nomimal-level data, with dependent measures, 109, 110*f*
Nominal scales, 4
Nonparametric techniques, 99–117
  chi-square as, 100–109, 103*f*–105*f*, 107*t*–108*t*
  for nominal-level data, with dependent measures, 109, 110*f*
  for ordinal data
    with dependent groups, 113–116, 114*f*, 115*f*
    with independent groups, 109–113, 111*f*–112*f*, 113*t*
  research questions for, 99
  type of data required for, 99–100, 100*t*
  vs. parametric techniques, 99–100, 100*t*
Nonrecursive models, of path analysis, 347–348
Normal curve, 53–55, 54*f*
  tests of significance using, one-tailed, 71, 72*f*
Normality, failures in, data transformation for, 58
Null hypothesis, 68
  false, 69
  within-group variation and, 144, 144*f*

O

Odds ratios, vs. relative risk, 291*t*–294*t*, 291–293
One-tailed hypothesis testing, 70–72, 71*f*–72*f*

One-tailed probability, 68, 411*t*–412*t*

ONEWAY program, of SPSS, 150

Ordinal data
  with dependent groups, 113–116, 114*f*, 115*f*
  with independent groups, 109–113, 111*f*–112*f*, 113*t*

Ordinal scales, 4
  bar graphs for, 10, 11*f*

Orthogonal coding, 262*t*, 262–263, 263*t*

Orthogonal contrasts, in one-way analysis of variance, 154–155, 155*f*–157*f*

Outliers, in descriptive statistics, 46, 48–49

Overidentified model, in path analysis, 350*f*, 350–351

P

Paired *t* tests, 131, 132*f*

Parameters, vs. statistics, 30

Parametric techniques, vs. nonparametric techniques, 99–100, 100*t*

Path analysis, 342–365
  assumptions underlying, 344–347, 345*f*–346*f*
    statistical, 346–347
    theoretical, 344–346, 345*f*
  causation in, 345–346
  compound paths in, identification of, 353–354
  computer-assisted, 354–362, 355*t*–361*t*, 357*f*–358*f*, 360*f*
    analysis of, 358*f*, 358–361, 359*t*–361*t*, 360*f*
    preparation for, 354–357, 355*t*–356*t*, 357*f*
  data required for, 344
  direct and indirect effects in, 351–354, 352*f*–353*f*, 359–361, 360*f*, 360*t*–361*t*
  endogenous variables in, 349*f*, 349–350
  exogenous variables in, 349*f*, 349–350
  identification in, 350*f*–352*f*, 350–351
  indirect and direct effects in, 348, 348*f*–349*f*
  limitations of, 361–362, 364
  models of, recursive and nonrecursive, 347–348
  path coefficients in, 350
  power in, 347
  presentation of data from, 362*t*, 362–364, 363*f*–364*f*
  regression in, 355*f*, 357, 357*f*, 363, 363*f*
  research questions for, 342–344, 343*f*

Robinson's model of, 343, 343*f*
  variables in, 347
    correlation among, 356*t*

Path coefficients, 350
  calculation of, 358

Peakedness, measures of, 42–43

Pearson correlation coefficient. *See* Correlation coefficient (*r*)

Pearson's skewness coefficient, 42

Pearson value, 105, 105*f*

Percentages, confidence intervals for, 85–86
  assumptions underlying, 86–87
  differences between, 90–93, 92*f*

Percentiles, 55–56, 56*f*

Phi
  in chi-square, 105*f*, 107
  as measure of relationship, 237

Pillai-Bartlett trace, 171

Planned comparisons, in one-way analysis of variance, 154–155, 155*f*–157*f*

Point-biserial formula, 238

Point estimates, 73–75
  information provided by, 94–96
  uncertainty of, 85–86

Polygons, 14, 16, 16*f*–17*f*
  use of, 16–19, 17*f*

Pooled *t* test, calculation of, 133, 133*t*

Population probability, 63

Positive relationship, 231–232, 232*f*, 233*t*

Post-hoc tests, in one-way analysis of variance, 151, 153*f*, 154

Power
  analysis of, in regression, 248–249
  in chi-square, 102
  in correlation, 227–228
  in factor analysis, 317
  in logistic regression, 294
  in multivariate analysis of variance, 170
  in one-way analysis of variance, 141
  in path analysis, 347
  in repeated measures analysis of variance, 204
  in structural equation modeling, 382
  in *t* tests, 126–128, 127*t*
  in two-way analysis of variance, 165, 168–169

Power analysis, in chi-square, 107, 107*t*

Predicted probabilities, in logistic regression, 300

Prediction equation, 252–254, 253*f*

Probabilities, predicted, in logistic regression, 300

Probability, 60–68, 61*f*, 64*f*, 66*t*
  axioms about, 61*f*, 61–62, 62*t*
  conditional, 65, 66*t*
  definition of, 62–65, 64*t*
  frequency, 62–64, 64*t*
  one-tailed, 68, 411*t*–412*t*
  population, 63
  rules of, 65–68
    addition, 67–68
    multiplication, 66–67
  subjective, 64–65
  two-tailed, 67–68, 411*t*–412*t*
Proxies, in structural equation modeling, 372–373
p values, 76, 90–93, 92*f*
  information provided by, 94–96

Q

Quartiles, 55
Quartimax, 323

R

R, transformation to z$_r$, 419*t*–420*t*
r. See Correlation coefficient (*r*)
Randomization, vs. random sampling, 88–89
Random sampling, 73
  confidence intervals and, 88
  vs. randomization, 88–89
Range, 40
Ratios, odds, vs. relative risk, 291*t*–294*t*, 291–293
Ratio variables, 5
  histograms for, 11–14, 13*f*–15*f*
  polygons for, 14, 16, 16*f*–17*f*
Raw data matrix, in factor analysis, 318
Recursive models, of path analysis, 347–348
Regression
  assumptions underlying, 247–248
  coding in, 259–265, 260*t*–264*t. See also* Coding
  computer-assisted, 256–258, 257*f*–259*f*
  correlation coefficient in, 257, 257*f*
  data required for, 247
  degrees of freedom in, 255

linear, 249–254, 250*f*–251*f*, 253*f*
  confidence intervals in, 254
  prediction equation in, 252–254, 253*f*
  standard scores in, 250*f*–251*f*, 250–252
logistic, 287–304
  b-weights in, 300–301
  chi-square in, 295, 300
  computer-assisted, 294–295, 296*f*–299*f*, 300–302
    coding for, 294–295
  data required for, 294
  discriminant function analysis, 288–289, 290*f*, 291
  example of, 302–304, 305*t*
  goodness of fit in, 295
  improvement in, 300
  odds ratios in, vs. relative risk, 291*t*–294*t*, 291–293
  power in, 294
  predicted probabilities in, 300
  research questions for, 293
  variables in, 287, 300–302
multicollinearity in, 268, 269*f*
multiple, 254–255
multiple comparisons among means in, 265
in path analysis, 355*f*, 357, 357*f*, 363, 363*f*
power analysis in, 248–249
research questions for, 246–247
sample size in, 248
selection of variables in, 265–268
  example of, 271*t*, 272–273
  hierarchical, 266
  methods of entry and, 267–268
  standard, 266
  stepwise, 266–267
significance testing in, 255–256
Regression line, 252–253, 253*f*
Regression weight, 260
Relationship, measures of, 237–239. *See also* Correlation coefficient (*r*)
  universal, 239
Relative chi-square, 377, 396*t*
Relative risk, vs. odds ratios, 291*t*–294*t*, 291–293
Residuals, analysis of, testing assumptions by, 270*f*–271*f*, 270–273
Risk, relative, vs. odds ratios, 291*t*–294*t*, 291–293
Robinson's path model, 343, 343*f*
Rotated factor matrices, in factor analysis, 321–322
Roy's greatest characteristic root, 171

S

Samples
  factors across, comparison of, confirmatory factor
      analysis for, 334
  random, 73
  selection of, 78–79
  size of, 78–79
    for chi-square, 102
    for factor analysis, 317
    for one-way analysis of variance, 141
    for regression, 248
    for repeated measures analysis of variance, 204
    in structural equation modeling, 381
    for t tests, 126–128, 127t
Sampling error, 88
Scales. *See* Measurement scales
Scatter, measures of, 36f, 36–41, 37t–38t, 40t. *See
      also* Variability, measures of
Scatter diagrams, 228, 229f
School of Nursing survey, of Boston College,
      421t–425t
Scores, standard, 56–58
SEM. *See* Structural equation modeling (SEM)
Separate t test, calculation of, 134
Shrinkage formula, 248
Significance
  of correlation coefficient, 235
  tests of
    confidence interval and, 75–77, 77f
    in regression, 255–256
    using normal curve, 71, 72f
Simple regression, 249–254, 250f–251f, 253f
6 x 6 correlation matrix, 312, 312t
Skewness, measures of, 41f, 41–42
Spearman rho, 238
Sphericity, Mauchly's test of, in repeated measures
      analysis of variance, 207, 209f
SPSS. *See also* under specific statistical methods
  frequency distributions produced by, 6–8, 7t–10t
  histograms produced by, 18f
  ONEWAY program of, 150
Standard deviation, 37t–38t, 37–39
  in normal curve, 54, 54f
  in standard error of mean, 59–60
Standard error of mean, 59–60
Standard scores, 56–58
  in regression, 250f–251f, 250–252
Statistical analysis, tailoring to specific problem, 89–90

Statistical errors, vs. statistical mistakes, 87–88
Statistical estimates, 73–78, 77f
Statistical inference, 73
Statistical mistakes, vs. statistical errors, 87–88
Statistical Package for the Social Sciences. *See* SPSS
Statistics, vs. parameters, 30
Structural equation modeling (SEM), 368–396
  assumptions in, 380–382
  coefficients in, 376–377
  computer examples of
    confirmatory factor analysis in, 383–386, 384f,
        385t
    goodness of fit in, 386–393, 387f–390f,
        388t–393t
  data required for, 379–380
  identification in, 378
  indicators in, 372–373
  Lagrange multiplier test in, 384–385, 385t, 389t,
      391t, 394t
  manifest variables in, 372–373
  measured variables in, 372–373
  measurement model for, 373–374, 375f
  model fit statistics in, 377–378, 378t
  modification indices in, 378–379
  multiple group analysis in, 379
  parameters in, 376–377
  power in, 382
  presentation of data in, 393–396, 395f, 396t
  proxies in, 372–373
  research questions for, 369–371, 370f–374f
  sample size in, 381
  theoretical constructs in, 374–376, 375f–376f
  unmeasured variables in, 374–375, 375f
  Wald test in, 384, 385t, 389t, 391t, 394t
Subjective probability, 64–65
Sum of squares, 32, 145–148, 146t–147t
Symmetry
  compound, in repeated measures analysis of vari-
      ance, 207
  measures of, 41f, 41–42

T

Tables
  construction of, 8–9
  descriptive statistics for, rounding of, 43
  frequency distribution in, 6–8, 7t–10t

interval scales in, 6
for univariate analysis, t*f*–10*t*, 6–9
Tolerance, of variables, 269
Transformed standard scores, 57–58
Trimmed mean, 48–49
T-scores, 57–58
t statistic, distribution of, 411*t*–412*t*
t tests, 122–134
   assumptions underlying, 125–126
   computer analysis of, 128, 129*f*, 130, 130*t*
   correlated, 131, 132*f*
   data required for, 124
   example of, 130, 131*t*
   pooled, calculation of, 133, 133*t*
   power in, 126–128, 127*t*
   research questions for, 123*t*, 123–124
   sample size for, 126–128, 127*t*
   sample size in, 126–128, 127*t*
   separate, calculation of, 134
   variables in, 125
   variance in, 125
Tukey's test of differences among means, 116*t*
Two-tailed hypothesis testing, 70–72, 71*f*–72*f*
Two-tailed probability, 67–68, 411*t*–412*t*
2 x 2 factorial design, 163, 163*t*

U

Underidentified model, in path analysis, 351,
   351*f*–352*f*
Univariate analysis, 6–21
   bar graphs for, 10–11, 11*f*–12*f*
   descriptive statistics for
      graphs using, 43–46, 44*f*–45*f*
      measures of central tendency as, 31–36, 32*t*,
         35*f*
      measures of skewness/symmetry as, 41*f*, 41–42
      measures of variability/scatter as, 36*f*, 36–41,
         37*t*–38*t*, 40*t*
      outliers in, 46, 48–49
      rounding for tables, 43
   histograms for, 11–19, 13*f*–15*f*, 18*f*–20*f*
   polygons for, 14–19, 16*f*–20*f*
   tables for, 6–9, 10*t*
Universal measure of relationship, 239
Unrotated factor matrix, in factor analysis, 318–321,
   319*t*

V

Variability, measures of, 36*f*, 36–41, 37*t*–38*t*, 40*t*
   comparison of, 41
   interpercentile, 39–40, 40*t*
   range as, 40
   standard deviation as, 37*t*–38*t*, 37–39
Variables
   dependent
      in multivariate analysis of variance, 170
      in one-way analysis of variance, 140
      in *t* tests, 125
   dichotomized, estimation of correlation coeffi-
      cient with, 238–239
   independent
      direct and indirect effects of, in path analysis,
         351–354, 352*f*–353*f*, 359–361, 360*f*,
         360*t*–361*t*
      in *t* tests, 125
   interval, 4–5
      histograms for, 11–14, 13*f*–15*f*
      polygons for, 14, 16, 16*f*–17*f*
      in tables, 6
   in logistic regression, 287, 300–302
   measured, in structural equation modeling,
      372–373
   in path analysis, 347
      correlation among, 356*f*
   ratio, 5
      histograms for, 11–14, 13*f*–15*f*
      polygons for, 14, 16, 16*f*–17*f*
   selection of, in regression, 265–268. *See also* Re-
      gression, selection of variables in
   tolerance of, 269
   unmeasured, in structural equation modeling,
      374–375, 375*f*
Variance
   multivariate analysis of, 169–172, 173*f*–177*f*, 178*t*
      advantages of, 169
      assumptions underlying, 170
      computer-assisted, 171–172, 173*f*–177*f*, 178*t*
      data required for, 169
      example of, 178*t*, 179
      power in, 170
      results of, 170–171
   one-way analysis of, 138–159
      and analysis of covariance, 192–193
      assumptions underlying, 140
      between-group variation in, 142, 142*f*

Variance, one-way analysis of (*continued*)
   computer-assisted, 150, 153*f*
   data required for, 139–140, 140*f*
   degrees of freedom in, 148
   displaying results of, 148–150, 149*t*
   multiple group comparisons in, 150–151, 153*f*
   orthogonal contrasts in, 154–155, 155*f*–157*f*
   planned comparisons in, 154–155, 155*f*–157*f*
   post-hoc tests in, 151, 153*f*, 154
   power in, 141
   research questions for, 139
   sample size for, 141
   source of, 141–145, 142*f*–144*f*
   sums of squares in, 145–148, 146*t*–147*t*
   V ratio in, 148–149
   within-group variation in, 142, 142*f*, 144*f*
  repeated measures analysis of, 202–217
   assumptions underlying, 204
   between-subjects effects in, 206, 208*f*–209*f*
   compound symmetry in, 207
   computer-assisted, 206–207, 208*f*–211*f*, 212
   data required for, 203–204
   example of, 216*f*, 216–217
   Mauchly's test of sphericity in, 207, 209*f*
   mixed design in, 205
   over time, 204–206, 205*f*
   power in, 204
   problems with, 213, 215*f*, 216
   research questions for, 202–203
   sample size in, 204
   within-subjects effects in, 211*f*–212*f*, 212–213,
    214*f*–215*f*
  in *t* tests, 125
   Levene's test for equality of, 128, 129*f*, 135*f*
  two-way analysis of, 162–169, 163*t*–164*t*,
    165*f*–167*f*, 168*t*
   assumptions underlying, 164
   computer-assisted, 165, 166*f*–167*f*, 168*t*,
    168–169
   data required for, 164, 164*t*, 165*f*
   power in, 165, 168–169
   research questions for, 162–164, 163*t*
Varimax, 323

Vectors, coding into, 259–260, 263, 263*t*
V ratio, in one-way analysis of variance, 148–149

W

Wald test, in structural equation modeling, 384,
    385*t*, 389*t*, 391*t*, 394*t*
Wilcoxon matched-pairs signed rank test, 113–116,
    115*f*
Wilks' lambda, 171
   in discriminant function analysis, 289
Winsorized mean, 49
Within-group variation, 142, 142*f*, 144*f*
   sum of squares for, 145
Within-subjects effects, in repeated measures analy-
    sis of variance, 211*f*–212*f*, 212–213,
    214*f*–215*f*
Wright's rules, for identification of compound paths,
    353–354

X

X^2 probability, distribution of, 409*t*–410*t*

Y

Yates' correction, in chi-square, 105*f*, 106

Z

z_r, transformation to r, 419*t*–420*t*
z scores, 56, 231*t*, 232
   and mean, normal curve between, 407*f*–408*f*
   in regression, 250*f*–251*f*, 250–252